ELEVENTH EDITION

W9-AZG-687

Handbook of

Nursing Diagnosis

LYNDA JUALL CARPENITO-MOYET, R.N., M.S.N., CRNP

Family Nurse Practitioner
ChesPenn Health Services
Chester, Pennsylvania

Nursing Consultant
Mickleton, New Jersey

LIPPINCOTT WILLIAMS & WILKINS
A **Wolters Kluwer** Company
Philadelphia · Baltimore · New York · London
Buenos Aires · Hong Kong · Sydney · Tokyo

Senior Acquisitions Editor: Quincy McDonald
Managing Editor: Michelle Clarke
Senior Production Editor: Marian A. Bellus
Director of Nursing Production: Helen Ewan
Senior Managing Editor / Production: Erika Kors
Art Director: Doug Smock
Manufacturing Manager: William Alberti
Indexer: Manjit Sahai
Compositor: Circle Graphics
Printer: R. R. Donnelley-Crawfordsville

ISBN 13: 978-0-7817-6130-7
ISBN 10: 0-7817-6130-1

11th Edition

Care has been taken to confirm the accuracy of the information presented and to describe generally accepted practices. However, the authors,
editors, and publisher are not responsible for errors or omissions or for
any consequences from application of the information in this book and
make no warranty, express or implied, with respect to the content of the
publication.

The authors, editors, and publisher have exerted every effort to ensure
that drug selection and dosage set forth in this text are in accordance
with the current recommendations and practice at the time of publication. However, in view of ongoing research, changes in government regulations, and the constant flow of information relating to drug therapy and
drug reactions, the reader is urged to check the package insert for each
drug for any change in indications and dosage and for added warnings
and precautions. This is particularly important when the recommended
agent is a new or infrequently employed drug.

Some drugs and medical devices presented in this publication have
Food and Drug Administration (FDA) clearance for limited use in restricted research settings. It is the responsibility of the health care provider to ascertain the FDA status of each drug or device planned for use
in his or her clinical practice.

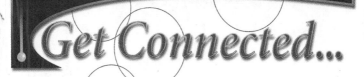

HOW TO USE THIS HANDBOOK

1. Collect data, both subjective and objective, from client, family, other health care professionals, and records.
2. Identify a possible pattern or problem.
3. Refer to the medical diagnostic category in Section II, and review the possible associated nursing diagnoses and collaborative problems. Select the possibilities.
4. After you have selected what physiological complications or collaborative problems are indicated to be monitored for onset or status changes, label them Potential Complications: (specify).
5. After you have determined which functional patterns are altered or at risk of altered functioning, review the list of nursing diagnoses under that pattern and select the appropriate diagnosis (refer to Table I-1).
6. If you select an actual diagnosis:
   a. Do you have signs and symptoms to support its presence? (Refer to Section I, Nursing Diagnoses, under the selected diagnosis.)
   b. Write the actual diagnosis in three parts: Label related to contributing factors as evident by signs and symptoms
7. If you select a risk diagnosis:
   a. Are risk factors present? Is this person or group more vulnerable than others in the same or a similar situation?
   b. Write the risk diagnosis in two parts: Label related to risk factors
8. If you suspect a problem but have insufficient data, gather the additional data to confirm or rule out the diagnosis. If this additional data collection must be done later or by other nurses, label the diagnosis *possible* on the care plan or problem list.*

*Specific focus assessment criteria questions, outcome criteria, and interventions for each nursing diagnosis category can be found in Carpenito-Moyet, L. J. (2006). *Nursing diagnosis: Application to clinical practice* (11th ed.). Philadelphia: Lippincott Williams & Wilkins.

TO OLEN, MY SON

for your wisdom and commitment to justice

for our quiet moments and embraces

for your presence in my life

   . . . I am grateful

for you are my daily reminder of what is

really important . . .

  love, health, and human trust

CONTENTS

How to Make an Accurate Nursing Diagnosis

To make an accurate nursing diagnosis, the nurse must:

1. Know the Nursing Diagnoses
2. Collect data that are valid and pertinent
3. Cluster the data
4. Differentiate nursing diagnoses from collaborative problems
5. Formulate nursing diagnoses correctly
6. Select priority diagnoses

Know the Nursing Diagnoses

Key Concepts

Nursing Diagnoses Components
Differentiate among Nursing Diagnoses

Nursing Diagnoses Components

To make a valid nursing diagnosis, the nurse must first have an understanding of the specific nursing diagnosis. To correctly diagnose fatigue, the signs and symptoms (characteristics) must be familiar.

The definition will help to differentiate one diagnosis from another. After the diagnosis has been validated, with defining characteristics, the nurse now needs to assess for factors that may have contributed to the problem occurring.

Collect Data That Are Valid and Pertinent

Key Concepts

Nursing-focused assessment
Screening versus focus assessment
Significance of data
Evaluation of data

Nursing-Focused Assessment

Nursing is defined as the diagnosis and treatment of human responses to actual or potential health problems and life situations (American Nurses Association, 1985; NANDA, 1998). The assessment format the nurse uses must be able to direct data collection on human responses ranging from skin condition and urinary function to spiritual health and self-care abilities. In other words, the nurses' knowledge of signs and symptoms for actual diagnoses, risk factors for risk diagnoses, or possible physiological complications directs the data collection. Nurses also use this knowledge to validate the accuracy of the diagnosis.

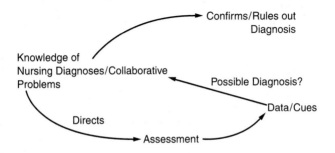

Screening Versus Focus Assessment

There are two types of assessments:

1. Screening: Collection of predetermined data, usually during initial contact
2. Focus: Collection of specific data as determined by the client, family, or situation

Frequently during first encounters with the client, the nurse will have broad screening assessment questions to determine how the person is functioning in various areas. Such questions might include the following:

• Do you have a problem sleeping?
• Do you have a problem with eating?
• How often do you have a bowel movement?
• Has any situation in your life been difficult for you to cope with?

If the person is complaining of a certain problem or has a specific concern, the nurse would limit the assessment (focus assessment). A limited assessment focus might include the following questions:

- Now tell me about your pain (Onset? Location? Severity? Duration? What helps? What aggravates?)
- What other symptoms do you have?
- How is this pain affecting sleep, eating, work, leisure?

In another situation, the nurse might be caring for a woman who has just had surgery, and complete a focus assessment of vital signs, wound appearance, intake, output, comfort level. In many situations, the nurse would not assess for problem nursing diagnoses, but instead would assess wellness and healthy lifestyles. For example, a healthy 42-year-old woman may be assessed for fiber content in diet.

Significance of Data

Beginning students will need to learn to determine whether data are significant in basic functional patterns or needs such as nutrition, safety, elimination, mobility, self-care. To recognize significant data, the nurse must first know what is expected or normal. For example, to determine whether a person has a nutritional problem, the nurse must first understand the food pyramid of five food groups, normal weight for height, and food preparation. In addition, the nurse needs to know that certain factors, such as nausea, poor dentures, sore mouth, or insufficient money, can interfere with food procurement, food preparation, eating, or metabolism.

Very simply, for assessment to be purposeful, the nurse has to know the following:

- What is the range of normal?
- What is the range of abnormal?
- What are the risk factors?

Evaluation of Data

The evaluation of data involves:

- Differentiating cues from inferences
- Ensuring validity
- Determining how much data are needed

Cues are facts that the nurse collects through interviewing, observing, examining, and reviewing the client record (e.g., vital signs, feelings, laboratory results). Inferences are judgments that the nurse makes about cues, such as the following:

Moist skin ⟍
Pale skin ―――――――――――→ Decreased blood volume
Rapid pulse ⟋

Validity is the extent to which data can be believed to be factual and true (Alfaro-LeFevre, 2002). Some data, such as decreasing blood pressure, are certain because there are agreed-upon standards. For situations in which criteria are not clear-cut, such as psychosocial responses, the nurse can increase the validity of the data or diagnosis by adding more evidence to support the inference. One defining characteristic may not be enough validation.

The judgments nurses make are only as valid as the data they use. Nurses can increase the validity or accuracy of data by verifying information.

Alfaro-LeFevre (2002) recommends several procedures to validate data:

- Recheck your own data.
- Ask someone to check.
- Compare subjective and objective data.
- Ask the client to verify.

Cluster the Data

Key Concepts
Knowledge of diagnostic categories
Sufficient number of cues
Differentiating one diagnosis from another
Tentative diagnosis (hypothesis)

Knowledge of Diagnostic Categories
Analysis of data is not possible unless you know which cues cluster or group to describe a diagnosis. In other words, you need to know which cues describe Powerlessness before you can recognize the cluster. Some diagnoses are very easy to confirm, such as Constipation or Impaired Skin Integrity. Often a single cue, such as "I have leg pain," can confirm a diagnosis of pain.

Other diagnoses, especially more complex psychosocial diagnoses such as Disturbed Body Image, may necessitate several nurse–client interactions before the diagnosis can be confirmed. Table 1, at the end of this introduction, lists nursing diagnoses under Functional Health Patterns.

Sufficient Number of Cues

One of the most difficult aspects of making accurate diagnoses is determining whether a sufficient number of cues are present to confirm an actual nursing diagnosis. The nurse should consult the list of defining characteristics for the diagnosis suspected. How many major characteristics are present? How many minor characteristics are present? Does the client confirm your suspected diagnosis? If you are still not confident, label the diagnosis Possible and collect more data or consult with a more experienced nurse.

Differentiating One Diagnosis From Another

Some diagnoses share some of the same defining characteristics, for example, Activity Intolerance, Fatigue, and Disturbed Sleep Pattern. Review the definitions and the author's notes for help. Determine what the focus of the interventions would be for the problem, for example, energy conservation techniques (Fatigue), promotion of sleep (Disturbed Sleep Pattern), or increasing endurance (Activity Intolerance). Sometimes this technique helps to clarify the diagnosis.

Tentative Diagnosis (Hypothesis)

The last cognitive activity in data analysis is the proposal of one or more likely diagnostic explanations for the clustered data. Sometimes only one diagnosis is proposed because the clustered data clearly support its presence. When more than one diagnosis is likely, the nurse should review the defining characteristics (for actual) or risk factors (for risk) for the tentative diagnosis. Systematically, the nurse should compare these signs, symptoms, or risk factors to the data assessed. If more data collection is needed, the nurse can proceed to this focused assessment. Another option is for the nurse to label the tentative diagnosis Possible if additional data collection is not realistic or feasible at this time. For example, some of the coping diagnoses require repetitive interactions for confirmation of the diagnosis.

Differentiate Nursing Diagnoses From Collaborative Problems

Key Concepts

Nursing diagnoses versus collaborative problems
Selection of collaborative problems

Nursing Diagnoses Versus Collaborative Problems

In 1983, Carpenito published the Bifocal Clinical Practice Model. In this model, nurses are accountable to treat two types of clinical judgments or diagnoses: nursing diagnoses and collaborative problems.

Nursing diagnoses are clinical judgments about individual, family, or community responses to actual or potential health problems/life processes. Nursing diagnoses provide the basis for selection of nursing interventions to achieve outcomes for which the nurse is accountable (NANDA, 1998).

Collaborative problems are certain physiological complications that nurses monitor to detect onset or changes in status. Nurses manage collaborative problems using physician-prescribed and nursing-prescribed interventions to minimize the complications of the events (Carpenito-Moyet, 2004).

Nursing interventions are classified as nurse-prescribed or physician-prescribed. Nurse-prescribed interventions are those that the nurse can legally order for nursing staff to implement. Nurse-prescribed interventions treat, prevent, and monitor nursing diagnoses. Nurse-prescribed interventions manage and monitor collaborative problems. Physician-prescribed interventions represent treatments for collaborative problems that the nurse initiates and manages. Collaborative problems require both nursing-prescribed and physician-prescribed interventions. Box 1 represents these relationships.

The following illustrates the types of interventions associated with the collaborative problem Potential Complications: Hypoxemia:

NP	1. Monitor for signs of acid–base imbalance.
NP/PP	2. Administer low flow oxygen as needed.
NP	3. Ensure adequate hydration.
NP	4. Evaluate the effects of positioning on oxygenation.
NP/PP	5. Administer medications as needed.

(NP: Nurse-prescribed; PP: Physician-prescribed)

⊙ BOX 1. RELATIONSHIP BETWEEN NURSING-PRESCRIBED INTERVENTIONS AND PHYSICIAN-PRESCRIBED INTERVENTIONS

Nursing-Prescribed Interventions

- Reposition q2h
- Lightly massage vulnerable areas
- Teach how to reduce pressure when sitting

Nursing Diagnoses

Risk for Impaired Skin Integrity related to immobility secondary to fatigue

Physician-Prescribed Interventions

Usually not needed

Nursing-Prescribed Interventions

- Maintain NPO state
- Monitor:
  Hydration
  Vital signs
  Intake/output
  Specific gravity
- Monitor electrolytes
- Maintain IV at prescribed rate
- Provide/encourage mouth care

Collaborative Problems

Potential Complication: Fluid and Electrolyte Imbalances

Physician-Prescribed Interventions

- IV (type, amount)
- Laboratory studies

Selection of Collaborative Problems

As mentioned earlier, collaborative problems are different from nursing diagnoses. The nurse makes independent decisions regarding both collaborative problems and nursing diagnoses. The decisions differ in that, for nursing diagnoses, the nurse prescribes the definitive treatment for the situation and is responsible for outcome achievement; for collaborative problems, the nurse monitors the client's condition to detect onset or status of physiological complications and manages the events with nursing and physician-prescribed interventions. Collaborative problems are labeled "Potential Complications" (specify), for example:

Potential Complication: Hemorrhage
Potential Complication: Renal Failure

The physiological complications that nurses monitor usually are related to disease, trauma, treatments, and diagnostic studies. The following examples illustrate some collaborative problems:

Situation	*Collaborative Problem*
Anticoagulant therapy	Potential Complication: Hemorrhage
Pneumonia	Potential Complication: Hypoxemia

Outcome criteria or client goals are used to measure the effectiveness of nursing care. When a client is not progressing to goal achievement or has worsened, the nurse must reevaluate the situation. Box 2 represents the questions to be considered. If none of these options is appropriate, the situation may not be a nursing diagnosis. For example:

Risk for Deficient Fluid Volume related to the effects of
  prolonged PTT secondary to anticoagulant therapy
Goal: The client will have hemoglobin >12.

✆ BOX 2. EVALUATION QUESTIONS

Is the diagnosis correct?
Has the goal been mutually set?
Is more time needed for the plan to work?
Does the goal need to be revised?
Do the interventions need to be revised?

Examine the questions in Box 2. Which option is appropriate? The answer is none. The nurse would initiate physician-prescribed orders if the client presented signs of bleeding. This situation is a collaborative problem, not a nursing diagnosis. For example:

Potential Complication: Bleeding
Goal: The nurse will manage and minimize episodes of bleeding.

Collaborative problems have nursing goals that represent the accountability of the nurse—to detect early changes and to co-manage with physicians. Nursing diagnoses have client goals that represent the accountability of the nurse—to achieve or maintain a favorable status after nursing care. Table 1 includes frequently used collaborative problems.

Some physiological complications, such as pressure ulcers and infection from invasive lines, are problems that nurses can prevent. Prevention is different from detection. Nurses do not prevent paralytic ileus but, instead, detect its presence early to prevent greater severity of illness or even death. Physicians cannot treat collaborative problems without nursing knowledge, vigilance, and judgment.

Formulate Nursing Diagnoses Correctly

Key Concepts

Types of nursing diagnoses
Diagnostic statements
Client validation
Clinical example
Actual nursing diagnoses
Clinical example

Types of Nursing Diagnoses

A nursing diagnosis can be actual, risk, or a wellness or syndrome type.

- Actual: An actual nursing diagnosis describes a clinical judgment that the nurse has validated because of the presence of major defining characteristics.
- Risk: A risk nursing diagnosis describes a clinical judgment that an individual/group is more vulnerable to

develop the problem than others in the same or a
similar situation because of risk factors.
- Wellness: A wellness nursing diagnosis is a clinical judgment about an individual, family, or community in transition from a specific level of wellness to a higher level of
wellness (NANDA, 1998).
- Syndrome: A syndrome diagnosis comprises a cluster of
actual or risk nursing diagnoses that are predicted to
present because of a certain situation or event.
- Possible nursing diagnosis is not a type of diagnosis as
are actual, risk, and syndrome. Possible nursing diagnoses are a diagnostician's option to indicate that some
data are present to confirm a diagnosis but are insufficient at this time.

Diagnostic Statements

The diagnostic statement describes the health status of an
individual or group and the factors that have contributed to
the status.

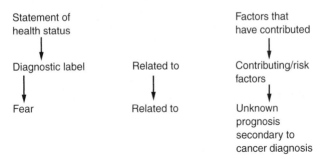

One-Part Statements

Wellness nursing diagnoses will be written as one-part
statements: Potential for Enhanced _____, e.g., Potential
for Enhanced Parenting. Related factors are not present for
wellness nursing diagnoses because they would all be the
same: motivated to achieve a higher level of wellness. Syndrome diagnoses, such as Rape Trauma Syndrome, have no
"related to" designations.

Two-Part Statements

Risk and possible nursing diagnoses have two parts. The
validation for a risk nursing diagnosis is the presence of risk
factors. The risk factors are the second part, as in:

Risk Nursing Diagnosis Related to Risk Factors

Possible nursing diagnoses are suspected because of the presence of certain factors.

The Following Are Examples of Two-Part Statements:

Risk for Impaired Skin Integrity related to immobility
  secondary to fractured hip
Possible Self-Care Deficit related to impaired ability to use
  left hand secondary to IV

Designating a diagnosis as possible provides the nurse with a method to communicate to other nurses that a diagnosis may be present. Additional data collection is indicated to rule out or confirm the tentative diagnosis.

Three-Part Statements

An actual nursing diagnosis consists of three parts.

Diagnostic label + contributing factors
                   + signs and symptoms

The presence of major signs and symptoms (defining characteristics) validates that an actual diagnosis is present. This is the third part. It is not possible to have a third part for risk or possible diagnoses because signs and symptoms do not exist.

The Following Are Examples of Three-Part Statements:

Anxiety related to unpredictable nature of asthmatic
  episodes as evident by statements of "I'm afraid I won't
  be able to breathe"
Urge Incontinence related to diminished bladder capacity
  secondary to habitual frequent voiding evident by inability to hold off urination after desire to void and report of
  voiding out of habit, not need

The presence of a nursing diagnosis is determined by assessing the individual's health status and ability to function. To guide the nurse who is gathering this information, a Screening Assessment Tool is included in the Appendix at the end of the book. This guide directs the nurse to collect data according to the individual's functional health patterns. Functional health patterns and the corresponding nursing diagnoses are listed in Table 1. If significant data are collected in a particular functional pattern, the next step is to check the related nursing diagnoses to see whether any of them are substantiated by the data that are collected.

Client Validation

The process of validating a nursing diagnosis should not be done in isolation from the client or family. Individuals are the experts on themselves. During assessments and interactions, nurses are provided a small glimpse of their clients. Diagnostic hunches or inferences about data should be discussed with clients for their input. Clients are given opportunities to select what they want assistance with, which problems are important to them, and which ones are not.

Clinical Example

After the screening assessment has been completed, the nurse applies each of these questions to each functional or need area:

- Is there a possible problem in a specific area?
- Is the person at risk (or high risk) for a problem?
- Does the person desire to improve his/her health?

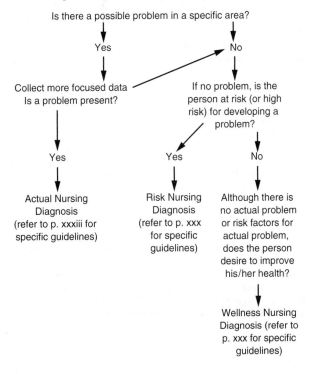

For example, after assessing a client's elimination pattern or need, the nurse would then analyze the data. Does this person have a possible problem with constipation or diarrhea? If yes, the nurse would then ask the person more focused questions to confirm the presence of the defining characteristics of constipation or diarrhea. If these defining characteristics are not present, then there is no actual diagnosis of Constipation or Diarrhea. Is there a risk diagnosis? To determine this, the nurse will assess for risk factors of constipation or diarrhea (listed under related/risk factors). If none of these are present, there is no risk for constipation or diarrhea.

Lastly, if there is no actual or at risk elimination nursing diagnosis, the nurse can ask whether the individual would like to improve his or her elimination patterns. If the answer is yes, the wellness diagnosis Potential for Enhanced Elimination is the appropriate choice.

Actual Nursing Diagnoses

Actual nursing diagnoses are written in two- or three-part statements:

1st part	2nd part	3rd part
Diagnostic Label	related to *factors that have caused or contributed*	as evident by *signs and symptoms in the individual that indicate the diagnosis is present*

Now that the defining characteristics have been confirmed to be present in the individual, you have:

Label:	Constipation
Causative/contributing factors:	related to inadequate fiber and fluid intake
Signs/symptoms: (defining characteristics)	as evident from reports of dry, hard stools, q 3–4 days

Clinical Example

As part of the screening assessment under nutrition you elicit:

Usual food intake	Usual fluid intake
Weight/height ratio	Current weight
Appearance of skin, nails, hair	

You then analyze the data to determine which data are within a normal range, and which are not.

- Are there sufficient servings of five food groups?
- Is there sufficient intake of calcium, protein, and vitamins?
- Is the fat intake <30% of total caloric intake?
- Does the person drink at least 6 to 8 cups of fluid besides coffee or soft drinks?
- Does the appearance of skin, hair, and nails reflect a healthy nutrition pattern?
- Is the person's weight within normal limits for height?

For example, in a specific person, Mr. Jewel, you find there is:

- Appropriate weight for height
- Insufficient fluid intake (4 8-oz. glasses of water/juice)
- Insufficient vegetable intake (two servings)
- Insufficient bread, cereal, rice, pasta intake (four servings)
- Dry skin and hair

From your assessment, you have confirmed that a nursing diagnosis is present because the person has signs or reports symptoms that represent those listed as defining characteristics under that specific diagnosis. These are usually the person's complaints.

At this point you have two parts of the diagnostic statement—the first and third but not the second:

Imbalanced Nutrition: less than body requirement related to _____, as evident from dry skin and hair, dietary intake (low in fiber, vegetables, complex CHO, and fluids)

Now you want to determine what has caused or contributed to Mr. Jewel's imbalanced nutrition. Look at the list of related factors or risk factors under Imbalanced Nutrition. Do any relate to Mr. Jewel's situation? Does Mr. Jewel think his diet is inadequate? If he says no, "lack of knowledge" would be the third part of your diagnostic statement. If he says yes, but it is not important to him to change his habits at his age, you will need to talk with him. Perhaps he has a problem with constipation or energy. Maybe a change of diet could help. When you are assured that Mr. Jewel understands the reasons for a balanced diet, but see that he has decided to continue his present diet, record his decision and your attempts to influence that decision.

Select Priority Diagnoses

Key Concepts

Priority criteria
Use of consultants/referrals

Priority Criteria

Nurses cannot treat all the nursing diagnoses and collaborative problems that an individual client, family, or community has. Attempts to do this will result in frustration for the nurse and the client. By identifying a priority set—a group of nursing diagnoses and collaborative problems that take precedence over other nursing diagnoses or collaborative problems—the nurse can best direct resources toward goal achievement. It is useful to differentiate priority diagnoses from those that are important, but not priority.

Priority diagnoses are those nursing diagnoses or collaborative problems that, if not managed now, will deter progress to achieve outcomes or will negatively affect the client's functional status.

Nonpriority diagnoses are those nursing diagnoses or collaborative problems for which treatment can be delayed to a later time without compromising present functional status. How does the nurse identify a priority set? In an acute-care setting, the client enters the hospital for a specific purpose, such as surgery or other treatments for acute illness.

- What are the nursing diagnoses or collaborative problems associated with the primary condition or treatments (e.g., surgery)?
- Are there additional collaborative problems associated with co-existing medical conditions that require monitoring (e.g., hypoglycemia)?
- Are there additional nursing diagnoses that, if not managed now, will deter recovery or affect the client's functional status (e.g., High Risk for Constipation)?
- What problems does the client perceive as priority?

Use of Consultants/Referrals

How are other diagnoses not on the diagnostic cluster selected for a client's problem list? Limited nursing resources and increasingly reduced client care time mandate that nurses identify important nursing diagnoses that can be addressed later and do not need to be included on the client's problem list. For example, for a client hospitalized after myocardial infarction who is 50 pounds overweight, the nurse would want to explain the effects of obesity on cardiac function and refer the client to community resources for a weight-reduction program after discharge. The discharge summary record would reflect the teaching and the referral; a nursing diagnosis related to weight reduction would not need to appear on the client's problem list.

Summary

Making accurate nursing diagnoses takes knowledge and practice. If the nurse uses a systematic approach to nursing diagnosis validation, then accuracy will increase. The process of making nursing diagnoses is difficult because nurses are attempting to diagnose human responses. Humans are unique, complex, and ever-changing; thus, attempts to classify these responses have been difficult.

REFERENCES

Alfaro-LeFevre, R. (2002). *Applying nursing diagnosis and nursing process: A step-by-step guide* (5th ed.) Philadelphia: Lippincott Williams & Wilkins.

American Nurses Association. (1985). *A nursing social policy statement.* Washington, DC: ANA.

Carpenito, L. J. (1983). *Nursing diagnosis: Application to clinical practice.* Philadelphia: J.B. Lippincott.

Carpenito-Moyet, L. J. (2004). *Nursing diagnosis: Application to clinical practice* (10th ed.). Philadelphia: Lippincott Williams & Wilkins.

North American Nursing Diagnosis Association. (1998–1999). *Taxonomy I* (rev. ed.). Philadelphia: NANDA.

Table 1 Conditions That Necessitate Nursing Care

Nursing Diagnoses*

1. **Health Perception—Health Management**
   Energy Field, Disturbed
   Growth and Development, Delayed
     Adult Failure to Thrive
     Growth, Risk for Delayed
     Development, Risk for Delayed
   Health Maintenance, Ineffective
   Surgical Recovery, Delayed
   Health Seeking Behaviors
   Injury, Risk for
     Risk for Suffocation
     Risk for Poisoning
     Risk for Trauma
   Injury, Risk for Perioperative Positioning
   Therapeutic Regimen Management, Effective
   Therapeutic Regimen Management, Ineffective
   Therapeutic Regimen Management, Ineffective: Family
   Therapeutic Regimen Management, Ineffective:
     Community
   Noncompliance
2. **Nutritional—Metabolic**
   Adaptive Capacity, Decreased: Intracranial
   Body Temperature, High Risk for Imbalanced
     Hypothermia
     Hyperthermia
     Thermoregulation, Ineffective
   Breastfeeding, Effective
   Breastfeeding, Ineffective
   Breastfeeding, Interrupted
   Deficient Fluid Volume
   Excess Fluid Volume
   Fluid Volume Imbalance, Risk for
   Infection, Risk for
   †Infection Transmission, Risk for
   Latex Allergy
     Latex Allergy, Risk for
   Nutrition, Imbalanced: Less Than Body Requirements
   Nutrition, Imbalanced: More Than Body Requirements
   Nutrition, Imbalanced: Potential for More Than Body
     Requirements
     Dentition, Impaired

(table continues on p. xxxviii)

Table 1 Conditions That Necessitate Nursing Care (continued)

Nursing Diagnoses*

Feeding Pattern, Ineffective Infant
Swallowing, Impaired
Protection, Ineffective
   Tissue Integrity, Impaired
      Oral Mucous Membrane, Impaired
      Skin Integrity, Impaired

3. **Elimination**
   Bowel Incontinence
   Constipation
      Constipation, Risk for
      Perceived Constipation
   Diarrhea
   Urinary Elimination, Impaired
      Urinary Retention
      Total Incontinence
      Functional Incontinence
      Reflex Incontinence
      Urge Incontinence
      Urge Incontinence, Risk for
      Stress Incontinence
      †Maturational Enuresis

4. **Activity—Exercise**
   Activity Intolerance
   Cardiac Output, Decreased
   Disuse Syndrome
   Diversional Activity Deficit
   Home Maintenance Management, Impaired
   Infant Behavior, Disorganized
   Infant Behavior, Risk for Disorganized
   Infant Behavior, Potential for Enhanced Organized
   Mobility, Impaired Physical
      Bed Mobility, Impaired
      Walking, Impaired
      Wheelchair Mobility, Impaired
      Wheelchair Transfer Ability, Impaired
   Peripheral Neurovascular Dysfunction, Risk for
   Respiratory Function, Risk for Impaired
      Dysfunctional Ventilatory Weaning Response
      Ineffective Airway Clearance
      Ineffective Breathing Patterns
      Impaired Gas Exchange

**Table 1 Conditions That Necessitate
Nursing Care** (continued)

Nursing Diagnoses*

      Sedentary Life Style
         Ventilation, Inability to Sustain Spontaneous
      †Self-Care Deficit Syndrome (Specify): (Feeding,
         Bathing/Hygiene, Dressing/Grooming, Toileting,
         Instrumental)
      Tissue Perfusion, Altered: (Specify) (Cerebral,
         Cardiopulmonary, Renal, Gastrointestinal, Peripheral)
      Wandering

5. **Sleep—Rest**
      Disturbed Sleep Pattern
      Sleep Deprivation

6. **Cognitive—Perceptual**
      Aspiration, Risk for
      †Comfort, Impaired
         Acute Pain
         Chronic Pain
         Pain
         Nausea
      †Confusion
         Acute Confusion
         Chronic Confusion
      Decisional Conflict
      Dysreflexia
         Dysreflexia, Risk for
      Environmental Interpretation Syndrome, Impaired
      Deficient Knowledge: (Specify)
      Risk for Aspiration
      Disturbed Sensory Perception: (Specify) (Visual,
         Auditory, Kinesthetic, Gustatory, Tactile, Olfactory)
      Thought Processes, Impaired
      Unilateral Neglect

7. **Self-Perception**
      Anxiety
      Death Anxiety
      Fatigue
      Fear
      Hopelessness
      Powerlessness
      Disturbed Self-Concept
         Disturbed Body Image

(table continues on p. xl)

**Table 1 Conditions That Necessitate
Nursing Care** (continued)

Nursing Diagnoses*

      Disturbed Personal Identity
      Disturbed Self-Esteem
         Chronic Low Self-Esteem
         Situational Low Self-Esteem
 8. **Role—Relationship**
      †Communication, Impaired
         Communication, Impaired Verbal
      Family Processes, Interrupted
      Family Processes, Dysfunctional: Alcoholism
      Grieving
         Grieving, Anticipatory
         Grieving, Dysfunctional
         Chronic Sorrow
      Loneliness, Risk for
      Parent/Infant/Child Attachment, Risk for Impaired
      Parenting, Impaired
      Parental Role Conflict
      Role Performance, Ineffective
      Social Interaction, Impaired
      Social Isolation
 9. **Sexuality—Reproductive**
      Sexual Dysfunction
      Sexuality Patterns, Ineffective
10. **Coping—Stress Tolerance**
      Adjustment, Impaired
      Caregiver Role Strain
      Coping, Ineffective Individual
         Defensive Coping
         Ineffective Denial
      Coping, Disabled Family
      Compromised Family Coping
      Readiness for Enhanced Family Coping
      Coping, Ineffective Community
      Readiness for Enhanced Community Coping
      Post-Trauma Response
         Post-Trauma Syndrome, Risk for
         Rape Trauma Syndrome
      Relocation Stress Syndrome
      †Self-Harm, Risk for:
         †Self-Abuse, Risk for
         Self-Mutilation, Risk for
      Suicide, Risk for
      Violence, Risk for

Table 1 Conditions That Necessitate Nursing Care (continued)

Nursing Diagnoses*

---

11. **Value—Belief**
      Religiosity, Impaired
        Impaired Religiosity, Risk for
      Spiritual Distress
        Spiritual Distress, Risk for
      Spiritual Well Being, Readiness for Enhanced

‡Collaborative Problems

Potential Complication: Cardiac/Vascular
    PC: Decreased Cardiac Output
    PC: Dysrhythmias
    PC: Pulmonary Edema
    PC: Cardiogenic Shock
    PC: Thromboembolic/Deep Vein Thrombosis
    PC: Hypovolemia
    PC: Peripheral Vascular Insufficiency
    PC: Hypertension
    PC: Congenital Heart Disease
    PC: Angina
    PC: Endocarditis
    PC: Pulmonary Embolism
    PC: Spinal Shock
    PC: Ischemic Ulcers

Potential Complication: Respiratory
    PC: Hypoxemia
    PC: Atelectasis/Pneumonia
    PC: Tracheobronchial Constriction
    PC: Pleural Effusion
    PC: Tracheal Necrosis
    PC: Ventilator Dependency
    PC: Pneumothorax
    PC: Laryngeal Edema

Potential Complication: Renal/Urinary
    PC: Acute Urinary Retention
    PC: Renal Failure
    PC: Bladder Perforation
    PC: Renal Calculi

(table continues on p. xlii)

Table 1 Conditions That Necessitate
Nursing Care (continued)

Nursing Diagnoses*

Potential Complication: Gastrointestinal/Hepatic/Biliary
- PC: Paralytic Ileus/Small Bowel Obstruction
- PC: Hepatic Failure
- PC: Hyperbilirubinemia
- PC: Evisceration
- PC: Hepatosplenomegaly
- PC: Curling's Ulcer
- PC: Ascites
- PC: Gastrointestinal Bleeding

Potential Complication: Metabolic/Immune/Hematopoietic
- PC: Hypoglycemia/Hyperglycemia
- PC: Negative Nitrogen Balance
- PC: Electrolyte Imbalances
- PC: Thyroid Dysfunction
- PC: Hypothermia (Severe)
- PC: Hyperthermia (Severe)
- PC: Sepsis
- PC: Acidosis (Metabolic, Respiratory)
- PC: Alkalosis (Metabolic, Respiratory)
- PC: Hypo/Hyperthyroidism
- PC: Allergic Reaction
- PC: Donor Tissue Rejection
- PC: Adrenal Insufficiency
- PC: Anemia
- PC: Thrombocytopenia
- PC: Opportunistic Infection
- PC: Polycythemia
- PC: Sickling Crisis
- PC: Disseminated Intravascular Coagulation

Potential Complication: Neurological/Sensory
- PC: Increased Intracranial Pressure
- PC: Stroke
- PC: Seizures
- PC: Spinal Cord Compression
- PC: Meningitis
- PC: Cranial Nerve Impairment (Specify)
- PC: Paralysis
- PC: Peripheral Nerve Impairment
- PC: Increased Intraocular Pressure

Table 1 Conditions That Necessitate Nursing Care (continued)

Nursing Diagnoses*

    PC: Corneal Ulceration
    PC: Neuropathies

Potential Complication: Muscular/Skeletal
    PC: Osteoporosis
    PC: Joint Dislocation
    PC: Compartmental Syndrome
    PC: Pathological Fractures

Potential Complication: Reproductive
    PC: Fetal Distress
    PC: Postpartum Hemorrhage
    PC: Pregnancy-Associated Hypertension
    PC: Hypermenorrhea
    PC: Polymenorrhea
    PC: Syphilis
    PC: Prenatal Bleeding
    PC: Preterm Labor

Potential Complication: Multisystem
    PC: Medication Therapy Adverse Effects
    PC: Adrenocorticosteroids Therapy Adverse Effects
    PC: Antianxiety Therapy Adverse Effects
    PC: Antiarrhythmia Therapy Adverse Effects
    PC: Anticoagulant Therapy Adverse Effects
    PC: Anticonvulsant Therapy Adverse Effects
    PC: Antidepressant Therapy Adverse Effects
    PC: Antihypertensive Therapy Adverse Effects
    PC: Beta-Adrenergic Blockers Therapy Adverse Effects
    PC: Calcium Channel Blockers Therapy Adverse Effects
    PC: Angiotensin-Converting Enzyme Therapy Adverse Effects
    PC: Antineoplastic Therapy Adverse Effects
    PC: Antipsychotic Therapy Adverse Effects

---

*The Functional Health Patterns were identified in Gordon, M. (1982). *Nursing diagnosis: Process and application.* New York: McGraw-Hill, with minor changes by the author.

†These diagnoses are not currently on the NANDA list but have been included for clarity and usefulness.

‡Frequently used collaborative problems are represented on this list. Other situations not listed here could qualify as collaborative problems.

Nursing Diagnoses

DEFINITION

Activity Intolerance: A reduction in one's physiologic capacity to endure activities to the degree desired or required (Magnan, 1987).

Ⓧ **AUTHOR'S NOTE**

Activity Intolerance is a diagnostic judgment that describes a person with compromised physical conditioning. This person can engage in therapies that increase strength and endurance. *Activity Intolerance* differs from *Fatigue* in that rest relieves *Activity Intolerance.* Moreover, the goal is to increase tolerance to activity; in *Fatigue,* the goal is to assist the person to adapt to the fatigue, not to increase endurance.

DEFINING CHARACTERISTICS
Major (Must be Present, One or More)
(Magnan, 1987)
During Activity
Weakness
Dizziness
Dyspnea

Three Minutes After Activity
Dizziness
Dyspnea
Exertional fatigue
Respiratory rate >24 breaths/min
Pulse rate >95 breaths/min

Minor (May be Present)
Pallor or cyanosis
Confusion
Vertigo

RELATED FACTORS

Any factors that compromise oxygen transport, physical deconditioning, or create excessive energy demands that outstrip the person's physical and psychological abilities can cause *Activity Intolerance.* Some common factors are listed below.

Pathophysiologic

Related to compromised oxygen transport system secondary to:

Cardiac

Congenital heart disease | Valvular disease
Cardiomyopathies | Dysrhythmias
Myocardial infarction | Angina
Congestive heart failure

Respiratory

Chronic obstructive | Bronchopulmonary dysplasia
pulmonary disease | Atelectasis

Circulatory

Anemia | Hypovolemia
Peripheral arterial disease

Related to increased metabolic demands secondary to:

Acute or chronic infection

Viral infection | Hepatitis
Mononucleosis

Endocrine or metabolic disorders
Chronic diseases

Renal | Inflammatory
Hepatic | Musculoskeletal
Cancer | Neurologic

Related to inadequate energy sources secondary to:

Obesity | Inadequate diet
Malnourishment

Related to compromised oxygen transport secondary to:

Hypovolemia

Treatment-Related

Related to increased metabolic demands secondary to:

Surgery | Treatment schedule
Diagnostic studies

Situational (Personal, Environmental)

Related to the deconditioning effects of bed rest

Related to inactivity secondary to depression, lack of motivation, sedentary lifestyle

Related to increased metabolic demands secondary to:

Assistive equipment (walkers, crutches, braces)

Extreme stress

Pain

Environmental barriers (e.g., stairs)

Climatic extremes (especially hot, humid climates)

Related to decreased available oxygen secondary to atmospheric pressure (e.g., recent relocation to high-altitude living)

Maturational

Older adults may experience decreased muscle strength and flexibility and sensory deficits. All these can undermine body confidence and may contribute directly or indirectly to *Activity Intolerance*.

NOC Activity Intolerance

Goals

The person will progress activity to (specify level of activity desired).

Indicators

- Identify factors that aggravate activity intolerance.
- Identify methods to reduce activity intolerance.
- Maintain blood pressure within normal limits 3 minutes after activity.

NIC Exercise Therapy, Joint Mobility Teaching, Prescribed Activity/Exercise

Generic Interventions

Monitor the Person's Response to Activity.

1. Take resting pulse, blood pressure, and respirations.

2. Consider rate, rhythm, and quality (if signs are abnormal—e.g., pulse >100—consult physician about the advisability of increasing activity).
3. Take vital signs immediately after activity; take pulse for 15 seconds, and multiply by 4 instead of for 1 full minute.
4. Have person rest for 3 minutes; take vital signs again. Compare findings with resting vital signs.
5. Discontinue the activity if the client responds to the activity with:
   • Reports of chest pain, dyspnea, vertigo, or confusion
   • Decrease in pulse rate
   • Failure of systolic rate to increase
   • Decrease in systolic blood pressure
   • Increase in diastolic rate of 15 mm Hg
   • Decrease in respiratory rate
6. Reduce the intensity, frequency, or duration of the activity if:
   • The pulse takes longer than 3 to 4 minutes to return within 6 beats of the resting pulse rate.
   • The respiratory rate increase is excessive after the activity.
   • Other signs of hypoxia are present (e.g., confusion, vertigo).

Progress the Activity Gradually.

For a person who is or has been on prolonged bed rest, begin range of motion at least twice a day.

Plan rest periods according to the person's daily schedule (rest periods may occur between activities).

Promote a sincere "can do" attitude to provide a positive atmosphere to encourage increased activity; convey to clients the belief that they can improve their mobility status. Acknowledge progress.

Allow person to set activity schedule and functional activity goals (if the goal is too low, make a contract: e.g., "If you walk halfway up the hall, I will play a game of cards with you").

Increase tolerance for the activity by having the client perform the activity more slowly, for a shorter period with more rest pauses, or with more assistance.

Gradually increase exercise tolerance by increasing the time out of bed by 15 minutes each day, three times a day.

Allow person to gauge the rate of the ambulation.

Encourage person to wear comfortable walking shoes (slippers do not support the feet properly).

Teach Energy Conservation Methods for Activities.

Take rest periods during activities, at intervals during the day, and 1 hour after meals.

Sit rather than stand when performing activities, unless this is not feasible.

When performing a task, rest every 3 minutes for 5 minutes to allow the heart to recover.

Stop an activity if fatigue or signs of cardiac hypoxia are present (increased pulse, dyspnea, chest pain).

Instruct the Person to Consult Physician and Physiatrist for a Long-Term Exercise Program or to Contact the American Heart Association for Names of Cardiac Rehabilitation Programs.

For Clients with Chronic Pulmonary Insufficiency:

Encourage conscious controlled-breathing techniques during increased activity and times of emotional and physical stress (techniques include pursed-lip and diaphragmatic breathing).

For pursed-lip breathing, the person should breathe in through the nose, then breathe out slowly through partially closed lips while counting to 7 and making a "poo" sound (often this is learned naturally by a person with progressive lung disease).

Teach diaphragmatic breathing:

Place your hands on the person's abdomen below the base of the ribs, and keep them there while the client inhales.

To inhale, the person should relax the shoulders, breathe in through the nose, and push the stomach outward against the nurse's hands, holding breath for 1 to 2 seconds to keep the alveoli open.

To exhale, the person should breathe out slowly through the mouth while the nurse applies slight pressure at the base of the ribs.

Practice several times; then have the person place his or her own hands at the base of the ribs and practice independently.

Instruct to practice this exercise a few times each hour.

Encourage gradual increase in daily activity to prevent "pulmonary crippling."

Encourage person to use adaptive breathing techniques to decrease the work of breathing.

Discuss physical barriers at home and at work (e.g., number of stairs) and ways of alternating expenditure of energy with rest pauses (place a chair in bathroom near sink to rest during daily hygiene).

Explain the importance of supporting arm weight to reduce the work of respiratory muscles (Breslin, 1992).

Teach how to increase unsupported arm endurance with lower extremity exercises performed during exhalation (Breslin, 1992).

Refer to Community Nurse for Follow-up if Needed.

Pediatric Interventions

Provide Age-Appropriate Games and Activities that Are Quiet and Challenging.

Sensory adventures (What does the hospital smell, sound, or look like?)

Telling and writing stories, creating collages, playing with puppets, playacting

Maternal Interventions

Explain the Causes of Fatigue and Dyspnea in Mid- to Late Pregnancy.

Changes in center of gravity

Increased weight

Pressure of enlarged uterus on diaphragm

Teach Energy Conservation Methods (Refer to Generic Interventions).

Adaptive Capacity, Decreased Intracranial

DEFINITION

Decreased Intracranial Adaptive Capacity: A clinical state in which intracranial fluid dynamic mechanisms that normally compensate for increases in intracranial volumes are compromised, resulting in repeated disproportionate increases in intracranial pressure in response to a variety of noxious and non-noxious stimuli.

ⓧ AUTHOR'S NOTE

This diagnosis represents increased intracranial pressure. It is a collaborative problem because it requires two disciplines to treat—nursing and medicine. In addition, it requires invasive monitoring for diagnosis. The collaborative problem Potential Complication: Increased Intracranial Pressure represents this clinical situation.

DEFINING CHARACTERISTICS

Major (Must be Present)

Repeated increases in intracranial pressure (ICP) of >10 mm Hg for >5 minutes after any of a variety of external stimuli.

Minor (May be Present)

Disproportionate increase in ICP after one environmental or nursing maneuver stimulus

Elevated P_2 ICP waveform

Volume pressure response test variation (volume–pressure ratio >2); pressure–volume index (<10)

Baseline ICP ≥10 mm Hg

Wide-amplitude ICP waveform

Adjustment, Impaired

DEFINITION

Impaired Adjustment: The state in which an individual is unable to modify his or her lifestyle or behavior in a manner consistent with a change in health status.

> #### ⊕ AUTHOR'S NOTE
>
> This diagnosis has presented problems in clinical use because of its lack of specificity. Generally speaking, are not most diagnoses a problem with adjustment? It is not clinically useful to have such a general diagnosis. The responses to illness and disabilities will be varied, and the nurse must clarify the response to be most helpful with treatment. Responses can be *Grieving, Anxiety, Fear,* and *Ineffective Coping.*
>
> If a client is attempting to manage the changes the illness or disability has caused but is having difficulty, the diagnosis *Ineffective Therapeutic Regimen Management* would be more useful.

DEFINING CHARACTERISTICS
Major (Must be Present)

Verbalization of nonacceptance of health status change or inability to be involved in problem-solving or goal-setting.

Minor (May be Present)

Lack of movement toward independence; extended period of shock, disbelief, or anger concerning health status change; lack of future-oriented thinking.

Anxiety

DEFINITION

Anxiety: The state in which an individual or group experiences feelings of uneasiness (apprehension) and activation of the autonomic nervous system in response to a vague, nonspecific threat.

 AUTHOR'S NOTE

Anxiety is a vague feeling of apprehension and uneasiness from a threat to one's value system or security pattern (May, 1987). The person may be able to identify the situation (e.g., surgery, cancer), but in actuality the threat to self relates to the uneasiness and apprehension enmeshed in the situation. The situation is the source of, but is not itself, the threat.

In contrast, fear is the feeling of apprehension to a specific threat or danger to which one's security patterns alert one (e.g., flying, heights, snakes). When the threat is removed, the fearful feeling dissipates (May, 1987).

Fear can exist without anxiety, and anxiety can be present without fear. Clinically, both may coexist in a person's response to a situation. An individual who is facing surgery may be fearful of pain and anxious about a possible cancer diagnosis.

DEFINING CHARACTERISTICS
Major (Must be Present)

Manifested by symptoms from three categories: physiologic, emotional, and cognitive; symptoms vary according to the level of anxiety.

Physiologic

Increased heart rate
Elevated blood pressure
Increased respiratory rate
Diaphoresis
Dilated pupils
Voice tremors/
  pitch changes
Trembling, twitching
Palpitations
Nausea or vomiting
Frequent urination
Diarrhea

Insomnia
Fatigue and weakness
Flushing or pallor
Dry mouth
Body aches and pains
  (especially chest,
  back, neck)
Restlessness
Faintness/dizziness
Paresthesias
Hot and cold flashes
Anorexia

Emotional

Person reports feelings of:
Apprehension
Helplessness
Nervousness
Lack of self-confidence

Losing control
Tension or being "keyed up"
Inability to relax
Anticipation of misfortune

Person exhibits:
Irritability/impatience
Angry outbursts
Crying
Tendency to blame others
Startle reaction

Criticism of self and others
Withdrawal
Lack of initiative
Self-deprecation
Poor eye contact

Cognitive

Inability to concentrate
  (inability to remember)
Lack of awareness of
  surroundings
Forgetfulness
Rumination
Orientation to past rather
  than to present or future

Blocking of thoughts
Hyperattentiveness
Preoccupation
Diminished learning ability
Confusion

RELATED FACTORS
Pathophysiologic

Any factor that interferes with the basic human needs for
  food, air, comfort, and security

Situational (Personal, Environmental)

Related to actual or perceived threat to self-concept secondary to:

Change in status and
  prestige
Failure (or success)
Loss of valued possessions

Ethical dilemma
Lack of recognition
  from others

Related to actual or perceived loss of significant others secondary to:

Death
Divorce
Cultural pressures

Moving
Temporary or permanent
  separation

Related to actual or perceived threat to biologic integrity secondary to:

Dying
Assault

Invasive procedures
Disease

Related to actual or perceived change in environment secondary to:

Hospitalization
Moving
Retirement

Safety hazards
Environmental pollutants

Related to actual or perceived change in socioeconomic status secondary to (e.g., unemployment, new job, promotion)

Related to idealistic expectations of self and unrealistic goals

Maturational

Infant/Child

Related to separation
Related to changes in peer relationships
Related to unfamiliar environment or persons

Adolescent

Related to threat to self-concept secondary to (e.g., sexual development, peer relationship changes)

Adult

Related to threat to self-concept or role status secondary to:

Pregnancy
Parenting

Career changes
Effects of aging

Older Adult

Related to threat to self-concept or role status secondary to:

Sensory losses   Financial problems
Motor losses   Retirement changes

NOC Anxiety Reduction, Coping, Impulse Control

Goals

The person will relate an increase in psychological and physiologic comfort.

Indicators

• Describe his or her own anxiety and coping patterns.
• Use effective coping mechanisms.

NIC Anxiety Reduction, Impulse Control Training,
Anticipatory Guidance

Generic Interventions

Assess Level of Anxiety:
Mild, Moderate, Severe, Panic.

Provide Reassurance and Comfort.

Stay with person.
Do not make demands or ask the person to make decisions.
  Sit in front of person.
Emphasize that all people feel anxious from time to time.
Speak slowly and calmly, using short, simple sentences.
Be aware of your own concern, and avoid reciprocal
  anxiety.
Convey a sense of empathic understanding (e.g., quiet
  presence, touch, allowing crying, talking).

Remove Excess Stimulation
(e.g., Take Person to Quieter Room);
Limit Contact with Others—Clients
or Family—Who Are Also Anxious.

**When Anxiety Is Diminished Enough
for Learning to Take Place, Assist
Person in Recognizing the Anxiety to
Initiate Learning or Problem-Solving.**

Encourage person to keep a diary (e.g., when client felt anxious, what was he or she doing or thinking? Who was with him or her?)

Assist to analyze diary to identify triggers.

Explore what alternative behaviors might have been used if coping mechanisms were maladaptive (e.g., assertiveness training).

**Teach Anxiety Interrupters to Use
When Stressful Situations Cannot
Be Avoided.**

Look up.

Control breathing.

Lower shoulders.

Slow thoughts.

Alter voice.

Give directions to self (out loud, if possible).

Exercise.

"Scruff your face"—change facial expression.

Change perspective—imagine watching the situation from a distance.

**Assist Person with Anger
(Thomas, 1989).**

Identify the presence of anger (e.g., feelings of frustration, anxiety, helplessness, irritability; verbal outbursts).

Recognize your reactions to client's behavior; be aware of your own feelings when working with angry individuals.

Do not interrupt; listen to grievance.

Encourage alternative problem-solving if expectations are not realistic or possible (e.g., "What can you do differently?").

Provide positive validation if possible.

Focus on what can be done, not on what was not done.

Explore consequences of explosive anger.

Elicit alternative behavior to violent behavior (e.g., "What could you do instead of punching the wall?").

Use "time-out" when needed (e.g., "I can see that we are not accomplishing anything. Let's try again when we are both less emotional.").

State limits clearly; tell person exactly what is expected
(e.g., "I cannot allow you to scream" [throw objects, etc.]).

When stating an unacceptable behavior, give an alternative (e.g., suggest a quiet room, physical exertion, a
chance for one-to-one communication).

Develop behavior modification strategies; discuss with all
personnel involved for consistency.

Interact with person when he or she is not demanding or
manipulative.

**Explore Interventions that Decrease
Anxiety (e.g., Music, Aromatherapy,
Relaxation Exercises, Guided Imagery,
Hydrotherapy, Thought-Stopping,
Massage) (Keegan, 2000).**

**If Appropriate, Provide Activities that
Can Reduce Tension (e.g., Physical
Activity, Games).**

**For Persons Identified as Having
Chronic Anxiety and Maladaptive
Coping Mechanisms, Refer for
Psychiatric Evaluation.**

🔹 Pediatric Interventions

**Explain Events Using Simple, Age-
Appropriate Terms and Illustrations;
Puppets; Dolls; and Sample
Equipment.**

**Allow Child to Wear Underwear and
Have Familiar Toys or Objects.**

**Assist Parents or Caregivers to
Manage Their Anxiety When
with Child.**

**Use the Following Nursing
Interventions to Help Children
Cope with Anxiety:**

Establish a trusting relationship.

Minimize separation from parents.

❖ Pediatric Interventions (cont'd)

Encourage expression of feelings.

Involve child in play.

Prepare child for new experiences (e.g., procedures, surgery).

Provide comfort measures.

Allow for regression.

Encourage parental involvement in care.

Allay parental apprehension, and provide parents with information (Wong, 2002).

Assist Child with Anger.

Encourage child to share anger (e.g., "How did you feel when you had your injection?" "How did you feel when Mary would not play with you?").

Tell child that being angry is okay (e.g., "I sometimes get angry when I can't have what I want.").

Encourage and allow child to express anger in acceptable ways (e.g., talking loud or running outside around the house).

▨ Maternal Interventions

Explore Fears and Concerns During Each Trimester (Reeder, 1997; Lugina et al., 2001).

First trimester

Ambivalence, new role expectations, uncertainty about adequacy

Second trimester

Success as a new mother

Third trimester

Feels unattractive; fears for own well-being, performance during labor, and well-being of fetus

Help Her and Her Partner Identify Unrealistic Expectations.

Acknowledge Her Anxiety and the Normalcy of It.

Maternal Interventions (cont'd)

**Discuss These Concerns with the
Woman Alone, Her Partner Alone,
and Then Together as Indicated.**

Geriatric Interventions

**Explore the Person's Worries
(e.g., Financial, Security, Health, Living
Arrangements, Crime, Violence).**

Death Anxiety

DEFINITION

Death Anxiety: The state in which an individual experiences
apprehension, worry, or fear related to death or dying.

⊚ AUTHOR'S NOTE

The inclusion of *Death Anxiety* in the NANDA classification creates a diagnostic category with the etiology in the
label. This opens the NANDA list to thousands of diagnostic labels with etiology, such as separation anxiety,
divorce anxiety, infidelity anxiety, failure anxiety, and
travel anxiety. Many diagnostic labels can take this
same path: fear as claustrophobic fear, diarrhea as traveler's diarrhea, decisional conflict as end-of-life decisional conflict.

> ⊗ **AUTHOR'S NOTE (continued)**
>
> This author recommends that etiology be deleted in the diagnostic label except for syndrome diagnoses, which require the etiology in the label. Syndrome diagnoses have no "related to" factors.

DEFINING CHARACTERISTICS

Worrying about the impact of one's own death on significant others

Feeling powerless over issues related to dying

Fear of loss of physical and/or mental abilities when dying

Anticipated pain related to dying

Deep sadness

Fear of the process of dying

Concerns of overworking the caregiver as terminal illness incapacitates self

Concern about meeting one's creator or feeling doubtful about the existence of a god or higher being

Total loss of control over any aspect of one's own death

Negative death images or unpleasant thoughts about any event related to death or dying

Fear of delayed demise

Fear of premature death because it prevents the accomplishment of important life goals

RELATED FACTORS

Impending death is the situation that causes this diagnosis. Additional factors can contribute to death anxiety.

Situational (Personal, Environmental)

Related to situational factors (anxiety)

Related to fear of being a burden

Related to fear of unmanageable pain

Related to fear of abandonment

Related to unresolved conflict (family, friends)

Related to fear that one's life lacked meaning

Related to social disengagement

Related to powerlessness and vulnerability

NOC Dignified Dying, Fear Control

Goals

The person will report diminished anxiety or fear.

Indicators

- Share his or her feelings regarding dying.
- Identify two activities that increase control and self-knowledge.

NIC Coping Enhancement, Emotional Support, Spiritual Support

Generic Interventions

Allow person to share his or her perceptions of the situation (e.g., "Share with me what you are experiencing.").

Encourage person to share his or her conflicts and concerns (e.g., "If you could fix something before you die, what would it be?" "What are you most concerned about?").

Explore person's relationship of spirituality and approaching death:
  Afterlife beliefs
  Search for meaning
  Relationship with greater Other

Explore the person's interpretation of suffering (e.g., punishment, testing bad luck, nature's course, will of greater Other, denial, redemption).

Encourage telling life stories and reminiscing.

Discuss leaving a legacy (e.g., donation, personal articles, taped message for survivors).

Encourage reflective activities (e.g., prayer, meditation, writing a journal).

Encourage person to return the gift of love to others (e.g., listening, praying for others, sharing personal wisdom gained from illness, creating legacy gifts) (Taylor, 2000).

Encourage friends and family to be emotionally and spiritually honest.

Explain advance directives and assist in process if desired.

Aggressively manage unrelieved symptoms (e.g., nausea, vomiting, pain).

Encourage person to reconstruct his or her worldview
(Taylor, 2000).
Allow to verbalize feelings about the meaning of death.
Advise that there are no right or wrong feelings.
Advise that his or her responses are choices.
Acknowledge the struggles.

Body Temperature, Risk for Imbalanced
Hyperthermia
Hypothermia
Thermoregulation, Ineffective

○ **AUTHOR'S NOTE**

Risk for Imbalanced Body Temperature includes those at
risk for hyperthermia, hypothermia, or ineffective thermoregulation. If the person is at risk for only one of the diagnoses (e.g., hypothermia but not hyperthermia), then it is
more useful to label the problem with the more specific
diagnosis (*Risk for Hypothermia*). If the person is at risk
for two or more of the diagnoses, then *Risk for Imbalanced
Body Temperature* is more appropriate. The focus of nursing care for these diagnoses is to prevent abnormal body
temperatures by identifying and treating those persons
with a normal temperature who demonstrate risk factors
that can be controlled by nursing-prescribed interventions (e.g., by removing or adding blankets or by controlling environmental temperature). If the alteration in
body temperature is related to a pathophysiologic complication that requires nursing and medical interventions,
then the problem should be labeled as a collaborative
problem (e.g., Potential Complication: Fever related to

> ⊚ **AUTHOR'S NOTE (continued)**
>
> atelectasis or Potential Complication: Severe Hypothermia related to hypothalamus injury). The focus of concern then becomes monitoring to detect and report significant temperature fluctuations and implementing collaborative interventions (e.g., a warming or cooling blanket) as ordered. (See also diagnostic considerations for *Hyperthermia* and *Hypothermia.*)

Body Temperature, Risk for Imbalanced

DEFINITION
Risk for Imbalanced Body Temperature: The state in which an individual is at risk of failing to maintain body temperature within normal range (36° to 37.5°C [98° to 99.5°F]).

RISK FACTORS
Major (Must be Present, One or More)
Presence of risk factors (see Related Factors)

RELATED FACTORS
Treatment-Related
Related to cooling effects of:
Parenteral fluid infusion, blood transfusion
Dialysis
Cooling blanket
Operating suite

Situational (Personal, Environmental)
Related to:
Exposure to cold, rain, snow, wind; exposure to heat, sun, humidity extremes

Inappropriate clothing for climate
Inability to pay for shelter, heat, or air-conditioning
Extremes of weight
Consumption of alcohol
Dehydration/malnutrition

Maturational
Related to ineffective temperature regulation secondary to extremes of age (e.g., newborn, older adult)

Hyperthermia

DEFINITION
Hyperthermia: The state in which an individual has or is at risk of having a sustained elevation of body temperature >37.8°C (100°F) orally or 38.8°C (101°F) rectally because of external factors.

DEFINING CHARACTERISTICS
Major (Must be Present)
Temperature >37.8°C (100°F) orally or 38.8°C (101°F)
   rectally
Skin warm to touch
Tachycardia

Minor (May be Present)
Flushed skin
Increased respiratory depth
Shivering/goose pimples
Feelings of warmth
   or coolness

Specific or generalized aches
   and pains (e.g., headache)
Malaise, fatigue, weakness
Loss of appetite
Sweating

RELATED FACTORS
Treatment-Related
Related to reduced ability to sweat secondary to (specify medication)

Situational (Personal, Environmental)
Related to:

Exposure to heat, sun   No access to air conditioning

Inappropriate clothing
  for climate

Related to decreased circulation secondary to:

Extremes of weight   Dehydration

Related to insufficient hydration for vigorous activity

Maturational
Related to ineffective temperature regulation secondary to age

NOC Thermoregulation

Goals

The person will maintain body temperature.

NIC Fever Treatment, Temperature Regulation, Environmental Management, Fluid Management

Indicators

- Identify risk factors for hyperthermia.
- Reduce risk factors for hyperthermia.

Generic Interventions (for Risk for Hyperthermia)

Teach the person the importance of maintaining an adequate fluid intake (≥2000 mL/d unless contraindicated by heart or kidney disease) to prevent dehydration.
Monitor intake and output.

See also *Deficient Fluid Volume.*

Assess whether clothing or bed covers are too warm for the environment or planned activity.
Teach the importance of increasing fluid intake during warm weather and exercise.
Recommended fluid replacement for moderate activities in hot weather (DeFabio, 2000):

78° to 84.9°F: 16 oz/hour
85° to 89.9°F: 24 oz/hour
>90°F: 32 oz/hour

Explain the need to avoid alcohol; caffeine; and large, heavy meals during hot weather.

Explain the need to wear loose-fitting clothing and to wear a hat or use an umbrella.

Avoid outdoor activity between 11 A.M. and 2 P.M.

Take cool baths or showers several times a day during heat waves. Do not use soap.

Teach the early signs of hyperthermia or heat stroke:
  Flushed skin
  Headache
  Fatigue
  Loss of appetite

❖ Pediatric Interventions

Determine if fever is drug-related (e.g., anticholinergics, amphetamines, epinephrine, acetaminophen [large doses], antihistamines [large doses], phenothiazines).

Explain to parents that fever is a protective measure and not harmful unless high (e.g., >41.1°C [100°F]).

Caution not to sponge, which causes extreme chilling.

⊙ Geriatric Interventions

Refer to *Ineffective Thermoregulation,* Geriatric Interventions.

DEFINITION

Hypothermia: The state in which an individual has or is at risk of having a sustained reduction of body temperature of <35.5°C (96°F) rectally because of increased vulnerability to external factors.

DEFINING CHARACTERISTICS*
Major (80% to 100%)

Reduction in body temperature <35.5°C (96°F) rectally
Cool skin
Pallor (moderate)
Shivering (mild)

Minor (50% to 79%)

Mental confusion, drowsiness, restlessness
Decreased pulse and respiration
Cachexia, malnutrition

RELATED FACTORS
Situational (Personal, Environmental)
Related to:

Exposure to cold, rain, snow, wind
Inappropriate clothing for climate
Inability to pay for shelter or heat

Related to decreased circulation secondary to:

Extremes of weight
Consumption of alcohol
Dehydration
Inactivity

NIC Thermoregulation

---

*Adapted from Carroll, S. M. (1989). Nursing diagnosis: Hypothermia. In R. M. Carroll-Johnson (Ed.), *Classification of nursing diagnoses: Proceedings of the eighth conference.* Philadelphia: J. B. Lippincott.

Maturational
Related to ineffective temperature regulation secondary to age

Goals

The person will maintain body temperature within normal limits.

> **NIC** Hypothermia Treatment, Temperature Regulation,
> Temperature Regulation: Intraoperative,
> Environmental Management

Indicators

- Identify risk factors for hypothermia.
- Reduce risk factors for hypothermia.

Generic Interventions
(for Risk for Hypothermia)

Teach Client to Reduce Prolonged Exposure to Cold Environment.

Explain the importance of wearing a hat, gloves, and warm socks and shoes to prevent heat loss.

Encourage the person to limit going outside when temperatures are very cold.

Acquire an electric blanket, warm blankets, or down comforter for bed.

Teach client to wear close-knit undergarments to prevent heat loss.

Consult with Social Services to Identify Sources of Financial Assistance, Warm Clothing, Blankets.

Teach the Early Signs of Hypothermia: Cool Skin, Pallor, Blanching, Redness.

Explain the Need to Drink 8 to 10 Glasses of Water Daily.

**Explain the Need to Avoid Alcohol in
Very Cold Weather.**

**Teach Person to Wear Extra Clothing
in the Morning When Metabolism Is
at Lowest Point.**

❖ ◉ Pediatric/Geriatric Interventions

**Explain to Family Members that
Newborns, Infants, and the Elderly Are
More Susceptible to Heat Loss (See
Also *Ineffective Thermoregulation*).**

**For Children and Elderly During
Surgery, Unless Hypothermia Is
Desired to Reduce Blood Loss,
Consider the Following Interventions
(Puterbough, 1991):**

Increase ambient temperature of operating room (OR)
  before case.
Use a portable radiant heating lamp to provide additional
  heat during surgery.
Cover with warm blankets when arriving in OR.
When possible, use a warming mattress.
During prepping and surgery, keep as much of body sur-
  face covered as possible.
Warm prep set, blood, fluids, anesthesia, irrigants.
Replace wet gowns and drapes with dry ones.
Keep head well covered.
Continue heat-conserving interventions postoperatively.

Thermoregulation, Ineffective

DEFINITION

Ineffective Thermoregulation: The state in which an individual experiences or is at risk of experiencing an inability to maintain normal body temperature in the presence of adverse or changing external factors.

⊚ AUTHOR'S NOTE

This diagnosis is indicated when the nurse can maintain or assist a client in maintaining a body temperature within normal limits by manipulating external factors (e.g., clothing) and environmental conditions. Persons who are at high risk for this diagnosis are the elderly and neonates. For those with temperature fluctuations because of disease, infections, or trauma, see *Impaired Comfort.*

DEFINING CHARACTERISTICS
Major (Must be Present)

Temperature fluctuations related to limited metabolic compensatory regulation in response to environmental factors.

RELATED FACTORS
Situational (Personal, Environmental)
Related to:

Fluctuating environmental temperatures
Cold or wet articles
Inadequate housing

Wet body surface
Inadequate clothing for weather (excessive, insufficient)

Maturational
Related to limited metabolic compensatory regulation secondary to age (e.g., neonate, older adult)

NOC Thermoregulation

Goals

The infant will have a temperature between 97.5°F and
98.6°F (36.4°C and 37°C).
The parent will explain techniques to avoid heat loss at
home.

NIC Temperature Regulation, Environmental Management,
Newborn Monitoring, Vital Sign Monitoring

Indicators

- List situations that increase heat loss.
- Demonstrate how to conserve heat during bathing.
- Demonstrate how to take infant's temperature.

❖ Pediatric Interventions

**Reduce or Eliminate the Sources of
Heat Loss in Infants.**

Evaporation
When bathing, provide a warm environment.
Wash and dry in sections to reduce evaporation.
Limit time in contact with wet clothing or blankets.

Convection
Avoid drafts (air conditioning, fans, windows, open portholes on isolette).

Conduction
Warm all articles for care (stethoscopes, scales, hands of
caregivers, clothes, bed linens).

Radiation
Limit objects in the room that absorb heat (metal).
Place crib or bed as far away from walls (outside) or win-
dows as possible.

Monitor Temperature of Infants.

If temperature is below normal:
Wrap in two blankets.
Put on head cap.

❖ Pediatric Interventions (cont'd)

Assess for environmental sources of heat loss.

If hypothermia persists for >1 hour, notify physician.

Assess for complications of cold stress: hypoxia, respiratory acidosis, hypoglycemia, fluid and electrolyte imbalances, weight loss.

If temperature is above normal:

Loosen blanket.

Remove cap, if on.

Assess environment for thermal gain.

If hyperthermia persists for >1 hour, notify physician.

Assess for Signs of Sepsis (Respiratory Function, Skin, Poor Feeding, Irritability, Signs of Localized Infections [Skin, Umbilicus, Circumcision, Eyes]).

Teach Caregiver Why Infant Is Vulnerable to Temperature Fluctuations (Cold and Heat).

Demonstrate how to conserve heat during bathing.

Instruct that it is not necessary to check temperature routinely at home.

Teach to check temperature if infant is hot, sick, or irritable.

ⓒ Geriatric Interventions

Explain age-related changes that interfere with thermoregulation (Miller, 2004):

  Cold (inefficient vasoconstriction, decreased cardiac output, decreased subcutaneous tissue, delayed and diminished shivering)

  Heat (delayed sweating response, diminished sweating response)

Explain that these changes will distort perception of environmental temperatures.

Investigate even a slight elevation of temperature. Use tympanic route for temperatures, not oral or axillary.

Teach how to prevent hypothermia and hyperthermia (refer to *Hypothermia, Hyperthermia*).

Bowel Incontinence

DEFINITION
Bowel Incontinence: The state in which an individual experiences a change in normal bowel habits characterized by involuntary passage of stool.

○○ AUTHOR'S NOTE

This diagnosis represents a situation in which nurses have multiple responsibilities. Clients experiencing bowel incontinence have various responses that disrupt functioning, such as embarrassment and skin problems related to the irritative nature of feces on skin.

For some spinal cord–injured persons, *Bowel Incontinence* related to lack of voluntary control over rectal sphincter would be descriptive.

DEFINING CHARACTERISTICS
Major (Must be Present)
Involuntary passage of stool

RELATED FACTORS
Pathophysiologic
Related to impaired rectal sphincter secondary to:
Diabetes mellitus
Anal or rectal surgery
Anal or rectal injury

Related to cognitive impairment
Related to overdistention of rectum secondary to chronic constipation or fecal impaction
Related to lack of voluntary sphincter control secondary to:

Progressive neuromuscular disorder	Spinal cord compression
	Multiple sclerosis
Spinal cord injury	Cerebrovascular accident

Related to impaired reservoir capacity secondary to:
Inflammatory bowel disease   Chronic rectal ischemia

Treatment-Related
Related to impaired reservoir capacity secondary to:
Colectomy   Radiation proctitis

Situational (Personal, Environmental)
Related to inability to recognize, interpret, or respond to rectal cues secondary to:
Depression   Cognitive impairment

NOC Bowel Continence, Tissue Integrity, Bowel Elimination

Goals

The person will evacuate a soft, formed stool every other day or every third day.

Indicators

- Relate bowel elimination techniques.
- Describe fluid and dietary requirements.

NOC Bowel Incontinence Care, Bowel Training, Bowel Management, Skin Surveillance

Generic Interventions

Assess Previous Bowel Elimination Patterns, Diet, and Lifestyle.

Determine Present Neurologic and Physical Status and Functional Level.

Plan a Consistent, Appropriate Time for Elimination:

Daily bowel program for 5 days or until a pattern develops; then bowel program every other day, morning or evening.

For Persons with Intact Sacral Reflex Center:

Position in an upright or sitting position if functionally able. If not functionally able (quadriplegic), position in left side–

lying position; use digital stimulation: gloves, lubricant, index finger (adults).

For the functionally able, use assistive devices: dil stick, digital stimulator, raised commode seat, and lubricant and gloves as appropriate.

For Persons with Upper Extremity Mobility and Those with Abdominal Musculature Innervation, Teach Bowel Elimination Facilitation Techniques as Appropriate.

Valsalva's maneuver
Forward bends
Sitting push-ups
Abdominal massage

For Persons with Absent Sacral Reflex Center:

Plan daily evacuation schedule, either morning or evening, with manual evacuation of rectal contents.
Position in upright or sitting position if functionally able.
Use assistive devices, raised commode seats, gloves, and lubricant as appropriate.
Teach bowel facilitation techniques:
  Valsalva's maneuver
  Forward bends
  Abdominal massage
  Sitting push-ups if person is functionally able

Maintain an Elimination Record of Bowel Schedule to Include Time, Stool Results, Method(s) Used, and Number of Involuntary Stools if Any.

Teach the Importance of High-Fiber Diet and Optimal Fluid Intake.

Cleanse Skin after Each Bowel Movement. Protect Intact Skin with an Ointment (e.g., Aluminum Paste). If Skin is Not Intact, Consult Clinical Nurse Specialist or Enterostomal Therapist.

Provide Physical Activity and Exercise Appropriate to Functional Level (e.g., Abdominal Exercises, Walking).

Teach Appropriate Use of Stool Softeners and Suppositories and Hazards of Enemas.

Teach Signs and Symptoms of Fecal Impaction and Constipation.

Provide Home Care Training for Those Who Can Be Functionally Independent with Bowel Program.

Breastfeeding, Effective

DEFINITION

Effective Breastfeeding: The state in which a mother-infant dyad exhibits adequate proficiency and satisfaction with the breastfeeding process.

ⓒ **AUTHOR'S NOTE**

This diagnosis reportedly represents a wellness diagnosis. The newly proposed NANDA wellness diagnosis is defined as "a clinical judgment about an individual, family or community in transition from a specific level of wellness to a higher level of wellness" (NANDA, 2001). This definition does not describe a mother-infant dyad seeking higher-level breastfeeding. Instead, it describes "adequate proficiency and satisfaction with the breastfeeding process."

ⓧ **AUTHOR'S NOTE (continued)**

In the management of the breastfeeding experience, the nurse will find three situations:

Ineffective Breastfeeding
Risk for Ineffective Breastfeeding
Effective Breastfeeding or *Readiness for Enhanced Breastfeeding*

Effective Breastfeeding can be used to describe correct and satisfying breastfeeding of a mother and child in the early weeks. The interventions would focus on teaching basic breastfeeding.

If the nurse, most likely in a community or private practice, has a mother who reports proficiency and satisfaction with the breastfeeding process and desires additional learning to achieve even greater proficiency and satisfaction, the nursing diagnosis of *Readiness for Enhanced Breastfeeding* is appropriate. The focus of this learning and continued support would not be to prevent *Ineffective Breastfeeding* or to maintain adequate proficiency and satisfaction but rather to promote enhanced, higher-quality breastfeeding.

DEFINING CHARACTERISTICS
Major (Must be Present, One or More)

Mother is able to position infant at breast to promote a successful latch-on response.

Infant is content after feeding.

Regular and sustained suckling/swallowing occurs at the breast.

Infant weight patterns are appropriate for age.

Effective mother-infant communication patterns (infant cues, maternal interpretation and response).

Minor (May be Present)

Signs and symptoms of oxytocin release (let-down or milk ejection reflex)

Adequate infant elimination patterns for age

Eagerness of infant to nurse

Maternal verbalization of satisfaction with the breastfeeding process

DEFINITION

Ineffective Breastfeeding: The state in which a mother, infant, or child experiences or is at risk of experiencing dissatisfaction or difficulty with the breastfeeding process.

DEFINING CHARACTERISTICS
Major (Must be Present, One or More)

Actual or perceived inadequate milk supply

Infant's inability to attach correctly onto breast

No signs of oxytocin release

Signs of inadequate infant intake

Nonsustained suckling at the breast

Insufficient emptying of each breast at each feeding

Persistence of sore nipples beyond the first week of breastfeeding

Infant exhibiting fussiness and crying within the first hour
after breastfeeding; unresponsive to other comfort
measures

Infant arching and crying at the breast, resisting
latching on

RELATED FACTORS
Physiologic
Related to difficulty of neonate to attach or suck secondary to:

Cleft lip/palate   Inverted nipples

Prematurity   Inadequate let-down reflex

Previous breast surgery

Situational (Personal, Environmental)

Related to maternal fatigue

Related to maternal anxiety

Related to maternal ambivalence

Related to multiple birth

Related to inadequate nutritional intake

Related to inadequate fluid intake

Related to history of unsuccessful breastfeeding
Related to nonsupportive partner/family
Related to lack of knowledge
Related to interruption in breastfeeding secondary to:
Ill mother
Ill infant

Related to work schedule and/or barriers in the work environment

NOC Breastfeeding, Establishment: Infant, Breastfeeding Establishment: Maternal, Breastfeeding Management

Goals

- The mother will report confidence in establishing satisfying, effective breastfeeding.
- The mother will demonstrate effective breastfeeding independently.

Indicators

- Identify factors that deter breastfeeding.
- Identify factors that promote breastfeeding.
- Demonstrate effective positioning.
- Have a relaxed, feeding infant.

NIC Breastfeeding Assistance, Lactation Counseling

Maternal Interventions

Assess for Factors Contributing to Difficulty or Dissatisfaction (Refer to Related Factors).

If Dissatisfied, Explore Specifics. Encourage Mother to Share Her

Maternal Interventions (cont'd)

**Concerns Openly. Evaluate Her
Fatigue Level, Knowledge, Anxiety,
Support System, and History
of Breastfeeding.**

Evaluate:

Mother's state (comfort, anxiety, position)
Infant's state (quiet, alert, crying, extremely hungry)
Let-down reflex
Baby at breast
Alignment
Areolar grasp
Areolar compression
Audible swallowing
Infant's intake and frequency of feedings
Infant's output (six to eight diapers per day, bowel move-
   ment daily)

Teach Management of Sore Nipples:

Decrease nursing time to 5 to 10 minutes per side.
   Start baby on nontender side first. Allow for more
   frequent, short feedings. Suggest alternate positions
   to rotate infant's grasps. Allow breasts to dry after each
   feeding.
Keep nursing pads dry.
Use breast cream only after breasts are dry.
Use breast shield as last measure, and remove after milk
   has let down.
Be sure infant's mouth is positioned correctly on the breast.

**If Symptoms of Mastitis or Breast
Abscess Develop (Increased Warmth,
Tenderness, Redness), Instruct
Mother to Contact Her Advanced
Practice Nurse or Physician.**

If Engorgement Occurs:

Massage breast before nursing by encircling breast with
   both hands and moving hands downward toward nipple.
   Use lotion if desired.

🐾 Maternal Interventions (cont'd)

Use heat before nursing (hot shower, hot pack).
If needed, massage breast again while infant is sucking in
  shorter sucks at end of feeding.
Use ice packs between feedings.
Wear a good support bra.
Use mild analgesics as needed.

**Respond to Concerns Regarding
Confidence and "Not Enough Milk."**

**If Supplementary Feedings Are Used,
Consider the Pouch and Tubing
Device to Continue Breastfeeding
and Prevent Nipple Confusion.**

**Support Mother's Decision to Continue
with Breastfeeding or to Discontinue.**

**If Breastfeeding Is Interrupted
(e.g., Illness, Maternal Employment):**

Allow mother to share her feelings.
Determine whether breastfeeding can be resumed if
  desired.

**Teach How to Express, Handle, Store,
and Transport Breast Milk Safely.**

**Provide Breast Pump, or Make
Mother Aware of Availability,
If Needed.**

**Encourage Verbal Expression
of Feelings.**

**Explore Feelings and Anticipation of
Problems. Older Child May Be
Jealous of Contact with Baby. Mother
Can Use This Time to Read to Older
Child.**

Maternal Interventions (cont'd)

Stress the Need for Rest:

Encourage mother to make herself and infant a priority.
Discuss temporary housekeeper.
Encourage mother to limit visits from relatives for first
  4 weeks.

**Provide Opportunities for Significant
Others to Ask Questions.**

**Initiate Referrals as Indicated
(Lactation Specialist,
La Leche League).**

Breastfeeding, Interrupted

DEFINITION

Interrupted Breastfeeding: A break in the continuity of the
breastfeeding process as a result of inability to put the baby
to breast for feeding or inadvisability of doing so.

> ○ AUTHOR'S NOTE
>
> This diagnosis represents a situation, not a response. If
> one examines the diagnosis *Ineffective Breastfeeding*,
> interrupted breastfeeding is listed as "related to." Nursing
> interventions do not treat the interruption but treat the
> effects of this interruption. The situation is interrupted
> breastfeeding; the responses can be varied. For example,
> if continued breastfeeding or use of a breast pump is
> contraindicated, the nurse will focus on the loss of this

> ⊛ **AUTHOR'S NOTE (continued)**
>
> breastfeeding experience, using the nursing diagnosis of *Grieving*. If breastfeeding is continued with expression and storage of breast milk, teaching, and support, the diagnosis will be *Risk for Ineffective Breastfeeding related to continuity problems* secondary to, for example, maternal employment. If difficulty is experienced, the diagnosis would be *Ineffective Breastfeeding related to interruption* secondary to (specify) and lack of knowledge. Refer to *Ineffective Breastfeeding* for interventions.

DEFINING CHARACTERISTICS
Major (Must be Present)
Infant does not receive nourishment at the breast for some or all of feedings.

Minor (May be Present)
Maternal desire to maintain lactation and provide (or eventually provide) her breast milk for her infant's nutritional needs

Separation of mother and infant

Lack of knowledge about expression and storage of breast milk

RELATED FACTORS
Maternal or infant illness

Prematurity

Maternal employment

Contraindications to breastfeeding (e.g., drugs, true breast milk jaundice)

Need to wean infant abruptly

Cardiac Output, Decreased

DEFINITION

Cardiac Output, Decreased: The state in which an individual experiences a reduction in the amount of blood pumped by the heart, resulting in compromised cardiac function.

⚭ AUTHOR'S NOTE

This diagnosis represents a situation in which nurses have multiple responsibilities. Individuals experiencing decreased cardiac output may present various responses that disrupt functioning, such as:

Activity Intolerance
Disturbed Sleep Pattern

They may be at risk for developing physiologic complications, such as:

Dysrhythmias
Cardiogenic shock
Congestive heart failure

I recommend that the nurse not use *Decreased Cardiac Output* but instead select another diagnosis that better describes the situation (see *Activity Intolerance*). By not using *Decreased Cardiac Output,* the nurse can more specifically describe the situations that nurses either treat as a nursing diagnosis or co-treat as a collaborative problem.

DEFINING CHARACTERISTICS

Low blood pressure	Vertigo
Rapid pulse	Edema (peripheral, sacral)
Dyspnea	Restlessness
Angina	Cyanosis
Dysrhythmia	Oliguria
Fatigability	

Caregiver Role Strain

DEFINITION

Caregiver Role Strain: A state in which an individual is experiencing physical, emotional, social, and/or financial burden(s) in the process of giving care to another.

ⓧ AUTHOR'S NOTE

There are 2.2 million unpaid home caregivers in the United States. These caregivers provide care for individuals of all ages, some across their entire life span (e.g., children with permanent disabilities). The care receivers have physical or mental disabilities. These disabilities can be temporary or permanent. Some disabilities are permanent but stable (e.g., blind child), whereas others signal progressive deterioration (e.g., Alzheimer's disease).

Caregiver Role Strain represents the burden of caregiving on the physical and emotional health of the caregiver and its effects on the family and social system of the caregiver and care receiver. *Risk for Caregiver Role Strain* can be a significant nursing diagnosis, because nurses can identify at-risk individuals and assist them to prevent this grave situation.

DEFINING CHARACTERISTICS
Expressed or observed

Reports insufficient time or physical energy
Difficulty performing caregiving activities required
Caregiving responsibilities interfere with other important
  roles (e.g., work, spouse, friend, parent)

Apprehension about the future for the care receiver's
  health and ability to provide care
Apprehension about care receiver's care when caregiver is
  ill or deceased
Depressed feelings, anger

RELATED FACTORS
Pathophysiologic
**Related to unrelenting or complex care requirements
secondary to:**

Debilitating conditions
  (acute, progressive)
Progressive dementia
Disability

Chronic mental illness
Unpredictable illness course
Addiction

Treatment-Related
Related to 24-hour care responsibilities
**Related to time (activities, e.g., dialysis, transporta-
tion)**

Situational (Personal, Environmental)
**Related to unrealistic expectations of caregiver by
care receiver**
Related to pattern of ineffective coping
Related to compromised physical health
Related to unrealistic expectations of self
Related to history of poor relationship
Related to history of family dysfunction
**Related to unrealistic expectations for caregiver by
others (society, other family members)**
Related to duration of caregiving required
Related to isolation
Related to insufficient respite
Related to insufficient recreation
Related to insufficient finances
Related to no or unavailable support

Maturational (Infant, Child, Adolescent)
**Related to unrelenting care requirements second-
ary to:**

Mental disabilities (specify)
Physical disabilities (specify)

NOC Caregiver Well-Being, Role Performance, Caregiver Endurance Potential, Family Coping, Family Integrity

Goals

The caregiver will report a plan to decrease his or her burden.

Indicators

- Share frustrations regarding caregiving responsibilities.
- Identify one source of support.
- Identify two changes that, if made, would improve daily life.

The family will establish a plan for weekly support or help.

- Relate an intent to listen without giving advice.
- Convey empathy to caregiver regarding daily responsibilities.

NIC Caregiver Support, Respite Care, Coping Enhancement, Family Mobilization, Mutual Goal Setting, Support System Enhancement, Anticipatory Guidance

Generic Interventions

Assess for Causative or Contributing Factors:

Poor insight into situation
Unrealistic expectations (caregiver, family)
Reluctance or inability to access help
Unsatisfactory caregiver–care receiver relationship
Insufficient resources (e.g., help, financial)
Social isolation
Insufficient leisure
Competing roles (spouse, parenting, work)

Evaluate Caregiver's and Others' Interpretation of the Situation. Re-evaluate Periodically (Winslow, 1999).

What information have they been told?
Do they expect the situation to continue as is, improve, or worsen?
Are they realistic?

**Provide Empathy, and Promote a
Sense of Competency.**

**Discuss the Effects of Present
Schedule and Responsibilities on:**

Physical health
Emotional status
Relationships

**Assist to Identify Activities for
Which Assistance Is Desired:**

Care receiver's needs
  (hygiene, food,
  treatments, mobility)
Meals
Transportation
Yard work
Respite
  (number of hours a week)

Laundry
House cleaning
Shopping, errands
Appointments
  (doctor, hairdresser)
House repairs
Money management

**Discuss with the Family
(Shields, 1992; Winslow, 1999):**

The importance of regularly acknowledging the burden of
  the situation for the caregiver
The benefits of listening without giving advice
The importance of emotional support:
  Regular phone calls
  Cards, letters
  Visits
The need to give caregiver "permission" to enjoy self
  (e.g., vacations, day trips)
The need to provide caregiver with opportunities to
  respond to "How can I help you?"

**Identify All Possible Sources of
Volunteer Help: Family (Siblings,
Cousins), Friends, Neighbors,
Church, Community Groups.**

Role-Play How to Ask for Help.

**Identify Community
Resources Available:**

Support groups   Counseling
Social service   Transportation
Home-delivered meals   Day care

🕑 Geriatric Interventions

If appropriate, discuss if and when an alternative source of
  care (e.g., nursing home, senior housing) may be indicated.
If elder abuse is suspected, refer to *Disabled Family Coping*.

Risk for Caregiver Role Strain

DEFINITION

Risk for Caregiver Role Strain: The state in which an individual is at high risk to experience physical, emotional, social, and/or financial burden(s) in the process of giving care
to another.

> ℃ AUTHOR'S NOTE
> Refer to *Caregiver Role Strain*.

RISK FACTORS

Presence of risk factors (refer to Related Factors)

RELATED FACTORS

Primary caregiver responsibilities for a recipient who requires regular assistance with self-care or supervision be-

cause of physical or mental disabilities in addition to one
or more of the following:

**Related to unrelenting or complex care requirements
secondary to:**
Care receiver characteristics
Unable to perform self-care activities
Not motivated to perform self-care activities
Cognitive problems
Psychological problems
Unrealistic expectations of caregiver
Caregiver/spouse characteristics
Pattern of ineffective coping
Compromised physical health
Unrealistic expectations of self

Related to history of poor relationship
Related to history of family dysfunction
**Related to unrealistic expectations for caregiver by
others (society, other family members)**
Related to duration of caregiving required
Related to isolation
Related to insufficient respite
Related to insufficient recreation
Related to insufficient finances
Related to no or unavailable support

NOC Refer to Caregiver Role Strain

Goals

The person will relate a plan on how to continue social activities despite caregiving responsibilities.

Indicators

- Identify activities that are important for self.
- Relate an intent to enlist the help of at least
  two people.

NIC Refer to Caregiver Role Strain

Generic Interventions

Explain the Causes of Caregiver Role Strain. Refer to *Caregiver Role Strain*. Assist with Anticipating the Effects of the Caregiving Role.

Stress the Importance of Daily Health-Promotion Activities:

Rest-exercise balance
Effective stress management
Low-fat, high-complex carbohydrate diet
Supportive social networks
Appropriate screening practices for age

See *Health Seeking Behaviors* for specific interventions.

Discuss the Need for Respite and Short-Term Relief.

Maintain a Good Sense of Humor; Associate with Others Who Laugh.

Caution About Spending Too Much Time Complaining, Which Is Depressing for All Involved and May Lead to Avoidance.

Advise to Initiate Phone Contacts or Visits with Friends or Relatives Rather Than Waiting for Others to Do It.

Emphasize the Importance of Respites to Prevent Isolating Behaviors That Foster Depression.

Discuss the Implications of Caring for Ill Family Member with All Family Members. Include:

Available resources (finances, environmental)
24-hour responsibility

Effects on other household members

Likelihood of progressive deterioration

Sharing of responsibilities (with other household members, siblings, neighbors)

Likelihood of exacerbating long-standing conflicts

Impact on lifestyle

Alternative or assistive options (e.g., community-based health care providers, life care centers, group living, nursing home)

Assist to Identify Activities for Which Assistance Is Desired:

Care receiver's needs (hygiene, food, treatments, mobility)

Meals

Transportation

Yard work

Respite (number of hours a week)

Laundry

House cleaning

Shopping, errands

Appointments (doctor, hairdresser)

House repairs

Money management

Identify Community Resources Available:

Support group

Social service

Home-delivered meals

Counseling

Transportation

Day care

Comfort, Impaired*
Acute Pain
Chronic Pain
Nausea

Comfort, Impaired

DEFINITION
Impaired Comfort: The state in which an individual experiences an uncomfortable sensation in response to a noxious stimulus.

> **ⓧ AUTHOR'S NOTE**
>
> This diagnosis, *Impaired Comfort,* can represent a variety of uncomfortable sensations, such as pruritus, immobility, or nothing by mouth (NPO) status. When an individual experiences nausea and vomiting, the nurse should assess whether *Nausea* or *Risk for Imbalanced Nutrition* is the appropriate category. Short-lived episodes of nausea or vomiting (e.g., postoperatively) can be best described with *Nausea related to nausea/vomiting* secondary to effects of anesthesia or analgesics. When the nausea/vomiting is at risk of compromising nutritional intake, use *Risk for Imbalanced Nutrition: Less Than Body Requirements related to nausea and vomiting* secondary to (specify).

DEFINING CHARACTERISTICS
Major (Must be Present)
The person reports or demonstrates discomfort (e.g., pain, nausea, vomiting, pruritus).

---

*This diagnosis is not currently on the NANDA list but has been included for clarity and usefulness.

Minor (May be Present)

Autonomic response to acute pain:
  Blood pressure increased
  Pulse increased
  Respirations increased
  Diaphoresis
  Dilated pupils
Guarded position
Facial mask of pain
Crying, moaning

RELATED FACTORS

Any factor can contribute to altered comfort. The most common are listed below.

Biopathophysiologic

Related to uterine contractions during labor
Related to trauma to perineum during labor and delivery
Related to involution of uterus and engorged breasts
Related to tissue trauma and reflex muscle spasms secondary to:

Musculoskeletal Disorders

Fractures	Arthritis
Contractures	Spinal cord disorders
Spasms	

Visceral Disorders

Cardiac	Intestinal
Renal	Pulmonary
Hepatic	

Vascular Disorders

Vasospasm	Phlebitis
Occlusion	Vasodilation (headache)
Cancer	

Related to inflammation of:

Nerve	Joint
Tendon	Muscle
Bursa	Juxtoarticular structures

Related to fatigue, malaise, and/or pruritus secondary to contagious disease:

Rubella	Mononucleosis
Chickenpox	Pancreatitis
Hepatitis	

Related to effects of cancer on (specify)

Related to abdominal cramps, diarrhea, and vomiting secondary to gastroenteritis, influenza, or gastric ulcers

Related to inflammation and smooth-muscle spasms secondary to renal calculi or gastrointestinal infections

Treatment-Related

Related to tissue trauma and reflex muscle spasms secondary to:

Surgery
Accidents
Burns
Diagnostic tests:
    Venipuncture
    Invasive scanning
    Biopsy

Related to nausea and vomiting secondary to chemotherapy, anesthesia, or side effects of (specify)

Situational (Personal, Environmental)

Related to fever
Related to immobility/improper positioning
Related to overactivity
Related to pressure points (tight cast, elastic bandage)
Related to allergic response
Related to chemical irritants
Related to unmet dependency needs
Related to severe repressed anxiety

Maturational

Related to tissue trauma secondary to:

Infancy: Colic
Infancy and early childhood: Teething, ear pain
Middle childhood: Recurrent abdominal pain, growing pains
Adolescence: Headaches, chest pain, dysmenorrhea

Acute Pain

DEFINITION

Acute Pain: The state in which an individual experiences and reports the presence of severe discomfort or an uncomfortable sensation lasting from 1 second to <6 months.

⚭ AUTHOR'S NOTE

The NANDA list contains *Pain* and *Chronic Pain.* For clarity and usefulness, the author has organized diagnoses associated with pain and discomfort under two levels:

Impaired Comfort
- *Acute Pain*
- *Chronic Pain*

DEFINING CHARACTERISTICS
Major (80% to 100%)

Communication of pain descriptors

Minor (60% to 79%)

Clenched jaws or fists
Altered ability to continue previous activities
Agitation
Anxiety
Irritability
Rubs painful part
Grunts
Unusual posture (knees to abdomen)
Physical inactivity or immobility
Problems with concentration
Changes in sleep patterns
Fear of reinjury
Withdraws when touched
Widely opened or tightly shut eyes
Pinched features
Nausea and vomiting

RELATED FACTORS

Refer to *Impaired Comfort*.

NOC Comfort Level, Pain Control

Goals

The person will relate relief after a satisfactory relief measure as evidenced by (specify).

Indicators

- Relate factors that increase pain.
- Relate interventions that are effective.
- Convey that others validate that the pain exists.

NIC Pain Management, Medication Management, Emotional Support, Teaching: Individual, Hot/Cold Application, Simple Massage

Generic Interventions

Reduce Lack of Knowledge:

Explain causes of the pain to the person, if known.
Relate how long the pain will last, if known.
Explain diagnostic tests and procedures in detail by relating the discomforts and sensations that will be felt, and approximate the length of time involved (e.g., "During the intravenous pyelogram, you might feel a momentary hot flash through your entire body.").

Provide Accurate Information to Reduce Fear of Addiction.

Relate Your Acceptance of the Person's Response to Pain:

Acknowledge the presence of the pain.
Listen attentively concerning the pain.
Convey that you are assessing the pain because you want to understand it better (not determine if it is really present).

Discuss the Reasons Why an Individual May Experience Increased or Decreased Pain (e.g., Fatigue [Increased] or Presence of Distractions [Decreased]).

Encourage family members to share their concerns privately (e.g., fear that the person will use pain for secondary gains if they give the person too much attention).

Assess whether the family doubts the pain, and discuss the effects of this on the person's pain and on the relationship.

Encourage the family to give attention also when pain is not exhibited.

Provide the Person with Opportunities to Rest During the Day and with Periods of Uninterrupted Sleep at Night (Must Rest When Pain Is Decreased).

Discuss with the Person and Family the Therapeutic Uses of Distraction as Well as Other Methods of Pain Relief.

Teach a Method of Distraction During Acute Pain (e.g., Painful Procedure) That Is Not a Burden (e.g., Count Items in a Picture; Count Anything in the Room, Such as Patterns on Wallpaper; Count Silently to Self; Breathe Rhythmically; Listen to Music, and Increase the Volume as the Pain Increases).

Teach Noninvasive Pain-relief Measures.

Relaxation

Instruct on techniques to reduce skeletal muscle tension, which will reduce the intensity of the pain.

Promote relaxation with a back rub, massage, or warm bath.

Teach a specific relaxation strategy (e.g., slow, rhythmic breathing or deep breath—clench fists—yawn).

Cutaneous Stimulation

Discuss the various methods of skin stimulation and their
effects on pain.

Discuss the following methods and the precautions:

Hot water bottle, warm tub

Electric heating pad, moist heat pack

Hot summer sun

Thin plastic wrap over painful area to retain body heat
(e.g., knee, elbow)

Cold towels (wrung out)

Cold-water immersion for small body parts

Ice bag, cold gel pack, ice massage

Explain the therapeutic uses of menthol preparations and
massage/back rub.

**Provide Optimal Pain Relief with
Prescribed Analgesics.**

**After Administering a Pain-relief
Medication, Return in 30 Minutes
to Assess Effectiveness.**

**Give Accurate Information to
Correct Family Misconceptions
(e.g., Addiction, Doubts about Pain).**

**Provide Individuals with
Opportunities to Discuss Their Fears,
Anger, and Frustrations in Private;
Acknowledge the Difficulty of the
Situation.**

◆ Pediatric Interventions

Assess the Child's Pain Experience:

Determine the child's concept of the cause of pain,
if feasible.

Ask the child to point to the area that hurts.

For children younger than 4 or 5 years, use Oucher Scale
of five faces from very happy (1) to crying (5).

For children older than 4 years, ask to rate the pain using
a scale of 0 to 5 (0 = no pain, 5 = worst pain).

❖ Pediatric Interventions (cont'd)

Ask the child what makes the pain better and what makes it worse.

Assess if fear or loneliness is contributing to the pain.

Promote Security with Honest Explanations and Opportunities for Choice.

Tell the truth. Explain:
  How much it will hurt
  How long it will last
  What will help the pain

Do not threaten (e.g., *do not* tell the child, "If you don't hold still, you won't go home.").

Explicitly explain and reinforce to the child that pain is not a means of punishment.

Explain to the parents that the child may cry more openly when they are present but that their presence is important for promoting trust.

Explain to the child that the procedure is necessary so he or she can get better, and it is important to hold still so the procedure can be done quickly.

Discuss with the parents the importance of truth-telling.
  Instruct parents to:
    Tell the child when they are leaving and when they will return.
    Relate to the child that they cannot take away the pain but that they will be there (except in circumstances when parents are not permitted to remain).

Allow the parents opportunities to share their feelings about witnessing their child's pain and their helplessness.

Prepare the Child for a Painful Procedure:

Discuss the procedure with the parents; determine what they have told the child.

Explain the procedure in words suited to the child's age and developmental level.

Relate the discomforts that will be felt (e.g., what the child will feel, taste, see, or smell).

❖ Pediatric Interventions (cont'd)

Encourage the child to ask questions before and during the
   procedure; ask the child to share with you what he or she
   thinks is going to happen and why.

Share with the child (who is old enough: older than
   3-½ years):

   You expect that the child will hold still and that such
      behavior will be pleasing to you.

   It is all right to cry or squeeze your hand if it hurts.

Arrange to have parents present for procedures (especially
   for children 18 months to 5 years).

**Explain to the Child That He or She
Can Be Distracted from the
Procedure If He or She Wishes. (The
Use of Distraction Without the Child's
Knowledge of the Impending
Discomfort Is Not Advocated Because
the Child Will Learn to Mistrust):**

Tell a story with a puppet.

Ask the child to name or count objects in a picture.

Ask the child to look at a picture, and to locate certain
   objects ("Where is the dog?").

Ask the child to tell you about a pet.

Ask the child to count your blinks.

Blow a party noisemaker.

**Provide the Child with Privacy
During the Painful Procedure;
Use a Treatment Room Rather
Than the Child's Bed.**

**Assist the Child with the Aftermath
of Pain:**

Tell the child when the painful procedure is over.

Pick up the small child to indicate that it is over.

Encourage the child to discuss the pain experience (draw
   or act out with dolls).

Encourage the child to perform the painful procedure
   under supervision using the same equipment on a doll.

❖ Pediatric Interventions (cont'd)

Praise the child for endurance, and convey that the pain was handled well, regardless of the child's behavior (unless the child was violent to others).

Give the child a souvenir of the pain (Band-Aid, badge for bravery).

Teach the child to keep a record of painful experiences and to place a star next to those for which he or she held still (e.g., gold stars on a paper for each injection or venipuncture).

❖ Maternal Interventions (Reeder et al., 1997)

Assess Contractions and Discomfort (Onset, Frequency, Duration, Intensity, Description of Discomfort).

Determine the Presence of Other Discomforts Not Related to Labor (e.g., Chronic or Recent Illness).

Assess Goals and Expectations Regarding:

Labor
Pain relief methods
Persons to be present
Medications

Explain Pain Relief Methods Available:

Relaxation techniques
Breathing patterns
Acupressure
Massage
Cold/heat applications
Positioning
Physical activities
Distraction
Medications

Maternal Interventions (Reeder et al, 1997) (cont'd)

Determine What Types of Methods Are Desired. Encourage Client to Try Several Methods.

Coach Her with the Method, and Include Her Labor Support Person.

Stand and Walk as Much as Possible During First Stage.

Change Positions at Least Every Hour.

For Backaches, Try Squatting, Kneeling, or an All-Fours Position (Hands and Knees).

Encourage Use of Heat (Bath, Showers, Heating Pad) for Lower Abdomen, Groin, Back, Perineum, or Thigh Pain.

For Back Pain, Apply Cold Pack to Back or Neck (20 to 30 Minutes).

If Mother Panics During Transition, Be Firm and Direct:
"I'm here, and I'm in charge."
"I'm here for you."
Make her look at you.
Hold her wrist.
Exaggerate your coaching breathing.

Assist Her with the Aftermath of Labor:
Praise her for her hard work.
Allow her to relive difficult moments.
Explain why pain increased.
Acknowledge support person's help.

Chronic Pain

DEFINITION
Chronic Pain: The state in which an individual experiences pain that is persistent or intermittent and lasts for >6 months.

DEFINING CHARACTERISTICS
Major (Must be Present)
The person reports that pain has existed for >6 months (may be the only assessment data present).

Minor (60% to 79%)
Disruption of social and family relationships
Irritability
Physical inactivity or immobility
Depression
Rubbing of painful part
Anxiety
"Beaten" look
Self-focusing
Skeletal muscle tension
Somatic preoccupation
Agitation
Fatigue
Decreased libido
Restlessness

RELATED FACTORS
Refer to *Impaired Comfort.*

> **NOC** Comfort Level, Pain Control, Pain: Disruptive Effects, Depression Control

Goals

The person will relate improvement of pain and an increase in daily activities as evidenced by (specify).

Indicators

- Relate that others validate that the pain exists.
- Practice selected noninvasive pain relief measures to manage the pain.

The child will demonstrate coping mechanism for pain and methods of controlling pain, as evidenced by an increase in play and usual activities of childhood, and (specify).

- Communicate improvement in pain verbally, by pain assessment scale, or by behavior (specify).
- Maintain usual family role and relationships throughout pain experience, as evidenced by (specify).

> **NIC** Pain Management, Medication Management, Exercise Promotion, Mood Management, Coping Enhancement

Generic Interventions

Refer to *Acute Pain*.

Assess the Effects of Chronic Pain on the Individual's Life.
Performance (job, role responsibilities)
Social interactions
Finances
Activities of daily living (sleeping, eating, mobility, sex)
Cognition/mood (concentration, depression)
Family unit (response of members)

Explore Expectations of Course of Pain, Treatment, and Side Effects; Clarify if Unrealistic.

Discuss the Effectiveness of Combining Physical and Psychological Techniques and Pharmacotherapy.

Discuss with the Individual and Family the Various Treatment Modalities Available (Family Therapy,

Group Therapy, Behavior
Modification, Biofeedback, Hypnosis,
Acupuncture, Exercise Program,
Cognitive Strategies).

Discuss the Suffering Caused by the
Pain Experience: Decreased
Endurance, Poor Appetite, Interrupted
Sleep, Diminished Enjoyment, Anxiety,
Fear, Difficulty Concentrating, and
Diminished Social and Sexual
Relationships

◆ Pediatric Interventions

Assess Pain Experiences by Using
Developmentally Appropriate
Assessment Scales and by
Assessing Behavior.

Set Goals for Pain Management with
Child and Family (Short- and
Long-Term), and Evaluate Regularly.

Promote the "Normal" Aspects
of the Child's Life: Play, School,
Relationships with Family,
Physical Activity.

Promote a Trusting Environment
for the Child and Family:
Believe the child's pain.
Encourage the child's perception that interventions are
    attempts to help.
Have the child, family, and nurse participate in controlling
    pain.

Use Interdisciplinary Team for Pain
Management as Necessary (e.g., Nurse,
Physician, Child Life Therapist,
Mental Health Therapist,
Occupational Therapist, Physical
Therapist, Nutritionist).

DEFINITION

Nausea: The state in which an individual experiences an unpleasant, wavelike sensation in the back of the throat, epigastrium, or throughout the abdomen that may or may not lead to vomiting.

DEFINING CHARACTERISTICS

Usually precedes vomiting, but may be experienced after vomiting or when vomiting does not occur

Accompanied by pallor, cold and clammy skin, increased salivation, tachycardia, gastric stasis, and diarrhea

Accompanied by swallowing movements affected by skeletal muscles

Reports "nausea" or "sick to my stomach"

RELATED FACTORS

Biopathophysiologic

Related to gastrointestinal irritation secondary to:

Acute gastroenteritis

Peptic ulcer disease

Irritable bowel syndrome

Pancreatitis

Migraine headaches

Pregnancy

Infections (e.g., food poisoning)

Drug overdose

Renal calculi

Motion sickness

Treatment-Related

Related to effects of chemotherapy, theophylline, digitalis, or antibiotics

Related to effects of anesthesia

Goals

The person will report decreased nausea.

NOC Comfort Level, Hydration, Nutritional Status

Indicators

- Name foods or beverages that do not increase nausea.
- Describe factors that increase nausea.

NIC Medication Management, Nausea Management, Fluid/ Electrolyte Management, Nutrition Management

Generic Interventions

Explain the Cause of the Nausea and the Duration if Known.

Encourage the Client to Eat Small, Frequent Meals and to Eat Slowly. Cool, Bland Foods and Liquids Are Usually Well Tolerated.

Eliminate Unpleasant Sights and Odors from the Eating Area.

Instruct the Client to Avoid:
Hot or cold liquids
Foods containing fat and fiber
Spicy foods
Caffeine

Encourage the Client to Rest in a Semi-Fowler's Position after Eating and to Change Position Slowly.

Teach Techniques to Reduce Nausea:
Restrict fluid with meals.
Avoid the smell of food preparation and other noxious stimuli.
Loosen clothing before eating.
Sit in fresh air or use a fan.
Avoid lying flat for at least 2 hours after eating.

Determine Etiology of Nausea and Consult with Nurse Practitioner or Physician for Treatment (Ladd, 1999):

Cough
Constipation
Urinary tract infection
Reflux disease
Electrolyte imbalance
Candidiasis
Increased intracranial pressure
Pharmaceutical agent
Anxiety

Teach How to Use Antiemetic Medications Aggressively Prior to and After Chemotherapy (Eckert, 2001).

Communication, Impaired*
Communication, Impaired Verbal

Communication, Impaired

DEFINITION

Impaired Communication: The state in which an individual experiences or is at high risk to experience difficulty exchanging thoughts, ideas, desires, wants, or needs with others.

---

*This diagnosis was developed by Rosalinda Alfaro-LeFevre and is not currently on the NANDA list; it has been included for clarity or usefulness.

> ⓧ **AUTHOR'S NOTE**
>
> *Impaired Communication* and *Impaired Verbal Communication* are diagnoses to describe people who desire to communicate but who are encountering problems. *Impaired Communication* may not be useful to describe a person for whom communication problems are a manifestation of a psychiatric illness or coping problem. If nursing interventions are focusing on reducing hallucinations, fear, or anxiety, the diagnosis of *Fear, Anxiety,* or *Disturbed Thought Processes* is more appropriate.

DEFINING CHARACTERISTICS
Major (Must be Present, One or More)
Impaired ability to speak or hear
Inappropriate or absent speech or response

Minor (May be Present)

Incongruence between verbal and nonverbal messages
Stuttering
Dysarthria
Aphasia

Slurring
Word-finding problems
Weak or absent voice
Statements of not understanding or being misunderstood

RELATED FACTORS
Pathophysiologic
Related to disordered, unrealistic thinking secondary to schizophrenic disorder, delusional disorder, psychotic or paranoid disorder
Related to impaired motor function of muscles of speech secondary to: or
Related to ischemia of temporal or frontal lobe secondary to:
Expressive or receptive aphasia
Cerebrovascular accident
Oral, facial trauma
Alzheimer's disease
Brain damage (e.g., birth/head trauma)
Central nervous system (CNS) depression/increased intracranial pressure

Tumor (head, neck, or spinal cord)
Chronic hypoxia/decreased cerebral blood flow
Quadriplegia
CNS diseases (e.g., myasthenia gravis, multiple sclerosis, muscular dystrophy)
Vocal cord paralysis

Related to impaired ability to produce speech secondary to:
Respiratory impairment (e.g., shortness of breath)
Laryngeal edema/infection
Oral deformities
Cleft lip or palate
Malocclusion or fractured jaw
Missing teeth
Dysarthria

Related to auditory impairment

Treatment-Related
Related to impaired ability to produce speech secondary to:
Endotracheal intubation
Tracheostomy/tracheotomy/laryngectomy
Surgery of the head, face, neck, or mouth
Pain (especially of the mouth or throat)

Situational (Personal, Environmental)
Related to decreased attention secondary to fatigue, anger, anxiety, or pain
Related to no access to hearing aid or malfunction of hearing aid
Related to psychological barrier (e.g., fear, shyness)
Related to lack of privacy
Related to loss of recent memory recall
Related to lack of interpreter

Maturational
Infant/Child
Related to inadequate sensory stimulation

Older Adult (Auditory Losses)
Related to hearing impairment
Related to cognitive impairments secondary to (specify)

NOC Communication Ability

Goals

The person will report improved satisfaction with ability to communicate.

Indicators

- Demonstrate increased ability to understand.
- Demonstrate improved ability to express self.
- Use alternative methods of communication, as indicated.

NIC Communication Enhancement, Active Listening, Socialization Enhancement

Generic Interventions

Use Factors that Promote Hearing and Understanding.

Talk distinctly and clearly, facing the person.

Minimize unnecessary sounds in the room.

  Have only one person talk.

  Be aware of background noises (e.g., close the door, turn off the television or radio).

Repeat, then rephrase, a thought if the person does not seem to understand the whole meaning.

Use touch and gestures to enhance communication.

If the person can understand only sign language, have an interpreter present as often as possible.

If the person is in a group (e.g., diabetes class), place him or her in front of the room near the teacher.

Approach the person from the side on which hearing is best (*i.e.,* if hearing is better with left ear, approach the person from the left).

If the person can lip-read, look directly at the person, and talk slowly and clearly.

Assess functioning of hearing aids (e.g., batteries).

Provide Alternative Methods of Communication:

Use pad and pencil, alphabet letters, hand signals, eye blinks, head nods, bell signals.

Make flash cards with pictures or words depicting frequently used phrases (e.g., "Wet my lips," "Move
my foot," glass of water, bedpan).

Encourage the person to point and to use gestures and
pantomime.

Provide a Nonrushed Environment.

Use normal loudness level, and speak unhurriedly in short
phrases.

Encourage the person to take plenty of time talking and to
enunciate words carefully with good lip movements.

Decrease external distractions.

Delay conversation when the person is tired.

Use Techniques to Increase Understanding:

Use uncomplicated one-step commands and directives.

Encourage the use of gestures and pantomime.

Match words with actions; use pictures.

Terminate conversation on a note of success (e.g., move
back to an easier item).

Use same words with same task.

Make a Concerted Effort to Understand When the Person is Speaking.

Allow enough time to listen if the person speaks slowly.

Rephrase the person's message aloud to validate it.

Respond to all attempts at speech even if they are unintelligible (e.g., "I do not know what you are saying. Can you
try to say it again?").

Ignore mistakes and profanity.

Do not pretend you understand if you do not.

Allow the person time to respond; do not interrupt. Supply
words only occasionally.

Teach Techniques to Improve Speech:

Ask the person to slow speech down and to say each word
clearly; provide an example.

Encourage the person to speak in short phrases.

Suggest a slower rate of talking or taking a breath before
beginning to speak.

Encourage the person to take time and concentrate on
forming the words.

Ask the person to write the message or to draw a picture if
verbal communication is difficult.
Ask questions that can be answered with a "yes" or "no."
Focus on the present; avoid topics that are controversial,
emotional, abstract, or lengthy.

**Verbally Address the Problem of
Frustration about Inability to
Communicate, and Explain that
Patience is Needed for the Nurse and
the Person Who is Trying to Talk.**

**Give the Person Opportunities to Make
Decisions about Care (e.g., "Do You
Want a drink?" "Would You Rather
Have Orange Juice or Prune Juice?").**

**Teach Techniques to Significant
Others and Repetitive Approaches
to Improve Communications.**

**If a Translator is Needed, Refer to
*Impaired Verbal Communication.***

**If the Person is Hearing-Impaired,
Refer to Geriatric Interventions.**

Geriatric Interventions

If the person can hear with a hearing aid, make sure that
it is on and functioning.
If the person can hear with one ear, speak slowly and
clearly into the good ear. (It is more important to speak
distinctly than to speak loudly.)
If the person can read and write, provide pad and pencil at
all times (even when going to another department).
If the person can understand only sign language, have an
interpreter with him or her as much as possible.
Write and speak all important messages.
Validate the person's understanding by asking questions
that require more than "yes" or "no" answers. Avoid asking, "Do you understand?"
Assess if cerumen impaction is impairing hearing.

Communication, Impaired Verbal

DEFINITION
Impaired Verbal Communication: The state in which an individual experiences or is at high risk to experience a decreased ability to speak but can understand others.

DEFINING CHARACTERISTICS
Major (Must be Present)
Inability to speak words but can understand others *or*
Articulation or motor planning deficits

Minor (May be Present)
Shortness of breath

RELATED FACTORS
See *Impaired Communication.*

NOC Communication: Expressive Ability

Goals

The person will demonstrate improved ability to express self.

Indicators

- Relate decreased frustration with communication.
- Use alternative methods as indicated.

NIC Active Listening, Communication Enhancement: Speech Deficit

Generic Interventions

Identify a method by which the person can communicate basic needs.
Provide alternative methods of communication.
  Use pad and pencil, alphabet letters, hand signals, eye blinks, head nods, bell signals.

Make flash cards with pictures or words depicting frequently used phrases (e.g., "Wet my lips," "Move my foot," glass of water, bedpan).

Encourage the person to point and to use gestures and pantomime.

Consult with speech pathologist for assistance in acquiring flash cards.

For individuals with dysarthria:

Reduce environmental noise.

Encourage the person to make a conscious effort to slow speech down and to speak louder (e.g., "Take a deep breath between sentences.").

Ask the person to repeat words that are unclear.

If the person is tired, ask questions that require only short answers.

If speech is unintelligible, teach the person to use gestures, written messages, and communication cards.

Do not alter your speech, tone, or type of message, because the person's ability to understand is not affected; speak on an adult level.

Verbally address the problem of frustration about inability to communicate, and explain that patience is needed for the nurse and the person who is trying to talk.

Write the method of communication that is used on the person's care plan.

Teach significant others techniques and repetitive approaches to improve communication.

Encourage the family to share feelings concerning communication problems.

Seek consultation with a speech pathologist early in treatment regimen.

For individuals with language barriers (Giger & Davidhizar, 1999):

Communicate in an unhurried, caring manner. Be polite and formal.

Speak in a low, moderate voice. Listen carefully; validate mutual understanding.

Use gestures and pictures.

Keep the message simple; do not use medical or technical terms.

If an interpreter is needed:

Clarify what language is spoken at home.

Attempt to use same gender and similar age as client.

Avoid interpreters from rival tribe, nation.

Ask to translate verbatim.

Use telephone translating system when necessary.

Confusion
Acute Confusion
Chronic Confusion

Confusion*

DEFINITION
Confusion: The state in which the individual experiences or is at risk of experiencing a disturbance in cognition, attention, memory, and orientation of an undetermined origin or onset.

> ⓐ **AUTHOR'S NOTE**
>
> This author has added *Confusion* to the diagnostic list to provide the nurse with an option when the origin, onset, or duration of the confusion is unknown. By providing this diagnostic option, the nurse can refrain from too quickly labeling the confusion as acute or chronic. Careful assessment is indicated. Until data collection is complete, the diagnosis can be written as *Confusion related to unknown etiology as evidenced by* (specify supporting data).

DEFINING CHARACTERISTICS
Major (Must be Present, One or More)
Disturbances of:

Consciousness	Memory
Attention	Orientation
Perception	Thinking

Minor (May be Present)
Misperceptions
Hypervigilance
Agitation

---

*This diagnosis is not currently on the NANDA list; it has been included for clarity and usefulness.

DEFINITION

Acute Confusion: The state in which there is an abrupt onset of a cluster of global, fluctuating disturbances in consciousness, attention, perception, memory, orientation, thinking, sleep-wake cycle, and psychomotor behavior (American Psychological Association, 2000).

DEFINING CHARACTERISTICS
Major (Some Must be Present)
Abrupt onset of:

Reduced ability to focus	Confusion
Disorientation	Restlessness
Incoherence	Fear
Anxiety	Excitement
Hypervigilance	

Symptoms worse at night or when fatigued

Minor (May be Present)

Illusions	Hallucinations
Delusions	Misperception of stimuli

RISK FACTORS

Presence of risk factors (see Related Factors)

RELATED FACTORS
Pathophysiologic

Related to abrupt onset of cerebral hypoxia or disturbance in cerebral metabolism secondary to (Miller, 2003):

Fluid and Electrolyte Disturbances

Dehydration	Hyponatremia/
Volume depletion	hypernatremia
Acidosis/alkalosis	Hypoglycemia/
Hypokalemia	hyperglycemia
Hypercalcemia	

Nutritional Deficiencies

Folate or vitamin B_{12}
  deficiency

Anemia

Niacin deficiency

Magnesium deficiency

Cardiovascular Disturbances

Myocardial infarction

Congestive heart failure

Dysrhythmias

Heart block

Temporal arteritis

Respiratory Disorders

Chronic obstructive
  pulmonary disease

Pulmonary embolism

Tuberculosis

Pneumonia

Infections

Sepsis

Meningitis, encephalitis

Urinary tract infection

Metabolic and Endocrine Disorders

Hypothyroidism

Hypopituitarism

Parathyroid disorders

Hypoadrenocorticism

Postural hypotension

Hypothermia/hyperthermia

Hepatic or renal failure

Central Nervous System Disorders

Multiple infarctions

Parkinson's disease

Neurosyphilis

Alzheimer's disease

Head trauma

Tumors

Seizures and postconvulsive
  states

Normal pressure
  hydrocephalus

Treatment-Related

Related to a disturbance in cerebral metabolism secondary to:

Surgery

Therapeutic drug intoxication (e.g., neuroleptics, narcotics)

General anesthesia

Side effects of medication:

  Diuretics

  Digitalis

  Propranolol

  Atropine

  Oral hypoglycemics

  Anti-inflammatory agents

  Barbiturates

  Methyldopa

  Disulfiram

  Lithium

  Phenytoin

  Antianxiety agents

Anticholinergics
Phenothiazines
Opiates

Over-the-counter cold,
cough, and sleeping
preparations

Situational (Personal, Environmental)
Related to disturbance in cerebral metabolism secondary to:
Withdrawal from alcohol
Withdrawal from sedatives, hypnotics
Heavy metal or carbon monoxide intoxication

Related to pain, bowel impaction, immobility, or depression
Related to chemical intoxications or medications (specify):

Alcohol
Amphetamines
Heroin

Cocaine
Hallucinogenics

> **NOC** Cognitive Orientation, Safety Behavior: Personal, Distorted Thought Control, Information Processing

Goals

The person will have diminished episodes of delirium.

Indicators

- Be less agitated.
- Participate in activities of daily living.
- Be less combative.

> **NIC** Delirium Management, Cognitive Stimulation, Calming Technique, Reality Orientation, Environmental Management: Safety

Generic Interventions

Assess for Causative and Contributing Factors.

Ensure that a thorough diagnostic workup has been completed.

Laboratory:
- Complete blood count, electrolytes, chemistry
- B_{12} and folate, thiamine
- Rapid plasma reagin (RPR)
- TSH, T_4
- Drug levels: alcohol, barbiturates
- Serum thyroxine and serum-free thyroxine
- Serum glucose and fasting blood sugar
- Urinalysis

Diagnostic:
- Electroencephalogram
- Computed tomography scan
- Electrocardiogram
- Chest x-ray, skull x-ray
- Spinal tap
- Psychiatric evaluation

**Promote Communication that
Contributes to the Person's
Sense of Integrity.**

Examine attitudes about confusion (in self, caregivers, significant others). Provide education to family, significant other(s), and caregivers regarding the situation and methods of coping.

Maintain standards of empathic, respectful care.

Attempt to obtain information that will provide useful and meaningful topics for conversations (likes, dislikes; interests, hobbies; work history). Interview early in the day.

Encourage significant others and caregivers to speak slowly with low voice pitch and at an average volume (unless hearing deficits are present), as one adult to another, with eye contact, and as if expecting person to understand.

Provide respect and promote sharing:

  Pay attention to what the person is saying.

  Pick out meaningful comments, and continue talking.

  Address the person by name, and introduce yourself each time a contact is made; use touch if welcomed.

  Use name the person prefers; avoid "Pops" or "Mom."

  Convey to the person that you are concerned and friendly (through smiles, an unhurried pace).

Use memory aids, if appropriate.

Provide Sufficient and Meaningful Sensory Input:

Keep person oriented to time and place.

Encourage family to bring familiar objects from home (e.g., photographs with nonglare glass, blanket).

Discuss current events, seasonal events (snow, water activities); share your interests (travel, crafts).

Assess if person can perform an activity with hands (e.g., latch rugs, wood crafts).

When teaching a task or activity (e.g., eating), break it into small, brief steps by giving only one instruction at a time.

Promote a Well Role:

Discourage the wearing of nightclothes during the day.

Encourage self-care and grooming activities.

Promote socialization during meals.

Plan an activity each day.

Encourage participation in decision-making.

Do Not Endorse Confusion:

Do not argue with person.

Never agree with confused statements.

Direct person back to reality; do not allow him or her to ramble.

Adhere to the schedule; if changes are necessary, advise person of them.

Avoid talking to coworkers about other topics in person's presence.

Provide simple explanations that cannot be misinterpreted.

Remember to acknowledge your entrance with a greeting and your exit with a closure. ("I will be back in 10 minutes.")

Avoid open-ended questions.

Replace five- or six-step tasks with two- or three-step tasks.

Promote Safety.

Ensure that the person carries identification.

Adapt the environment so the person can pace or walk if desired.

Keep the environment uncluttered.

Keep medications, cleaning solutions, and other toxic chemicals in inaccessible places.

If the person cannot manipulate the call button, use another method (e.g., bell, extension from bed call system).

Discourage Use of Restraints; Explore Alternatives (Quinn, 1994; Rateau, 2000).

If the person's behavior disrupts treatment (e.g., nasogastric tube, urinary catheter, intravenous line), reevaluate whether treatment is appropriate.

Evaluate if restlessness is associated with pain. If analgesics are used, adjust dosage to reduce side effects.

Put the person in a room with others who can help watch him or her.

Enlist aid of family or friends to watch the person during confused periods.

Give the person something to hold (e.g., a stuffed animal).

Chronic Confusion

DEFINITION

Chronic Confusion: A state in which the individual experiences an irreversible, long-standing, and/or progressive deterioration of intellect and personality.

DEFINING CHARACTERISTICS
Major (Must be Present, One or More)

Cognitive or intellectual losses

Loss of memory

Loss of time sense

Inability to make choices, decisions

Inability to problem-solve, reason

Altered perceptions

Loss of language abilities

Poor judgment

Affective or personality losses

Loss of affect

Diminished inhibition

Increasing self-preoccupations

Loss of tact,
  control of temper
Loss of recognition
  (others, environment, self)

Psychotic features
Antisocial behavior
Loss of energy reserve

Cognitive or planning losses
Loss of general ability to plan.
Impaired ability to set goals, plan

Progressively lowered stress threshold
Purposeful wandering
Violent, agitated, or anxious behavior
Purposeless behavior
Withdrawal or avoidance behavior
Compulsive repetitive behavior

RELATED FACTORS
Pathophysiologic (Hall, 1991)
Related to progressive degeneration of the cerebral cortex secondary to:
Alzheimer's disease
Multi-infarct disease (MID)
Combination of senile dementia of Alzheimer's type
  and MID

Related to disturbance in cerebral metabolism, structure, or integrity secondary to:
Pick's disease
Creutzfeldt-Jakob disease
Toxic substance injection
Degenerative neurologic disease
Brain tumor
Huntington's chorea
End-stage diseases:
  AIDS
  Cancer
  Cardiac failure
  Cirrhosis
  Renal failure
  Chronic obstructive pulmonary disease
Psychiatric disorders

NOC Cognitive Ability, Cognitive Orientation, Distorted
Thought Control

Goals

The person will participate to maximum level of independence in a therapeutic milieu.

Indicators

- Has decreased frustration
- Has diminished episodes of combativeness
- Has decreased use of restraints
- Increases hours of sleep at night
- Stabilizes or gains weight

NIC Surveillance: Safety, Emotional Support, Environmental Management, Fall Prevention, Calming Technique

Generic Interventions

Refer to Interventions under
Acute Confusion.

Observe the Person to Determine Baseline Behaviors (Hall, 1994):

Client's best time of day
Response time to a simple question
Amount of distraction tolerable
Judgment ability
Insight into own disability
Signs/symptoms of depression
Usual routine

Promote a Sense of Integrity (Miller, 2004):

Adapt communication to the ability level of the person. It may be necessary to use very simple sentences and to present one idea at a time.

Avoid "baby talk" and a condescending tone of voice.

If the person does not understand, repeat the sentence using the same words.

Use positive statements; avoid "don'ts."

Unless a safety issue is involved, do not argue with the person.

Avoid general questions such as, "What would you like to do?" Instead ask, "Do you want to go for a walk or work on your rug?"

Be sensitive to the feelings the person is trying to express.

Avoid questions you know he or she cannot answer.

If possible, demonstrate to reinforce verbal communication.

Use touch to gain attention or show concern, unless a negative response is elicited.

Maintain good eye contact and pleasant facial expressions.

Determine which sense dominates the person's perception of the world (auditory, kinesthetic, olfactory, or gustatory).

Communicate through the preferred sense.

Promote Safety:

Ensure that the person carries identification.

Adapt the environment so that the person can pace or walk if desired.

Keep the environment uncluttered.

Keep medications, cleaning solutions, and other toxic chemicals in inaccessible places.

If person cannot manipulate the call button, use another method (e.g., bell, extension from bed call system).

Discourage Use of Restraints; Explore Alternatives (Quinn, 1994).

If person's behavior disrupts treatment (e.g., nasogastric tube, urinary catheter, intravenous line), re-evaluate whether treatment is appropriate.

Intravenous therapy:
- Camouflage the tubing with loose gauze.
- If dehydration is a problem, institute a regular schedule for offering oral fluids.
- Use sites that are least restrictive.

Urinary catheters:
- Evaluate causes of incontinence; institute specific treatment depending on type. Refer to *Impaired Urinary Elimination.*
- Place urinary collection bag at end of bed with catheter between legs rather than draped over legs. Velcro bands can hold catheter against leg.

Gastrointestinal tubes:
- Check frequently for pressure against nares.

- Camouflage gastrostomy tube with a loosely applied abdominal binder.
- If the person is pulling out tubes, use mitts instead of wrist restraints.

Evaluate if restlessness is associated with pain. If analgesics are used, adjust dosage to reduce side effects.

Put person in a room with others who can help watch him or her.

Enlist aid of family or friends to watch the person during confused periods.

Give the person something to hold (e.g., stuffed animal).

Ensure Physical Comfort and Maintenance of Basic Health Needs (e.g., Elimination, Nutrition, Bathing, Toileting, Hygiene, Grooming, Safety). Refer to Individual Nursing Diagnoses to Assist a Cognitively Impaired Person with Self-Care.

Use Various Modalities to Promote Stimulation.

Music therapy

Provide soft, familiar music during meals.

Play music to individuals that they preferred in their younger years.

Recreation therapy

Encourage arts and crafts (knitting and crocheting).

Suggest creative writing.

Provide puzzles.

Organize group games.

Remotivation therapy

Topics for remotivation sessions are based on suggestions from group leaders and the interest of the group. Examples are pets, bodies of water, canning fruits and vegetables, transportation, holidays (Janssen & Giberson, 1988).

Use associations and analogies:

"If ice is cold, then fire is . . . ?"

"If day is light, then night is . . . ?"

Sensory training

Stimulate vision (with brightly colored items of different shapes; pictures, color decorations, kaleidoscopes).

Stimulate smell (with flowers, coffee, cologne).

Stimulate hearing (ring a bell, play records).

Stimulate touch (sandpaper, velvet, steel wool pads, silk, stuffed animals).

Stimulate taste (spices, salt, sugar, sour substances).

Reminiscence therapy (Smith, 1990; Burnside & Haight, 1994)

Consider instituting reminiscence therapy on a one-to-one or group basis. Discuss purpose and goals with client care team. Prepare yourself well before initiating. Refer to Burnside and Haight (1994) for specific protocols for one-to-one and group reminiscence.

Implement Techniques to Lower the Stress Threshold in Individuals in Middle or Later Stages of Dementia (Hall & Buckwalter, 1987; Miller, 2004).

Reduce competing or excessive stimuli.

Plan and maintain a consistent routine.

Focus on the person's ability level.

Reduce fatigue and anxiety.

Allow for wandering.

Be alert to the individual's expressions of fatigue or increasing anxiety, and immediately reduce stimuli.

Discuss the Proposed Benefits of Selected Nutrients: Zinc, Choline, Lecithin, Selenium, Magnesium, Beta Carotene, Folic Acid, and Vitamins C and E (Miller, 2004).

Constipation
Perceived Constipation
Risk for Constipation

Constipation

DEFINITION

Constipation: The state in which an individual experiences stasis of the large intestine, resulting in infrequent (two or less weekly) elimination and/or hard, dry feces.

DEFINING CHARACTERISTICS
Major (Must be Present, One or More)

Hard, formed stool *and/or*
Defecation fewer than three times a week
Prolonged and difficult defecation

Minor (May be Present)

Decreased bowel sounds
Reported feeling of rectal fullness
Reported feeling of pressure in rectum
Straining and pain on defecation
Palpable impaction
Feeling of inadequate emptying

RELATED FACTORS
Pathophysiologic
Related to defective nerve stimulation, weak pelvic floor muscles, and immobility secondary to:

Spinal cord lesions
Spinal cord injury
Spina bifida
Dementia
Cerebrovascular accident, stroke
Neurologic diseases (multiple sclerosis, Parkinson's disease)

Related to decreased metabolic rate secondary to:
Obesity
Pheochromocytoma
Diabetic neuropathy
Hypopituitarism
Uremia
Hypothyroidism
Hyperparathyroidism

Related to decreased response to urge to defecate secondary to:
Affective disorders

Related to pain on defecation (e.g., hemorrhoids, back injury)
Related to decreased peristalsis secondary to hypoxia (cardiac, pulmonary)
Related to failure to relax anal sphincter or high resting pressure in the anal canal secondary to:
Multiple vaginal deliveries
Chronic straining

Treatment-Related
Related to side effects of (specify):
Antacids (calcium, aluminum)
Iron
Barium
Aluminum
Aspirin
Phenothiazines
Calcium
Anticholinergics
Anesthetics
Narcotics (codeine, morphine)
Diuretics
Antiparkinsonian agents

Related to effects of anesthesia and surgical manipulation on peristalsis
Related to habitual laxative use
Related to mucositis secondary to radiation

Situational (Personal, Environmental)
Related to decreased peristalsis secondary to: e.g., immobility, pregnancy, stress, lack of exercise

Related to irregular evacuation patterns
Related to cultural or health beliefs
Related to lack of privacy
Related to inadequate fiber in diet
Related to fear of rectal or cardiac pain
Related to faulty appraisal
Related to inadequate fluid intake
Related to inability to perceive bowel cues

NOC Bowel Elimination, Hydration, Symptom Control

Goals

The person will report bowel movements at least every 2 to 3 days.

Indicators

• Describe components for effective bowel movements.
• Explain rationale for lifestyle change(s).

NIC Bowel Management, Fluid Management, Constipation/ Impaction Management

Generic Interventions

Teach the Importance of a Balanced Diet.

Review list of foods high in bulk:
    Fresh fruits with skins
    Bran, dried beans
    Nuts and seeds
    Whole-grain breads and cereals
    Cooked fruits and vegetables
    Fruit juices
Include approximately 800 g of fruits and vegetables (about four pieces of fresh fruit and large salad) for normal daily bowel movement.
Gradually increase amount of bran as tolerated (may add to cereals, baked goods, etc.). Explain the need for fluid intake with bran.

Encourage Daily Intake of at least 2 L of Fluids—8 to 10 Glasses—Unless Contraindicated. Limit Coffee to Two to Three Cups per Day.

Recommend a Glass of Warm Water to Be Taken 30 Minutes Before Breakfast; This May Act As Stimulus to Bowel Evacuation.

Establish a Regular Time for Elimination. Use a Commode Chair or Toilet Instead of Bedpan, if Possible.

Assist Person to Normal Semisquatting Position to Allow Optimal Use of Abdominal Muscles and Effect of Force of Gravity.

Teach How to Massage along Lower Abdomen Gently While on Toilet.

Teach the Importance of Responding to Urge to Defecate.

If Fecal Impaction Is Present, Instill Warm Mineral Oil, and Retain It for 20 to 30 Minutes. Using a Well-Lubricated Glove, Break Up Hard Stool, and Remove Pieces.

Monitor for Vagal Stimulation (Dizziness, Slow Pulse).

Explain the Hazards of Enema and Non–Bulk-Producing Laxative Use (Refer to <u>Perceived Constipation</u>).

Explain How to Use Bulk-Producing Laxatives (e.g., Psyllium Hydrophilic Mucilloid [Metamucil, Effersyllium Citracel, FiberCon]).

Emphasize the Need for Regular Exercise.
Suggest walking.

If walking is prohibited:

Teach client to lie in bed or sit on chair, and bend one knee at a time to chest (10 to 20 times each knee) three or four times a day.

Teach client to sit in chair or lie in bed, and turn torso from side to side (10 to 20 times) 6 to 10 times a day.

Reduce Rectal Pain, if Possible, by Instructing Person in Corrective Measures:

Gently apply a lubricant to anus to reduce pain on defecation.

Apply cool compresses to area to reduce itching.

Take sitz bath or soak in tub of warm water (43° to 46°C) for 15-minute intervals if soothing.

Take stool softeners or mineral oil as an adjunct to other approaches.

Consult with physician concerning use of local anesthetics and antiseptic agents.

Protect the Skin from Contamination:

Evaluate the surrounding skin area.

Cleanse properly with nonirritating agent (e.g., use gentle motion; use soft tissues following defecation).

Suggest a sitz bath following defecation.

Gently apply protective emollient or lubricant.

Initiate Health Teaching if Indicated.

Teach methods to prevent rectal pressure, which contributes to hemorrhoids.

Avoid prolonged sitting and straining at defecation.

Soften stools (e.g., low-roughage diet, high fluid intake).

🐢 Pediatric Interventions

Discuss some causes of constipation in infants and children (underfeeding; high-protein, low-carbohydrate diet; lack of roughage; dehydration).

If bowel movements are infrequent with hard stools:

With infants, add corn syrup to feeding or fruit to diet. Avoid apple juice or sauce.

With children, add bran cereal, prune juice, fruits, and vegetables.

Persistent constipation should be evaluated medically.

Maternal Interventions

Explain the risks of constipation in pregnancy and post-partum (Reeder, 1997).

Decreased gastric motility

Prolonged intestinal time

Pressure of enlarging uterus

Distended abdominal muscles (postpartum)

Relaxation of intestines (postpartum)

Explain aggravating factors for hemorrhoid development (straining at defecation, constipation, prolonged standing, wearing constrictive clothing).

If the woman has a history of constipation, discuss how to use bulk-producing laxatives to keep stool soft. Advise patient to avoid other types of laxatives (e.g., stimulants, mineral oil).

Postdelivery, assess bowel sounds, presence of abdominal distention, hemorrhoids, perineal swelling, and if passing flatus.

Postdelivery, provide relief from pain of hemorrhoids, episiotomy, or perineal lacerations.

Consider the need for stool softeners, laxative, or rectal suppository. Promote defecation 2 to 3 days postdelivery.

Refer to *Constipation*.

Geriatric Interventions

Discuss that individual bowel patterns vary (e.g., three times a day to three times a week).

Discuss medication that can contribute to constipation (anticholinergics, narcotics, iron sulfate, psychotropic medications, aluminum and calcium antacids, tricyclic antidepressants, overuse of antidiarrheals).

Perceived Constipation

DEFINITION

Perceived Constipation: The state in which an individual self-prescribes the daily use of laxatives, enemas, or suppositories to ensure a daily bowel movement.

DEFINING CHARACTERISTICS (MCLANE & MCSHANE, 1986)
Major (80% to 100%)

Expectation of a daily bowel movement with the resulting overuse of laxatives, enemas, and/or suppositories

Expected passage of stool at the same time every day

RELATED FACTORS
Pathophysiologic

Related to faulty appraisal secondary to: e.g., obsessive-compulsive disorders, central nervous system (CNS) deterioration, depression

Situational (Personal, Environmental)

Related to inaccurate information secondary to: e.g., cultural beliefs, family beliefs

NOC Bowel Elimination, Health Beliefs: Perceived Threat

Goals

The person will verbalize acceptance of bowel movements every 2 or 3 days.

Indicators

- Do not use laxatives regularly.
- Relate the causes of constipation.
- Describe the hazards of laxative use.
- Relate an intent to increase fiber, fluid, and exercise in daily life as instructed.

> **NIC** Bowel Movement Health Education, Behavior Modification, Nutrition Management

Generic Interventions

Explore with person his or her bowel patterns and expectations.

Gently explain that bowel movements are needed every 2 to 3 days, not daily.

Explain the hazards of regular laxative, enema, or suppository use:

Temporary relief

Impaired nutrient metabolism, riboflavin, calcium, magnesium, zinc, potassium

Water deficiency

Malabsorption of fat-soluble vitamins A, D, E, and K

Diarrhea-constipation cycle

Possible interactions with other medications (e.g., diuretics, digoxin [Lanoxin])

Teach the importance of a balanced diet (refer to *Constipation*).

Encourage intake of at least 6 to 10 glasses of water (unless contraindicated).

Recommend drinking a glass of warm water 30 minutes before breakfast; this may act as a stimulus to bowel evacuation.

Establish a regular time for elimination.

Emphasize the need for regular exercise.

Suggest walking.

If walking is prohibited:

Teach client to lie in bed or sit on chair, and bend one knee at a time to chest (10 to 20 times each knee) three or four times a day.

Teach client to sit in chair or lie in bed, and turn torso from side to side (20 to 30 times) 6 to 10 times a day.

Emphasize that normal bowel function is possible without laxatives, enemas, or suppositories.

Risk for Constipation

DEFINITION

Risk for Constipation: The state in which an individual is at high risk of experiencing stasis of the large intestine, resulting in infrequent elimination and/or hard, dry feces.

RISK FACTORS

Refer to *Constipation.*

Goals

The person will report continued satisfactory bowel movements every 1 to 3 days.

Indicators

Identify the effects of fluid, fiber, and activity on bowel elimination.

Generic Interventions

Refer to *Constipation.*

Coping, Ineffective

DEFINITION

Ineffective Coping: The state in which the individual experiences or is at risk of experiencing an inability to manage internal or environmental stressors adequately because of inadequate resources (physical, psychological, behavioral, or cognitive).

> #### ✪ AUTHOR'S NOTE
>
> This diagnosis can be used to describe a variety of situations in which an individual does not adapt effectively to stressors. Examples can be isolating behaviors, aggression, and destructive behavior. If the response is inappropriate use of the defense mechanisms of denial or defensiveness, the diagnosis *Ineffective Denial* or *Defensive Coping* can be used instead of *Ineffective Coping*.

DEFINING CHARACTERISTICS
(Vincent, 1985)
Major (Must be Present, One or More)
Verbalization of inability to cope or ask for help *or*
Inappropriate use of defense mechanisms *or*
Inability to meet role expectations

Minor (May be Present)
Chronic worry, anxiety
Reported difficulty with life stressors

Ineffective social participation
Destructive behavior toward self or others
High incidence of accidents
Frequent illnesses
Verbal manipulation
Inability to meet basic needs
Nonassertive response patterns
Change in usual communication pattern
Substance abuse

RELATED FACTORS
Pathophysiologic
Related to chronicity of condition or complex self-care regimens
Related to changes in body integrity secondary to:
Loss of body part
Disfigurement secondary to trauma

Related to altered affect caused by changes secondary to:
Body chemistry
Tumor (brain)
Intake of mood-altering substance
Mental retardation

Treatment-Related
Related to separation from family and home (e.g., hospitalization, confinement to a nursing home)
Related to disfigurement caused by surgery
Related to altered appearance owing to drugs, radiation, or other treatment

Situational (Personal, Environmental)
Related to increased food consumption in response to stressors
Related to changes in physical environment secondary to:
War   Poverty
Natural disaster   Homelessness
Relocation   Inadequate finances
Seasonal work
  (migrant worker)

Related to disruption of emotional bonds secondary to:

Death

Separation or divorce

Desertion

Relocation

Jail

Foster home

Orphanage

Educational institution

Institutionalization

Related to sensory overload secondary to:

Factory environment

Urbanization: crowding, noise pollution, excessive activity

Related to inadequate psychological resources secondary to:

Poor self-esteem

Excessive negative beliefs about self

Negative role-modeling

Helplessness

Lack of motivation to respond

Related to culturally related conflicts with (specify):

Premarital sex

Abortion

Maturational

Child or Adolescent
Related to:

Inconsistent methods of discipline

Fear of failure

Childhood trauma

Parental substance abuse

Parental rejection

Repressed anxiety

Panic level of anxiety

Poor impulse control

Poor social skills

Peer rejection

Adolescent
Related to inadequate psychological resources to adapt to:

Physical and emotional
  changes

Independence from family

Relationships

Sexual awareness

Educational demands

Career choices

Young Adult
Related to inadequate psychological resources to adapt to:

Career choices	Marriage
Educational demands	Parenthood
Leaving home	

Middle Adult
Related to inadequate psychological resources to adapt to:

Physical signs of aging	Problems with relatives
Career pressures	Social status needs
Child-rearing problems	Aging parents

Older Adult
Related to inadequate psychological resources to adapt to:

Physical changes	Retirement
Changes in financial status	Response of others to older
Changes in residence	persons

> **NOC** Coping, Self Esteem, Social Interaction Skills

Goals

The person will make decisions and follow through with appropriate actions to change provocative situations in personal environment.

Indicators

- Verbalize feelings related to emotional state.
- Identify his or her coping patterns and the consequences of the behavior that results.
- Identify personal strengths and accept support through the nursing relationship.

> **NIC** Coping Enhancement, Counseling, Emotional Support, Active Listening, Assertiveness Training, Behavior Modification

Generic Interventions

Assess Individual's Present Coping Status.

Determine onset of feelings and symptoms and their correlation with events and life changes.

Assess ability to relate facts.

Listen carefully, and observe facial expressions, gestures, eye contact, body positioning, tone and intensity of voice.

Determine risk of client inflicting self-harm, and intervene appropriately (see *Risk for Self-Harm*).

Offer Support as Person Talks:

Reassure that the feelings he or she has must be difficult.

When person is pessimistic, attempt to provide a more hopeful, realistic perspective.

If Person Is Angry (Thomas, 1998):

Maintain an environment with low levels of stimuli.

Explore why the person is angry.

Do not argue or become defensive.

Focus on what can be done rather than what has not been done.

Offer options to increase sense of control.

Acknowledge that everyone gets angry, but certain actions are not acceptable.

If violence is a risk, refer to *Risk for Violence.*

Encourage a Self-Evaluation of His or Her Own Behavior:

"Did that work for you?"

"How did it help?"

"What did you learn from that experience?"

Assist the Person to Solve Problems in a Constructive Manner:

What is the problem?

Who or what is responsible for the problem?

What are the options? (Make a list.)

What are the advantages and disadvantages of each option?

Discuss Possible Alternatives (i.e., Talk about the Problem with Those Involved, Try to Change the Situation, or Do Nothing and Accept the Consequences).

Assist the Individual to Identify Problems that Cannot Be Controlled Directly and Help Him or Her to Practice Stress-Reducing Activities for Control (e.g., Exercise Program, Yoga).

Instruct the Person in Relaxation Techniques; Emphasize the Importance of Setting 15 to 20 Minutes Aside Each Day to Practice Relaxation.

Mobilize the Person into a Gradual Increase in Activity.

Find Outlets that Foster Feelings of Personal Achievement and Self-Esteem.

Provide Opportunities to Learn and Use Stress Management Techniques (e.g., Jogging, Yoga).

Establish a Network of Persons Who Understand the Situation.

For Depression-Related Problems Beyond the Scope of Nurse Generalists, Refer to Appropriate Professionals (Marriage Counselor, Psychiatric Nurse Therapist, Psychologist, Psychiatrist).

Prepare for Problems that May Occur after Discharge:

Medications—schedule, cost, misuse, side effects
Increased anxiety
Sleep problems
Eating problems—access, decreased appetite
Inability to structure time

Family/significant other conflicts
Follow-up—forgetting, access, difficulty organizing time

◆ Pediatric Interventions (Wong, 2003)

Establish eye contact before giving instructions.
Set firm, responsible limits.
State rules simply; do not lecture.
Maintain regular routine.
Advise parents to avoid disagreeing with each other in child's presence.
Maintain a calm, simple environment.
If hyperactive, provide for periods of activity using large muscles.
Provide immediate and constant feedback.
Advise parents to consult with educational professionals for educational programming.

Defensive Coping

DEFINITION

Defensive Coping: The state in which an individual repeatedly presents falsely positive self-evaluation as a defense against underlying perceived threats to positive self-regard.

DEFINING CHARACTERISTICS (Norris & Kunes-Connell, 1987) Major (80% to 100%)

Denial of obvious problems/weaknesses
Projection of blame/responsibility
Rationalization of failures

Hypersensitivity to slight criticism
Grandiosity

Minor (50% to 79%)

Superior attitude toward others
Difficulty in establishing or maintaining relationships
Hostile laughter or ridicule of others
Difficulty in testing perceptions against reality
Lack of follow-through or participation in treatment
  or therapy

RELATED FACTORS

See *Chronic Low Self-Esteem, Powerlessness,* and *Impaired Social Interaction.*

NOC Acceptance: Health Status, Self Esteem, Social Interaction Skills

Goals

The person will report or demonstrate less defensive behavior.

Indicators

- Identify defensive responses.
- Establish realistic goals in concert with caregivers.
- Work effectively toward achieving these goals.

NIC Coping Enhancement, Emotional Support, Self Awareness Enhancement, Environment Management, Presence Active Listening

Generic Interventions

Reduce Demands on the Individual if Stress Levels Increase.

Establish a Dialogue Stance that Will Reduce Defensiveness and Increase Effective Actions:

Maintain a neutral, matter-of-fact tone with a consistent positive regard. Ensure that all staff relate in a consistent fashion with consistent expectations.

Focus on simple here-and-now, goal-directed topics when encountering the client's defenses.

Encourage the client to express goals, and establish agreement with the client in at least one or two areas.

Do not defend or dwell on the client's negative projections or displacements.

Disengage from disagreement.

Do not challenge distortions or unrealistic/grandiose self-expressions. Try instead to redirect the conversation toward more neutral topics or more realistic topics about which some agreement has already been established.

Encourage the person to evaluate his or her own progress.

Identify for the person actions that have interfered with achieving established goals.

Practice role-playing less defensive responses to difficult situations.

Evaluate interactions, progress, and approach with other team members to ensure overall consistency within the treatment milieu.

Work to Establish a Therapeutic Relationship with the Client to Decrease the Need to Defend and Permit a More Direct Addressing of Underlying, Related Factors (See *Chronic Low Self-Esteem*).

Validate the client's reluctance to trust in the beginning.

Engage the client in diversional, non–goal-directed, non-competitive activities (e.g., relaxation therapy, games, outing).

Encourage self-expression of neutral themes, positive reminiscences, and so forth.

Encourage other means for self-expression (e.g., writing or art) if verbal interaction is difficult or if another means is an area of personal strength.

Listen passively to some grandiose or negative self-expression to reinforce your "positive regard."

Ineffective Denial

DEFINITION

Ineffective Denial: The state in which the individual minimizes or disavows symptoms or a situation to the detriment of his or her health.

> ⊕ **AUTHOR'S NOTE**
>
> This type of denial differs from the denial in response to a loss. The denial in response to an illness or loss is necessary to maintain psychological equilibrium and is beneficial. *Ineffective Denial* is not beneficial when the individual will not participate in regimens to improve health or the situation (e.g., denial of substance abuse). If the cause of the *Ineffective Denial* is not known, *Ineffective Denial related to unknown etiology* can be used; for example, *Ineffective Denial related to unknown etiology as manifested by repetitive refusal to admit that barbiturate use is a problem.*

DEFINING CHARACTERISTICS
(Lynch & Phillips, 1989)
Major (Must be Present, One or More)

Delays seeking or refuses health care attention to the detriment of health

Does not perceive personal relevance of symptoms or danger

Minor (May be Present)

Does not admit fear of death or invalidism

Minimizes symptoms

Displaces source of symptoms to other areas of the body

Unable to admit impact of disease on life pattern

Makes dismissive gestures or comments when speaking of distressing events

Displaces fear of impact of the condition

Displays inappropriate affect

106

RELATED FACTORS
Pathophysiologic
Related to inability to consciously tolerate the consequences of any chronic or terminal illness

Treatment-Related
Related to prolonged treatment with no positive results

Situational/Psychological
Related to inability to tolerate consciously the consequences of:

Drug use
Alcohol use
Smoking
Obesity
Loss of spouse/significant
  other

Financial crisis
Feelings of negative
  self-concept, inadequacy,
  guilt, loneliness, despair,
  failure
Loss of job

Related to feelings of increased anxiety/stress; need to escape personal problems, anger, and frustration
Related to feelings of omnipotence
Related to culturally permissive attitudes toward alcohol/drug use

Biologic/Genetic
Related to family history of alcoholism

NOC See Ineffective Coping

Goals

The person will use alternative coping mechanism instead of denial.

Indicators

- Acknowledges the source of anxiety or stress.
- Uses problem-focused coping skills.

NIC See Ineffective Coping

Generic Interventions

Provide opportunities to share fears and anxieties.

Focus on present response.

Assist in lowering anxiety level (see *Anxiety* for additional interventions).

Avoid confronting person on use of denial.

Carefully explore with person his or her interpretation of the situation.

  Reflect self-reported cues used to minimize the situation (e.g., "a little," "only").

  Identify recent detrimental behavior, and discuss the effects of this behavior on health.

Emphasize strengths and past successful coping.

Provide positive reinforcement for any expressions of insight.

Do not accept rationalization or projection. Be polite, caring, but firm.

If substance abuse is present (Smith-DiJulio, 1998):

  Review observations and findings with client and family.

  Present evidence of damage (physical, social, financial, spiritual, familial).

  Establish goals.

  Provide self-help manuals or other pamphlets.

  Acquire commitment to keep daily log of alcohol/drug use.

  At next visit:

  • Review log.

  • Review progress.

  • Refer those who are dependent and desire to continue abstinence.

  • Explain why women are more affected by alcohol than are men.

Coping, Ineffective Community

DEFINITION

Ineffective Community Coping: The state in which a community's pattern of activities for adaptation and problem-solving are unsatisfactory for meeting the demands or needs of the community.

○ **AUTHOR'S NOTE**

This diagnosis is useful for nurses who practice with aggregates. An aggregate is a group of persons "who have in common one or more personal or environmental characteristics" (Williams, 1977). Therefore, an aggregate can be the population of a small town, high school girls, or Hispanic men with hypertension.

This diagnosis may be more frequently used as a risk diagnosis than an actual one. Nurses practicing with community aggregates would identify risk factors that could cause *Ineffective Community Coping*. The focus would be on assisting the community to prevent the diagnosis.

DEFINING CHARACTERISTICS
Major (Must be Present, One or More)
Failure of community to meet its own expectations
Unresolved community conflicts
Expressed difficulty in meeting demands for change
Expressed vulnerability

Minor (May be Present)

Angry	Bitter
Indifferent	Apathetic
Helpless	Hopeless
Overwhelmed	

RISK FACTORS
Presence of risk factors (see Related Factors)

RELATED FACTORS
Situational (Personal, Environmental)
Related to lack of knowledge of resources
Related to inadequate communication patterns
Related to inadequate community cohesiveness
Related to inadequate problem-solving
Related to inadequate community resources
Related to inadequate law enforcement services
Related to overwhelming community destruction secondary to:

Flood	Hurricane
Earthquake	Epidemic

Related to traumatic effects of airplane crash, large fire, industrial disaster, or environmental accident
Related to threat to community safety (e.g., murder, rape, kidnapping, robberies)
Related to sudden rise in community unemployment

Maturational
Related to inadequate resources for children, adolescents, working parents, or older adults

NOC	Community Competence, Community Health Status, Community Risk Control

Goals
The community will engage in effective problem-solving.

Indicators
- Identify problem.
- Access information to improve coping.
- Use communication channels to access assistance.

NIC	Community Health Development, Environmental Risk Protection, Program Development, Risk Identification

Generic Interventions
Assess for causative or contributing factors.
  Lack of knowledge of available resources
  Inadequate problem-solving
  Inadequate communication links
  Overwhelming, multiple stressors
  Threat to community safety
Provide opportunities (e.g., schools, churches, synagogues, town hall) for community members to face and discuss the situation and demonstrate acceptance of their anger, withdrawal, or denial.
Do not offer false reassurance. Emphasize their ability to cope effectively.
Explore techniques that may improve coping. Elicit suggestions from group.

Discuss resources that can be accessed. Prepare the group
  to accept outside help:
  Emergency shelter, funds, food, clothes
  Counseling
  Transportation
  Health care
Plan how to access isolated persons in the community.
Establish a method to access information and support (e.g.,
  local health department, hospital, churches, synagogues,
  community center).
Initiate referrals as indicated:
  Counseling
  Public assistance

Coping, Readiness for Enhanced Community

DEFINITION

Readiness for Enhanced Community Coping: A state in which
a community's pattern for adaptation and problem-solving is
satisfactory for meeting the demands or needs of the community, but the community desires to improve management of
current and future problems or stressors.

> ### ⓧ AUTHOR'S NOTE
>
> This diagnosis can be used to describe a community that
> desires to improve an already effective pattern of coping.
> For a community to be able to be assisted to a higher
> level of functioning, its basic needs for food, shelter,
> safety, a clean environment, and a supportive network
> must be addressed first. When these needs are met,
> programs can focus on higher functioning, such as well-
> ness and self-actualization. Community programs can

> ⊛ **AUTHOR'S NOTE** (continued)
>
> be designed after a community assessment and because of community requests. Community programs can focus on enhancing health promotion, with topics related to optimal nutrition, weight control, regular exercise programs, constructive stress management, social support, role responsibilities, and preparing for and coping with such life cycle events as retirement, parenting, or pregnancy.

DEFINING CHARACTERISTICS
Major (Must be Present)
Successful coping with a previous crisis

Minor (May be Present)
Active planning by community for predicted stressors

Active problem-solving by community when faced with issues

Agreement that community is responsible for stress management

Positive communication among community members

Positive communication between community/aggregates and larger community

Programs available for recreation and relaxation

Resources sufficient for managing stressors

RISK FACTORS
Presence of risk factors (see Related Factors)

RELATED FACTORS
Situational (Personal, Environmental)
Related to availability of community programs to augment (specify):
Nutritional status
Weight control
Stress management
Exercise program
Self-actualization
Social support

Maturational

Related to availability of community programs to augment coping with life cycle events; for example:

Aging

Adolescence

Pregnancy

Parenting

Retirement

"Empty nest"

NOC Community Competence, Community Health Status, Community Risk Control

Goals

The community will provide programs to improve well-being.

Indicators

• Identify health promotion needs.
• Access resources needed.
• Develop programs based on needs assessment.

NIC Program Development, Risk Identification, Community Health Development, Environmental Risk Protection

Generic Interventions

Meet with Influential Members of the Target Population to Determine Health Promotion Needs:

For what needs could the nursing agency develop services?

How can the agency promote or market the services to motivate people to use them?

Will enough members of the targeted population use the service?

Based on past programming, what improvements can be made for the future?

Are similar services provided by another agency or organization (hospital, religious)?

Plan the Development of Programs Targeted for a Specific Population.

**Delineate the Geographic Area to Be
Served and the Site of the Program.**

**Develop Detailed Program Objectives
and the Evaluation Framework to Be
Used: Content, Time Needed, Ideal
Teaching Method for Targeted Group,
Teaching Aids (e.g., Large-Print
Materials).**

**Establish Resources Needed
and Sources:**

Space
Transportation facilities
Optimal day of week, time of year
Supplies, audio/video equipment
Financial (budgeted, donations)

Market the Program:

Media (e.g., newspaper, television, radio)
Posters (food market, train station)
Flyers (distribute in school to home)
Word of mouth (religious organizations, community clubs,
    schools)
Guest speakers (community clubs, schools)

**Provide Program, and Evaluate
Whether the Desired Results
(Objectives) Were Achieved:**

Number of participants
Actual expenditures versus budgeted
Participant evaluations
Revisions for future programs

Family Coping, Readiness for Enhanced

DEFINITION

Family Coping, Readiness for Enhanced: Effective management of adaptive tasks by a family member involved with the individual's health challenge and who is now exhibiting the desire and readiness for enhanced health and growth in regard to self and in relation to the client.

> ### ⚏ AUTHOR'S NOTE
>
> This diagnosis describes a family that seeks the opportunity to adapt together to changes and to have a sense of control over outcomes.

DEFINING CHARACTERISTICS

Family member attempts to describe the growth impact of a crisis on his or her own values, priorities, goals, or relationships.

Family member moves in the direction of a health-promoting and enriching lifestyle that supports and monitors maturational processes, audits and negotiates treatment programs, and generally chooses experiences that optimize wellness.

Individual expresses interest in making contact on a one-to-one basis or in a mutual-aid group with another person who has experienced a similar situation.

RELATED FACTORS

See *Health-Seeking Behaviors* and *Interrupted Family Processes.*

Generic Interventions

See also *Interrupted Family Processes.*

Compromised Family Coping

DEFINITION

Compromised Family Coping: The state in which a usually supportive primary person (family member or close friend) is providing insufficient, ineffective, or compromised support, comfort, assistance, or encouragement that may be needed by the client to manage or master adaptive tasks related to his or her health challenge.

> ⓐ **AUTHOR'S NOTE**
>
> This nursing diagnosis describes situations that are similar to the diagnosis *Interrupted Family Processes.* Until clinical research differentiates this category from the preceding ones, use *Interrupted Family Processes.*

DEFINING CHARACTERISTICS
Subjective

Client expresses or confirms a concern or complaint about a significant other's response to his or her health problem.

Significant other describes preoccupation with personal reactions (e.g., fear, anticipatory grief, guilt, anxiety) to client's illness, disability, or other situational or developmental crises.

Significant other describes or confirms an inadequate understanding or knowledge base that interferes with effective assistive or supportive behaviors.

Objective

Significant other attempts assistive or supportive behaviors with less-than-satisfactory results.

Significant other withdraws or enters into limited or temporary personal communication with the client in times of need.

Significant other displays protective behavior disproportionate (too little or too much) to the client's abilities or need for autonomy.

RELATED FACTORS

See *Interrupted Family Processes.*

DEFINITION

Disabled Family Coping: The state in which a family demonstrates, or is at risk to demonstrate, destructive behavior in response to an inability to manage internal or external stressors due to inadequate resources (physical, psychological, or cognitive).

⊚ AUTHOR'S NOTE

The diagnosis *Disabled Family Coping* describes a family that has a history of demonstrating destructive overt or covert behavior or that has adapted detrimentally to a stressor. This diagnosis differs from *Interrupted Family Processes,* which describes a family that usually functions constructively but is challenged by a stressor that has altered or may alter its functioning. Sustained *Interrupted Family Processes* may progress to *Disabled Family Coping.* This diagnosis requires long-term care by a nurse specialist. The interventions in this book are for nurses in a short-term relationship.

DEFINING CHARACTERISTICS
Major (Must be Present, One or More)

Abusive or neglectful care of client
Decisions/actions that are detrimental to family well-being
Neglectful relationships with other family members

Minor (May be Present)

Distortion of reality regarding the client's health problem
Intolerance
Rejection
Abandonment
Desertion
Agitation
Depression

Aggression
Hostility
Impaired restructuring of family unit

RELATED FACTORS

Related to impaired ability to fulfill role responsibilities secondary to any acute or chronic illness

Situational (Personal, Environmental)

Related to impaired ability to manage stressors constructively secondary to:
Substance abuse
Negative role-modeling
History of ineffective relationship with own parents
History of abusive relationships with parents

Related to unrealistic expectations of child by parent
Related to unrealistic expectations of parent by child
Related to unmet psychosocial needs of child by parent
Related to unmet psychosocial needs of parent by child

Goals

The person will set short-term and long-term goals for change.

Indicators

- Appraise coping behaviors that are unhealthy for family members.
- Relate expectations for self and family.
- Relate community resources available.

Generic Interventions

Assist Family to Evaluate Past and Present Family Functioning.

Provide All Family Members an Opportunity to Discuss their Appraisal of the Situation.

Discourage Blaming, but Allow Ventilation of Anger.

Clarify Feelings of Members.

**Assist Family with Appraisal
of the Situation:**

What is wrong?
What are the causes?
Who has contributed to the problem?
What are the options?
What are the advantages/disadvantages of each option?
What activity could be added to the family?

**If Indicated, Ask Members to
Consider the Problem from the
Perspective of Another
Family Member.**

**If a Member Is Ill, Assist Family to
Have More Realistic Expectations.**

If Domestic Abuse Is Suspected:

Know your state's laws regarding domestic abuse
 (e.g., mandatory reporting).
Provide an opportunity to validate abuse and talk about
 feelings.
Be direct and nonjudgmental:
  "How do you handle stress?"
  "How does your partner or caregiver handle stress?"
  "How do you and your partner argue?"
  "Are you afraid of your partner?"
  "Have you ever been hit, pushed, or injured by your
   partner?"
Encourage a realistic appraisal of the situation; dispel
 guilt and myths:
  "Violence is not normal for most families."
  "Violence may stop, but it usually becomes increasingly
   worse."
  "Alcohol and drugs do not cause violence."
  "The victim is not responsible for the violence."
  "You do not deserve this."
  "You have a right to be protected."
Provide options, but allow family members to make a
 decision at their own pace.
Discuss the importance of a "safety plan." For specifics of a
 safety plan, refer to a hotline or programs specific for
 domestic violence.

Provide a list of community agencies available to victim
  and abuser (emergency and long-term):
    Hotlines
    Legal services
    Shelters
    Counseling agencies
Discuss the availability of the social service department for
  assistance.
Consult with the legal resources in the community, and
  familiarize the victim with the state laws regarding:
    Eviction of abuser
    Counseling
    Temporary support
    Protection orders
    Criminal law
    Types of police interventions
Document findings and dialogue for possible future
  court use.

🔸 Pediatric Interventions

**Report Suspected Cases
of Child Abuse.**

**Know your state's child abuse laws
and procedures for reporting child
abuse (e.g., Bureau of Child Welfare,
Department of Social Services, Child
Protective Services).**

Maintain an objective record:

Description of injuries
Record conversations with parents and child using
  quotations
Description of behaviors, not interpretation (e.g., avoid
  "angry father"; instead, write "Father screamed at child,
  'If you weren't so bad, this wouldn't have happened.'")
Description of parent-child interactions (e.g., shies away
  from mother's touch)
Nutritional status
Growth and development compared with age-related norms

🔹 Pediatric Interventions (cont'd)

Provide the Child with Acceptance and Affection.

Assist Child with Grieving if Foster Home Placement Is Necessary.

Allow Opportunities for Child to Ventilate Feelings.

Provide Interventions that Promote Parents' Self-Esteem and Sense of Trust.

Tell them it was good that they brought the child to the hospital.
Promote their confidence by presenting a warm, helpful attitude and acknowledging any competent parenting activities.
Provide opportunities for parents to participate in their child's care (e.g., feeding, bathing).

Refer Abusive Parents to Community Agencies and Professionals for Counseling.

Disseminate Information to the Community (e.g., Parent-School Organizations, Radio, Television, Newspaper) About the Problem of Child Abuse.

🔘 Geriatric Interventions

Identify Suspected Cases of Elder Abuse; Observe For:

Failure to adhere to therapeutic regimens
Evidence of malnutrition, dehydration
Bruises, swelling, lacerations, burns, bites
Pressure ulcers
Caregiver not allowing nurse to be alone with elder

⬤ Geriatric Interventions (cont'd)

If Abuse Suspected
(Anetzberger, 1987):

Know your state's laws regarding elder abuse.
Consult with supervisor for procedures.
Maintain an objective record, including:
  Description of injuries
  Conversations with elder and caregivers
  Description of behaviors
  Nutritional, hydration status
Consider the elder's right to choose to live at risk of harm,
  providing he or she is capable of making that choice.
Do not initiate an action that could increase the elder's
  risk of harm or antagonize the abuser.
Respect the elder's right to secrecy and the right for self-
  determination.

Disseminate Information to
Community Regarding Prevention.

Decisional Conflict

DEFINITION
Decisional Conflict: The state in which an individual or group
experiences uncertainty about a course of action when the
choice involves risk, loss, or challenge.

DEFINING CHARACTERISTICS
(HILTUNEN, 1987)
Major (80% to 100%)
Verbalization of uncertainty about choices

Verbalization of undesired consequences of alternative
  actions being considered
Vacillation between alternative choices
Delayed decision-making

Minor (50% to 79%)

Verbalized feeling of distress while attempting a decision
Self-focusing
Physical signs of distress or tension (e.g., increased heart
  rate, increased muscle tension, restlessness) whenever
  the decision comes within focus of attention
Questioning personal values and beliefs while attempting
  to make a decision

RELATED FACTORS

Many situations can contribute to *Decisional Conflict,* particularly those that involve complex medical interventions
of great risk. Any decisional situation can precipitate conflict for an individual; thus, the examples listed below are not
exhaustive but reflect situations that may be problematic and
possess factors that increase the difficulty.

Treatment-Related
**Related to risks versus benefits of (specify test, treat-
ment):**
Surgery
Tumor removal   Joint replacement
Cataract   Hysterectomy
  Laminectomy   Transplant
  Orchiectomy   Cesarean section
  Cosmetic Surgery
Diagnostics
  Amniocentesis   X-rays
Ultrasonography
Chemotherapy
Radiation
Dialysis
Mechanical ventilation
Enteral feedings
Intravenous hydration
Use of medications during labor
HIV antiviral therapy

Situational (Personal, Environmental)
Related to risks versus benefits of:

Personal

Marriage
Separation
Divorce
Parenthood
Birth control
Artificial insemination
Adoption
Circumcision
Foster home placement

Institutionalization
  (child, parent)
Breastfeeding versus
  bottle-feeding
Abortion
Sterilization
Nursing home placement
Transport from rural
  facilities
In vitro fertilization

Work/Task

Career change
Relocation

Business investments
Professional ethics

Related to lack of relevant information
Related to confusing information
Related to:

Disagreement within support systems
Inexperience with decision-making
Unclear personal values/beliefs
Conflict with personal values/beliefs
Resignation
Family history of poor prognosis
Hospital environment—loss of control
Ethical dilemmas of:
  Quality of life
  Cessation of life-support systems
  "Do not resuscitate" orders
  Termination of pregnancy
  Organ transplant

Maturational
Adolescent
Related to risks versus benefits of:

Peer pressure
Sexual activity
Alcohol/drug use
Illegal/dangerous
  situations

Career choice
Use of birth control
Whether to continue
  a relationship
College

Adult
Related to risks versus benefits of:

Career change   Relocation
Retirement

Older Adult
Related to risks versus benefits of:

Retirement   Nursing home placement

> **NOC** Decision Making, Information Processing, Participation: Health Care Decisions

Goals

The person will make an informed choice.

Indicators

- Relate the advantages and disadvantages of choices.
- Share fears and concerns regarding choices and responses of others.
- Define what would be most helpful to support the decision-making process.

> **NIC** Decision-Making Support, Mutual Goal Setting, Learning Facilitation, Health System Guidance, Anticipatory Guidance, Patient Rights Protection, Value Clarification, Anxiety Reduction

Generic Interventions

Establish a trusting and meaningful relationship that promotes mutual understanding and caring.
Facilitate a logical decision-making process.
  Assist the person in recognizing what the problem is, and clearly identify that a decision needs to be made.
  Explore what the outcomes of not deciding would be.
  Have the person make a list of all the possible alternatives or options.
  Help identify the probable outcomes of the various alternatives.
  Help the person to face fears.
  Correct misinformation.

Aid in evaluating the alternatives based on actual or
potential threats to beliefs/values.

Encourage the person to make a decision.

Encourage the person's significant others to be involved in
the entire decision-making process.

Assist the individual in exploring personal values and relationships that may have an impact on the decision.

Support the individual making informed decision, even if
decision conflicts with own values. Consult spiritual
leader.

Actively reassure the person that the decision is his or
hers to make and that he or she has the right to do so.

Do not allow others to undermine the person's confidence
in making own decision.

Collaborate with family members to clarify the process.

Pediatric Interventions

Include children and adolescents in decision-making process.

Geriatric Interventions

Ensure that older adult is involved in decisions.

Facilitate communication among the elder, family, and
professionals.

If needed, use simple explanations, and provide the pros
and cons of the decision.

DEFINITION
Diarrhea: The state in which an individual experiences or is at risk of experiencing frequent passages of liquid stool or unformed stool.

DEFINING CHARACTERISTICS
Major (Must be Present, One or More)
Loose, liquid stools *and/or*
Increased frequency of stools (more than three times a day)

Minor (May be Present)
Urgency
Cramping/abdominal pain
Increased frequency of bowel sounds
Increased fluidity or volume of stools

RELATED FACTORS
Pathophysiologic
Related to malabsorption or inflammation secondary to:

Gastritis	Crohn's disease
Peptic ulcer	Colon cancer
Diverticulitis	Spastic colon
Ulcerative colitis	Celiac disease (sprue)
	Irritable bowel

Related to lactase deficiency
Related to increased peristalsis secondary to increased metabolic rate (hyperthyroidism)
Related to dumping syndrome
Related to infectious process secondary to:

Trichinosis	Shigellosis
Dysentery	Typhoid fever
Cholera	Infectious hepatitis
Malaria	*Microsporidia*
Cryptosporidium	

Related to excessive secretion of fats in stool secondary to liver dysfunction

Related to inflammation and ulceration of gastro-intestinal mucosa secondary to high levels of nitrogenous wastes (renal failure)

Treatment-Related

Related to malabsorption or inflammation secondary to surgical intervention of the bowel
Related to side effects of (specify):

Thyroid agents
Antacids (magnesium hydroxide)
Laxatives
Stool softeners
Antibiotics
Cancer chemotherapeutic agents
Analgesics
Cimetidine
Iron sulfate
Antivirals (HIV)

Related to high-solute tube feedings

Situational (Personal, Environmental)

Related to stress or anxiety
Related to irritating foods (fruits, bran cereals)
Related to change in water or food secondary to travel
Related to change in bacteria in water
Related to bacteria, virus, or parasite to which no immunity is present
Related to increased caffeine consumption

Maturational

Infant: Related to breast milk

NOC Bowel Elimination, Electrolyte and Acid/Base Imbalance, Fluid Balance, Hydration, Symptom Control

Goals

The person will report less diarrhea.

Indicators

- Describe contributing factors when known.
- Explain rationale for interventions.

NIC Bowel Management, Diarrhea Management, Electrolyte Management, Nutrition Management, Enteral Tube Feeding

Generic Interventions

Assess for Causative or Contributing Factors: Tube Feedings, Dietary Indiscretions/Contaminated Foods, Food Allergies, Foreign Travel, Fecal Impaction.

Reduce Diarrhea:
Discontinue solids.
Ingest clear liquids (fruit juices, Gatorade, broth).
Avoid milk products, fat, high-fiber foods (whole-grain products, fresh fruits and vegetables).
Gradually add semisolids and solids (crackers, yogurt, rice, bananas, applesauce).

Increase Oral Intake to Maintain a Normal Urine-Specific Gravity (Pale Yellow Urine).

Encourage Fluids High in Potassium and Low in Sugar (Water, Apple Juice, Flat Ginger Ale).

Caution Against Use of Very Hot or Very Cold Liquids.

Explain to Client and Significant Others the Interventions Required to Prevent Future Episodes.

If Related to Tube Feedings (Fuhrman, 1999):
Change to continuous-drip tube feedings.
Administer more slowly if signs of gastrointestinal intolerance occur.
If refrigerated, warm in hot water to room temperature.
Dilute strength of feeding temporarily.
Follow tube feeding with specified amount of water to ensure hydration.

Teach Precautions to Take When Traveling to Foreign Lands (Bennett, 2002):
Avoid foods served cold, salads, milk, fresh cheese, cold cuts, and salsa.

Drink carbonated or bottled beverages; avoid ice.

Peel fresh fruits and vegetables.

Consult with primary health care provider for treatment
of traveler's diarrhea by prophylactic use of bismuth
subsalicylate (e.g., Pepto-Bismol), 30 to 60 mL qid during travel and 2 days after return, or antimicrobials.
Avoid opiate-containing antidiarrheals (e.g., Lomotil,
Imodium).

**Explain How to Prevent Transmission
of Infection (Handwashing; Proper
Storing, Cooking, and Handling
of Food; Foods at Picnics).**

◆ Pediatric Interventions

For Breastfed Infants:

Discontinue solids.

Offer clear liquid supplements.

Continue breastfeeding.

For Formula-Fed Infant
or Milk-Fed Child:

Discontinue formula, milk products, and solid foods.

Avoid high-carbohydrate fluids (e.g., soft drinks, gelatin,
fruit juices, caffeinated drinks, chicken or beef broth).

Use oral rehydration solutions (e.g., Pedialyte, Lytren,
Infalyte, Resol) (Larson, 2000). Provide 60 to 80 mL/kg
over a 2-hour period for mild to moderate diarrhea.

Gradually add plain solids (Jell-O, bananas, rice, cereal,
crackers).

Gradually return to regular diet (except milk products) after
36 to 48 hours; after 3 to 5 days, gradually add milk products (half-strength skim milk to full-strength skim milk to
half-strength whole milk to full-strength whole milk).

Gradually introduce formula (half-strength formula to full-
strength formula).

**Explain the BRAT Diet (Bananas,
Rice, Applesauce, Tea, and Toast) to
Counter the Effects of Diarrhea.**

🌑 Geriatric Interventions

Determine if impaction is present; if so, remove it (refer to *Constipation* for specific interventions).

Monitor closely for hypovolemia and electrolyte imbalance (potassium, sodium).

Disuse Syndrome

DEFINITION

Disuse Syndrome: The state in which an individual is experiencing or at risk for deterioration of body systems or altered functioning as a result of prescribed or unavoidable musculoskeletal inactivity.

⊗ AUTHOR'S NOTE

Disuse Syndrome represents an individual experiencing or at risk for the adverse effects of immobility. Syndrome nursing diagnoses should not be written as *Risk,* because clustered under them are risk and actual diagnoses. *Disuse Syndrome* identifies an individual as vulnerable to certain complications and experiencing altered functioning in a health pattern. In most situations, syndrome diagnoses do not require causative or contributing factors (*i.e., Disuse Syndrome related to spinal cord injury*). When the causative or contributing factors to *Disuse Syndrome* are personal, environmental, or maturational, it may be useful to specify the related factors.

⊛ **AUTHOR'S NOTE (continued)**

If an individual who is immobile manifests the signs and symptoms of *Impaired Skin Integrity* or another diagnosis, the specific diagnosis should be used. The nurse should continue to use *Disuse Syndrome* so that deterioration of the other body systems does not occur.

DEFINING CHARACTERISTICS

Presence of a cluster of actual or risk nursing diagnoses related to inactivity:

Risk for Impaired Skin Integrity
Risk for Constipation
Risk for Impaired Respiratory Function
Risk for Impaired Peripheral Tissue Perfusion
Risk for Infection
Risk for Activity Intolerance
Risk for Impaired Physical Mobility
Risk for Injury
Risk for Disturbed Sensory Perception
Powerlessness
Disturbed Body Image

RELATED FACTORS (OPTIONAL)
Pathophysiologic
Related to:

Decreased sensorium
Unconsciousness
Neuromuscular impairment
 Multiple sclerosis   Muscular dystrophy
 Parkinsonism   Partial or total paralysis
 Guillain-Barré syndrome   Spinal cord injury
Musculoskeletal conditions
 Fractures   Rheumatic diseases
End-stage disease
 AIDS   Cardiac disease
Renal disease   Cancer
Psychiatric/mental health disorders
Major depression   Severe phobias
 Catatonic state

Treatment-Related
Related to:

Surgery (amputation,
 skeletal)
Mechanical ventilation

Traction/casts/splints
Prescribed immobility
Invasive vascular lines

Situational (Personal, Environmental)
**Related to depression, fatigue, debilitated state, or
pain**

Maturational
Newborn, Infant, Child, or Adolescent
Related to:

Down syndrome
Legg-Calvé-Perthes disease
Spina bifida
Autism
Mental/physical disability

Osteogenesis imperfecta
Cerebral palsy
Risser turnbuckle jacket
Juvenile arthritis

Older Adult
Related to:

Decreased motor agility
Muscle weakness

Presenile dementia

NOC Endurance, Immobility Consequences: Physiological,
Immobility Consequences: Psycho-Cognitive, Mobility Level

Goals

The person will not experience complications of immobility.

Indicators

- Display intact skin/tissue integrity; maximum pulmonary function; maximum peripheral blood flow; full range of motion; bowel, bladder, and renal functioning within normal limits.
- Use social contacts and activities when possible.
- Explain rationale for treatments.
- Make decisions regarding care when possible.
- Share feelings regarding immobile state.

NIC Activity Therapy, Energy Management, Mutual Goal Setting,
Exercise Therapy, Fall Prevention, Pressure Ulcer
Prevention, Body Mechanism Connection, Skin Surveillance
Positioning, Coping Enhancement, Decision-Making Support

Generic Interventions

Assist to reposition, turning frequently from side to side
(hourly if possible).

Encourage deep breathing and controlled coughing exercises five times every hour.

Auscultate lung fields every 8 hours.

Maintain usual pattern of bowel elimination. Refer to *Constipation* for specific interventions.

Prevent pressure ulcers.

  Use repositioning schedule that relieves vulnerable area
    most often.

  Turn the person or instruct the person to turn or shift
    weight every 30 minutes to 2 hours.

  Keep bed as flat as possible to reduce shearing forces;
    limit Fowler's position to 30 minutes at a time.

  Use foam blocks or pillows to provide a bridging effect.

  Use enough personnel to lift person up in bed or chair.

Observe for erythema and blanching, and palpate for
warmth and tissue sponginess with each position change.

Do not massage reddened areas.

Refer to *Impaired Skin Integrity* for additional interventions.

Elevate extremity above the level of the heart (may be contraindicated if severe cardiac or respiratory disease is
present).

Perform range-of-motion exercises (frequency to be determined by condition of the individual).

Position the person in alignment to prevent complications.

Provide a daily intake of fluid of 2000 mL or greater (unless
contraindicated); refer to *Deficient Fluid Volume* for specific interventions.

Provide weight-bearing when possible (e.g., tilt table).

Encourage the person to share feelings and fears regarding
restricted movement.

Encourage the person to wear own clothes rather than
pajamas.

Include the individual in planning schedule for daily routine.

Be creative; vary the physical environment and daily routine when possible.

Provide opportunities for the individual to control decisions.

◆ Pediatric Interventions

Provide the child with play appropriate for condition.

Encourage the child to share feelings regarding immobilization.

Encourage the child to keep a diary of experiences.

If possible, provide the child with lunchmates (e.g., staff, other children).

Deficient Diversional Activity

DEFINITION

Deficient Diversional Activity: The state in which an individual or group experiences or is at risk of experiencing decreased stimulation from or interest in activities that promote enjoyment of life.

DEFINING CHARACTERISTICS
Major (Must be Present)

Observed or statements of boredom/depression from inactivity

Minor (May be Present)

Frequent expression of unpleasant thoughts or feelings
Yawning or inattentiveness
Flat affect

Body language (shifting of body away from speaker)
Restlessness/fidgeting
Weight loss or gain
Hostility

RELATED FACTORS
Pathophysiologic
Related to difficulty accessing or participating in enjoyable activities secondary to communicable disease or pain

Situational (Personal, Environmental)
Related to unsatisfactory social behaviors
Related to no peers or friends
Related to monotonous environment
Related to confinement
Related to lack of motivation
Related to difficulty accessing or participating in enjoyable activities secondary to:
Excessive long hours of work
No time for leisure activities
Career changes (e.g., teacher to homemaker, retirement)
Children leaving home ("empty nest")
Disability
Decreased sensory perception (e.g., blindness, hearing loss)
Multiple role responsibilities

Maturational
Infant/Child
Related to lack of appropriate stimulation, toys, peers

Older Adult
Related to difficulty accessing or participating in enjoyable activities secondary to:

Sensory motor deficits	Lack of peer group
Lack of transportation	Limited finances
Fear of crime	Confusion

NOC Leisure Participation, Social Involvement

Goals

The person will report participating in at least one enjoyable activity each day.

Indicators

- Relate improved satisfaction with current activity level.
- Identify enjoyable activities that can enhance quality of life.

NIC Recreation Therapy, Socialization Enhancement, Self-Esteem Enhancement

Generic Interventions

Stimulate motivation by showing interest and encouraging sharing of feelings and experiences.

Help the person to work through feelings of anger and grief.

Vary daily routine when possible (e.g., give bath in the afternoon so that the person can watch a special show or talk with a visitor who drops in).

Include the individual in planning daily schedule.

Plan time for visitors.

Be creative; vary the physical environment when possible.

Place the person near a window or take outside, if possible.

Discuss previously enjoyed hobbies. Consult with recreational or occupational therapist.

Provide reading material, radio, television, books-on-tape.

Plan an activity daily to give person something to look forward to, and always keep your promises.

Discourage the use of television as the primary source of recreation unless it is highly desired.

Consider using a volunteer to spend time reading to the person or helping with an activity.

If appropriate, enlist the person to help others with an activity.

In an institutional setting:

  Encourage participation in recreational therapy.
  Praise involvement.
  Allow the person to choose which recreational activities are of interest.
  Focus on capabilities, not deficits.
  Consider using reminiscence, music, or pet therapy.
  Organize book discussions.

◆ Pediatric Interventions

Provide an environment with accessible playthings that suit the child's developmental age, and ensure that they are well within reach.

Encourage family to bring in child's favorite playthings, including items from nature that will help to keep the real world alive (e.g., goldfish; leaves in the fall).

Dysreflexia
Risk for Dysreflexia

Dysreflexia

DEFINITION

Dysreflexia: The state in which an individual with a spinal cord injury at T6 or above experiences or is at risk of experiencing a potential life-threatening uninhibited sympathetic response of the nervous system to a noxious stimulus.

> ⓧ **AUTHOR'S NOTE**
>
> This is a situation that the nurse or client can prevent or treat. If the nurse's initial treatment does not abate the symptoms, medical treatment is imperative. An individual does not experience dysreflexia as a continued state but rather is at risk for it, so if it is experienced, it must be abated. Thus, *Risk for Dysreflexia* better describes the clinical situation than does *Dysreflexia*.

DEFINING CHARACTERISTICS
Major (Must be Present, One or More)
Individual with spinal cord injury at T6 or above with:

Paroxysmal hypertension (sudden periodic elevated blood pressure in which systolic pressure is >140 mm Hg and diastolic is >90 mm Hg)

Bradycardia (pulse rate <60) or tachycardia (>100 beats/min)

Diaphoresis (above the injury)

Red splotches on the skin (above the injury)

Pallor (below the injury)

Headache (a diffuse pain in different portions of the head and not confined to any nerve distribution area)

Apprehension

Minor (May be Present)
Chilling

Conjunctival congestion

Horner's syndrome (contraction of the pupil, partial ptosis of the eyelid, enophthalmos, and sometimes loss of sweating over the affected side of the face)

Paresthesia

Pilomotor reflex

Blurred vision

Nasal congestion

Chest pain

Metallic taste in the mouth

RELATED FACTORS
Pathophysiologic
Related to visceral stretching and irritation secondary to:

Bowel

Constipation	Fecal impaction
Acute abdominal condition	Hemorrhoids
Gastric ulcers	Anal fissure

Bladder

Distended bladder	Infection
Urinary calculi	

Cutaneous

Pressure ulcers	Insect bites
Burns	Ingrown toenails
Sunburn	Blister

Reproductive

Menstruation	Epididymitis
Pregnancy or delivery	Uterine contraction
Vaginal infection	Vaginal dilation

Related to stimulation of skin (abdominal, thigh)
Related to spastic sphincter
Related to deep vein thrombosis

Treatment-Related
Related to visceral stretching secondary to:
Removal of fecal impaction
Clogged or nonpatent catheter
Visceral stretching and irritation secondary to surgical
  incision
Catheterization, enema

Situational (Personal, Environmental)
Related to lack of knowledge of
prevention or treatment
Related to visceral stretching
secondary to:
Sexual activity
Menstruation
Boosting
Pregnancy or delivery
Submergence in cold water

NOC Neurological Status, Neurological Status: Autonomic,
     Vital Signs Status

Goals

The individual/family will prevent or respond to early signs/
symptoms.

Indicators

- State factors that cause dysreflexia.
- Describe the treatment for dysreflexia.
- Relate when emergency treatment is indicated.

NIC Dysreflexia Management, Vital Signs Monitoring, Emergency
     Care, Medication Administration

Generic Interventions

If signs of dysreflexia occur:

    Stand person up, or sit person up, or raise head of bed.

    Lower legs.

    Loosen all constrictive clothing, appliances.

Check for distended bladder.

If catheterized:

    Check catheter for kinks or compression.

    Irrigate with only 30 mL saline very slowly.

    Replace catheter if it will not drain.

If not catheterized, insert catheter using an anesthetic ointment and remove 500 mL, then clamp for 15 minutes; repeat cycle until bladder is drained.

For fecal impaction:

    First apply dibucaine hydrochloride ointment (Nupercaine) to the anus and 1 inch (2.54 cm) into the rectum.

    Gently check rectum with a well-lubricated glove.

    Insert rectal suppository, or gently remove impaction.

Assess for other causes:

    Skin stimulation: spray lesion with a topical anesthetic agent.

    Other stimuli: these include cold draft, objects that pressure skin.

    Bladder infection: send urine for culture.

Continue to monitor blood pressure every 3 to 5 minutes.

Immediately consult physician for pharmacologic treatment if hypertension or noxious stimuli are not eliminated.

Teach signs and symptoms and treatment of dysreflexia to person and family.

Teach when immediate medical intervention is warranted.

Explain what situations can trigger dysreflexia (menstrual cycle, sexual activity, bladder or bowel routines).

Advise consultation with physician for long-term pharmacologic management if individual is very vulnerable.

Document how frequently episodes occur and precipitating factor(s).

Provide with printed instructions to guide actions during crisis or to show other health care personnel (e.g., dentists, gynecologists) (Kavchak-Keyes, 2000).

Advise athletes with high spinal cord injury about the danger of boosting (binding their legs, distending bladder to increase norepinephrine levels) (McClain, 1999).

Risk for Dysreflexia

DEFINITION

Risk for Dysreflexia: The state in which an individual with a spinal cord injury at T7 or above is at risk of experiencing a potential for life-threatening uninhibited sympathetic response of the nervous system to a noxious stimulus.

RISK FACTORS

Refer to Related Factors in *Dysreflexia.*

RELATED FACTORS

Refer to Related Factors in *Dysreflexia.*

Goals

Refer to *Dysreflexia.*

Generic Interventions

Teach signs and symptoms and treatment of dysreflexia to person and family.

Teach when immediate medical intervention is warranted.

Explain what situations can trigger dysreflexia (menstrual cycle, sexual activity, bladder or bowel routines).

Teach to observe for early signs of bladder infections and skin lesions (pressure ulcers, ingrown toenails).

Advise consultation with physician for long-term pharmacologic management if individual is very vulnerable.

Disturbed Energy Field

DEFINITION

Disturbed Energy Field: The state in which a disruption of the flow of energy surrounding a person's being results in a disharmony of the body, mind, and/or spirit.

> **AUTHOR'S NOTE**
>
> This addition to the NANDA list is unique for two reasons. It represents a specific theory (human energy field theory), and the interventions used require specialized instruction and supervised practice. Meehan (1991) recommends:
>
> - At least 6 months' experience in professional practice in an acute care setting
> - Guided learning by a nurse with at least 2 years' experience
> - Conformance with practice guidelines
> - Thirty hours of instruction in the theory and practice
> - Thirty hours of supervised practice with relatively healthy individuals
> - Successful completion of written and practice evaluations
>
> This diagnosis may be considered unconventional by some. Perhaps each nurse needs to be reminded that there are many theories, philosophies, and frameworks of nursing practice, just as there are many definitions of clients and practice settings; some nurses practice on street corners with homeless persons, whereas others practice in an office attached to their home. Nursing diagnoses should not represent only the practices of nurses in the mainstream practice setting (acute care, long-term care, and home health). Rather than criticize a diagnosis as having little applicability to one's own practice, perhaps we should celebrate the diversity among us. Fundamentally, nurses are all connected as each of us and all of us seek to improve the condition of clients, families, groups, and communities.

DEFINING CHARACTERISTICS
Perception of changes in patterns of the energy flow, such as:

Temperature change
Warmth   Coolness

Visual changes
Image   Color

Disruption of the field
Vacant   Hole
Spike   Bulge

Movement
Wave   Spike
Tingling   Dense
Flowing

Sounds
Tone   Words

RELATED FACTORS
Pathophysiologic
Related to slowing or blocking of energy flows secondary to: illness (specify), injury, or pregnancy

Treatment-Related
Related to slowing or blocking of energy flows secondary to: immobility, labor and delivery, or perioperative experience

Situational (Personal, Environmental)
Related to the slowing or blocking of energy flows secondary to pain, anxiety, fear, or grieving

Maturational
Related to age-related developmental difficulties or crises (specify)

NOC Spiritual Well-Being, Well-Being

Goals

The person will report relief of symptoms after therapeutic touch.

NIC Therapeutic Touch, Spiritual Support

Indicators

- Report increased sense of relaxation.
- Report a decrease in pain, using a scale of 0 to 10 before and after therapies.
- Have slower, deeper respirations.

Generic Interventions

The following phases of therapeutic touch are learned separately but are rendered concurrently. The presentation of these interventions is for the purpose of describing the process for nurses who do not practice therapeutic touch. This discussion may help nurses support colleagues who practice therapeutic touch and initiate referrals. As discussed previously, preparing for therapeutic touch requires specialized instruction that is beyond the scope of this book.

Explain therapeutic touch, and obtain verbal permission.

Prepare the client and environment for therapeutic touch.

Provide as much privacy as possible.

Give the person permission to stop the therapy at any time.

Allow the person to assume a comfortable position (e.g., lying or sitting on a bed or couch).

Shift from a direct focus on the environment to an inner focus, which is perceived as the center of life within the nurse (centering).

Assess by scanning the person's energy field for openness and symmetry (Krieger, 1979).

Move hands, palms toward the person, at a distance of 2 to 4 inches over the person's body from head to feet, in a smooth, light movement.

Sense the cues to energy imbalance (e.g., warmth, coolness, tightness, heaviness, tingling, emptiness).

Facilitate a rhythmic flow of energy by moving hands more vigorously from head to toe (unruffling/clearing).

Focus intent on the specific repatterning of areas of imbalance and impeded flow. Using your hands as focal points, move the hands in gentle, sweeping movements from head to feet one time.

Encourage the person to provide feedback.

Document the procedure and the feedback.

Environmental Interpretation Syndrome, Impaired

DEFINITION

Impaired Environmental Interpretation Syndrome: Consistent lack of orientation to person, place, time, or circumstances for more than 3 to 6 months, necessitating a protective environment.

> ### ⊚ AUTHOR'S NOTE
>
> *Impaired Environmental Interpretation Syndrome* describes an individual who needs a protective environment because of consistent lack of orientation to person, place, time, or circumstances. This diagnosis is described under *Chronic Confusion* and *Risk for Injury.* Interventions focus on maintaining maximum level of independence and preventing injury. Until clinical research differentiates this diagnosis from the aforementioned diagnoses, use *Chronic Confusion* or *Risk for Injury,* depending on the data presented.

DEFINING CHARACTERISTICS
Major (Must be Present, One or More)
Consistent disorientation in known and unknown environments
Chronic confusional states

Minor (May be Present)
Loss of occupation or social functioning from memory decline
Slow in responding to questions

Inability to reason
Inability to concentrate
Inability to follow simple directions or instructions

RELATED FACTORS
Dementia (Alzheimer's disease, multi-infarct dementia, Pick's disease, AIDS dementia)

Parkinson's disease
Huntington's disease
Depression
Alcoholism

Family Processes, Interrupted
Family Processes, Dysfunctional:
    Alcoholism

Family Processes, Interrupted

DEFINITION

Interrupted Family Processes: The state in which a normally supportive family experiences or is at risk to experience a stressor that challenges its previously effective functioning ability.

> **⊙ AUTHOR'S NOTE**
>
> The nursing diagnosis *Interrupted Family Processes* describes a family that usually functions optimally but is challenged by a stressor that has altered or may alter the family's function. This diagnosis differs from *Disabled Family Coping*, which describes a family that has a pattern of destructive behavioral responses. Unsuccessful resolution of a problem can change *Interrupted Family Processes* to *Disabled Family Coping*.

DEFINING CHARACTERISTICS
Major (Must be Present, One or More)

Family system cannot or does not:
Adapt constructively to crisis
Communicate openly and effectively among family members

Minor (May be Present)

Family system cannot or does not:
Meet physical needs of all its members
Meet emotional needs of all its members
Meet spiritual needs of all its members

Express or accept a wide range of feelings
Seek or accept help appropriately

RELATED FACTORS

Any factor can contribute to *Interrupted Family Processes*.
  Some common factors are listed below.

Treatment-Related
Related to:
Disruption of family routines owing to time-consuming
  treatments (e.g., home dialysis)
Physical changes owing to treatments of ill family
  member
Emotional changes in all family members owing to treat-
  ments of ill family member
Financial burden of treatments for ill family member
Hospitalization of ill family member

Situational (Personal, Environmental)
Related to loss of family member:

Death   Incarceration
Going away to school   Desertion
Separation   Hospitalization
Divorce

**Related to gain of family member (e.g., birth, adoption,
marriage, elderly relative)**
Related to losses associated with:

Poverty   Change in family roles
Disaster   Working mother
Relocation   Retirement
Economic crisis   Birth of child with defect

Related to conflict (moral, goal, cultural)
Related to breach of trust among members
**Related to social deviance by family member (e.g.,
crime)**

NOC   Family Coping, Family Environment: Internal, Family
      Normalization: Parenting

Goals

The family members will maintain a functional system of
mutual support for each other.

Indicators
- Frequently verbalize feelings to professional nurse and each other.
- Identify appropriate external resources available.

> **NIC** Family Involvement Promotion, Coping Enhancement, Family Integrity Promotion, Family Therapy, Counseling, Referral

Generic Interventions

Assist the family with appraisal of the situation.

What is at stake? Encourage the family to have a realistic perspective by providing accurate information and answers to questions.

What are the choices? Assist the family to reorganize roles at home and set priorities to maintain family integrity and reduce stress.

Where is help available? Direct the family to community agencies, home health care organizations, and sources of financial assistance as needed (see *Impaired Home Maintenance* for additional interventions).

Create a private and supportive hospital environment for the family.

Acknowledge strengths to the family when appropriate:
"I can tell you are a very close family."
"You know just how to get your mother to eat."
"Your brother means a great deal to you."

Involve family members in care of ill member when possible (feeding, bathing, dressing, ambulating).

Involve family members in patient care conferences when appropriate.

Encourage family to acquire substitutes to care for the ill person to provide the family with time away.

Encourage verbalization of guilt, anger, blame, hostility, and subsequent recognition of feelings in family members.

Aid family members to change their expectations of the ill member in a realistic manner.

Provide the family with anticipatory guidance as illness continues:

Inform parents of the effects of prolonged hospitalization on children (appropriate to developmental age).

Prepare family members for signs of depression, anxiety, and dependency, which are a natural part of the illness experience.

Enlist help of other professionals when problems extend beyond realm of nursing (e.g., social worker, clinical psychologist, nurse therapist, clinical specialist, psychiatrist, child care specialist).

Family Processes, Dysfunctional: Alcoholism

DEFINITION

Dysfunctional Family Processes: Alcoholism: The state in which the psychosocial, spiritual, economic, and physiologic functions of the family members and system are chronically disorganized because of the effects of alcohol abuse.

✪ AUTHOR'S NOTE

Alcoholism is a family disease. This nursing diagnosis represents the consequences of the disturbed family dynamics related to alcohol abuse by a family member. The NANDA definition of *Interrupted Family Processes* is "the state in which a family that normally functions effectively experiences a dysfunction" (NANDA, 1992, p. 41). The alcoholic family does not have a history of effective functioning. The diagnosis *Disabled Family Coping* would be more descriptive of the alcoholic family. The diagnosis could be stated as *Dysfunctional Family Coping: Alcoholism.* Further assessments will determine the effects of alcoholism on physical, psychological, spiritual, financial, and developmental aspects of the family unit. If clinical research validates that alcoholism affects all of these dimensions in all or most families, the diagnosis *Alcoholic Family Process Syndrome* may prove very useful.

DEFINING CHARACTERISTICS
(Lindeman et al., 1994)
Major (80% to 100%)
Behaviors
Loss of control of drinking
Denial of problems
Alcohol abuse
Impaired communication
Rationalization
Broken promises
Inability to meet emotional needs of members
Manipulation
Inappropriate expression of anger
Dependency
Refusal to get help
Blaming
Enabling behaviors
Ineffective problem-solving skills
Inadequate understanding or knowledge of alcoholism
Criticizing

Roles and Relationships
Deterioration in family relationships
Disturbed family dynamics
Marital problems
Ineffective spouse communication
Disruption of family roles
Inconsistent parenting
Family denial
Intimacy dysfunction
Closed communication systems

Feelings
Decreased self-esteem
Anger
Frustration
Powerlessness
Tension
Suppressed rage
Anxiety
Repressed emotions
Responsibility for
   alcoholic's behavior
Embarrassment
Hurt
Unhappiness
Guilt
Emotional isolation
Vulnerability
Worthlessness
Shame
Loneliness
Mistrust
Hopelessness
Rejection

Minor (50% to 79%)

Behaviors
Inability to express or accept wide range of feelings
Orientation toward tension relief rather than achievement
  of goals
Family's special occasions are alcohol-centered
Escalating conflict
Lying
Failure to send clear messages
Inability to get help or receive help appropriately
Ineffective decision-making
Contradictory, paradoxical communication
Failure to deal with conflict constructively
Harsh self-judgment
Isolation
Difficulty having fun
Inability to adapt to change
Immaturity
Power struggles
Stress-related physical illnesses
Lack of reliability
Disturbances in academic performance in children
Disturbances in concentration
Chaos
Substance abuse other than alcohol
Difficulty with life cycle transitions
Verbal abuse of spouse or parent
Failure to accomplish current or past developmental tasks

Feelings
- Being different from
    other persons
- Depression
- Hostility
- Fear
- Emotional control by
    others
- Confusion
- Dissatisfaction
- Self-blaming
- Unresolved grief
- Loss
- Feeling misunderstood
- Abandonment
- Confused love and pity
- Moodiness
- Failure
- Being unloved
- Lack of identity

Roles and Relationships
Triangulating family relationship
Inability to meet spiritual needs of family members

Reduced ability of family members to relate to each other for mutual growth and maturation
Lack of skills necessary for relationships
Lack of cohesiveness
Disrupted family rituals or no family rituals
Family unable to meet security needs of members
Does not demonstrate respect for individuality of its members
Decreased sexual communication
Low perception of parental support
Pattern of rejection
Neglected obligations

RELATED FACTORS

Because the cause of this diagnosis is alcohol abuse by a family member, no related factors are needed.

NOC Family Coping, Family Functioning, Substance Abuse Consequences

Goals

The family will acknowledge the alcoholism in the family.
The family will set short- and long-term goals.

Indicators

- Relate the effects of alcoholism on the family unit and individuals.
- Identify destructive response patterns.
- Describe resources available for individual and family therapy.

NIC Coping Enhancement, Referral, Family Process Maintenance, Substance Abuse Treatment, Family Integrity Promotion, Limit-Setting Support Group

Generic Interventions

Establish a Trusting Relationship.

Be consistent; keep promises.
Be accepting and noncritical.
Do not pass judgment on what is revealed.
Focus on family member responses.

Allow the Family as Individuals and as a Group to Share Their Pent-Up Feelings.

Emphasize that Family Members Are Not Responsible for the Person's Drinking.

Explore the Family's Beliefs About their Situation and their Goals.

Discuss characteristics of alcoholism. Review a screening test that outlines characteristics of alcoholism (e.g., the Michigan Alcoholism Screening Test).

Discuss causes, and correct misinformation.

Assist to establish short- and long-term goals.

Discuss Ineffective Methods Families Use:

Hiding alcohol or car keys

Anger, silence, threats, crying

Making excuses for work, family, or friends

Bailing the person out of jail

Assist Family Members to Gain Insight into the Effects of their Attempts to Control the Drinking:

Does not stop drinking

Increases family anger

Removes the responsibility for drinking from the person

Prevents the person from suffering the consequences of his or her drinking behavior

Emphasize that Helping the Alcoholic Means First Helping Themselves.

Focus on changing their response.

Allow the person to be responsible for his or her drinking behavior.

Describe activities that will improve their life as individuals and as a family.

Initiate one stress-management technique (e.g., aerobic exercises, assertiveness course, walking, meditation, relaxation breathing).

Plan time as a family together outside the home (e.g., museum, zoo, picnic). If the alcoholic person is included, the person must contract not to drink during the activity and agree on a consequence if he or she does.

Discuss with the Family that, During Recovery, Their Usual Family Dynamics Will Be Dramatically Changed.

Discuss the Possibility of Relapse and the Contributing Factors.

If Additional Family or Individual Nursing Diagnoses Exist, Refer to *Child Abuse* **or** *Domestic Violence* **Under** *Disabled Family Coping.*

Initiate Health Teaching Regarding Community Resources and Referrals as Indicated.
Al-Anon
Alcoholics Anonymous
Family therapy
Individual therapy
Self-help groups (e.g., adult children of alcoholics)

Fatigue

DEFINITION
Fatigue: The self-recognized state in which an individual experiences an overwhelming sustained sense of exhaustion and decreased capacity for physical and mental work that is not relieved by rest.

> ⊙ **AUTHOR'S NOTE**
>
> Fatigue is different from tiredness. Tiredness is a transient, temporary state from lack of sleep, improper nutrition, sedentary lifestyle, or a temporary increase in work or social responsibilities. Fatigue is a pervasive, subjective, drained feeling that cannot be eliminated. Persons with fatigue are taught energy-conservation techniques. *Activity Intolerance* is different from *Fatigue* in that the person with *Activity Intolerance* will be assisted to increase endurance to progress and increase activity. The person with chronic fatigue will not return to the previous level of functioning.

DEFINING CHARACTERISTICS
(Voith et al., 1987)
Major (80% to 100%)
Verbalization of an unremitting and overwhelming lack of
  energy
Inability to maintain usual routines
Verbalization of distress

Minor (50% to 79%)
Perceived need for additional energy to accomplish routine
  tasks
Increase in physical complaints
Emotionally labile or irritable
Impaired ability to concentrate
Decreased performance
Lethargic or listless
Sleep disturbances

RELATED FACTORS
Many factors can cause fatigue. It may be useful to combine
related factors, such as related to muscle weakness, build-
up of waste products, inflammatory process, and infections
secondary to AIDS.

Pathophysiologic
Related to:
Acute infections (e.g., mononucleosis, hepatitis, viruses)
Chronic infections (Epstein-Barr)
Pregnancy

Related to inadequate tissue oxygenation secondary to:
Congestive heart failure
Chronic obstructive lung disease
Anemia
Peripheral vascular disease

Related to biochemical changes secondary to:
Endocrine/metabolic disorders

Diabetes mellitus	Pituitary disorders
Hypothyroidism	Addison's disease

Chronic diseases (e.g., renal failure, cirrhosis, Lyme disease)

Related to muscle wasting secondary to:

Myasthenia gravis	Parkinson's disease
Multiple sclerosis	AIDS
Amyotrophic lateral sclerosis	

Related to hypermetabolic state, competition between body and tumor for nutrients, anemia, and stressors associated with cancer
Related to nutritional deficits or changes in nutrient metabolism secondary to:

Nausea	Side effects of medications
Vomiting	Gastric surgery
Diarrhea	Diabetes mellitus

Related to chronic inflammatory process secondary to:

AIDS	Cirrhosis
Arthritis	Inflammatory bowel disease
Lupus erythematosus	Renal failure
Hepatitis	

Treatment-Related
Related to biochemical changes secondary to:
Chemotherapy
Radiation therapy
Side effects if (specify)

Related to surgical damage to tissue and anesthesia
Related to increased energy expenditure secondary to, for example, amputation, gait disorder, use of walker, crutches

Situational (Personal, Environmental)
Related to prolonged decreased activity and deconditioning secondary to:

Anxiety

Fever

Diarrhea

Pain

Social isolation

Nausea/vomiting

Depression

Obesity

Related to excessive role demands
Related to overwhelming emotional demands
Related to extreme stress
Related to sleep disturbance

Maturational
Child/Adolescent
Related to hypermetabolic state secondary to:

Mononucleosis   Fever

Related to chronic insufficient nutrients secondary to:

Obesity   Excessive dieting

Eating disorders

Related to effects of newborn care on sleep patterns and need for continuous attention
Related to hypermetabolic state during first trimester

NOC Activity Tolerance, Endurance, Energy Conservation

Goals

The person will participate in activities that stimulate and balance physical, cognitive, affective, and social domains.

Indicators

- Discuss the causes of fatigue.
- Share feelings regarding the effects of fatigue on his or her life.
- Establish priorities for daily and weekly activities.

NIC **Mutual Goal Setting, Socialization Enhancement**

Generic Interventions

Explain the causes of the person's fatigue.

Allow expression of feelings regarding the effects of fatigue on the person's life.

Assist the individual to identify strengths, abilities, interests.

Instruct the individual to record fatigue levels each hour during a 24-hour period (select a usual day).

Ask individual to rate fatigue 0 to 10 using the Rhoten (1982) fatigue scale (0 = not tired, peppy; 10 = total exhaustion).

Record the activities at the time of each rating.

Together, analyze the 24-hour fatigue levels:

Times of peak energy

Times of exhaustion

Activities associated with increasing fatigue

Assist the individual to identify what tasks can be delegated.

Plan the important tasks during periods of high energy.

Assist the individual to identify priorities and eliminate nonessential activities.

Teach energy conservation techniques:

Place work items within easy reach.

Reduce trips up and down stairs.

Distribute difficult tasks throughout the week.

Rest before difficult tasks, and stop before fatigue ensues.

Install grab rails.

Eat small meals (five times daily).

Request drivers instead of driving.

Delegate or barter for household chores.

Explain the psychological and physiological benefits of exercise, and discuss what is realistic.

Provide significant others with opportunities to discuss their feelings in private.

Explain the effects of conflict and stress on energy levels.

Assist to learn effective coping skills (e.g., sharing, assertiveness, relaxation techniques).

Refer to community services (Meals on Wheels, housekeeper).

Maternal Interventions

Explain the reason for fatigue in first and third trimesters:
    Increased basal metabolic rate
    Changes in hormonal levels
    Anemia
    Increased cardiac output (third trimester)
Emphasize the need for naps and 8 hours of sleep.
Discuss the importance of exercise (e.g., walking).
Advise to avoid overexertion.
For postpartum women, discuss factors that increase
  fatigue (Gardner & Campbell, 1991):
    Labor more than 30 hours, difficult labor, or reports of
      high labor pain
    Hemoglobin <10 g/dL or postpartum hemorrhage
    Preexisting chronic disease
    Episiotomy, tear, or cesarean section
    Sleeping difficulties
    Ill neonate or a congenital anomaly
    Nonsupportive partner
    Dependent children at home
    Child care problems
    Unrealistic expectations

Geriatric Interventions

Consider if chronic fatigue is the consequence of late-life
  depression.
Refer individual suspected of depression for evaluation.

Fear

DEFINITION
Fear: The state in which an individual or group experiences a feeling of physiologic or emotional disruption related to an identifiable source that is perceived as dangerous.

> ⊛ **AUTHOR'S NOTE**
> See *Anxiety.*

DEFINING CHARACTERISTICS
Major (Must be Present, One or More)
Feelings of dread, fright, apprehension, alarm
Behaviors of avoidance; narrowing of focus on danger; and deficits in attention, performance, control, and self-assurance

Minor (May be Present)
Verbal reports of panic, obsessions
Behavioral acts of:

Crying	Dysfunctional immobility
Aggression	Compulsive mannerisms
Escape	Increased questioning/
Hypervigilance	verbalization

Visceral-somatic activity
Musculoskeletal

Trembling	Fatigue/weakness of limbs
Muscle tightness	

Cardiovascular

Palpitations	Increased blood pressure
Rapid pulse	

Respiratory

Shortness of breath	Increased rate

Gastrointestinal

Anorexia	Diarrhea/urge to defecate
Nausea/vomiting	Dry mouth/throat

Genitourinary
Urinary frequency/urgency

Skin
Flush/pallor   Paresthesia
Sweating

Central Nervous System/Perceptual
Syncope   Absentmindedness
Insomnia   Nightmares
Lack of concentration   Dilated pupils
Irritability

RELATED FACTORS

Fear can occur as a response to a variety of health problems, situations, or conflicts. Some common sources are indicated below.

Pathophysiologic
Related to perceived immediate and long-term effects of:

Loss of body part   Cognitive impairment
Loss of body function   Long-term disability
Disabling illness   Terminal disease
Sensory impairment

Treatment-Related
Related to loss of control and unpredictable outcome secondary to:

Hospitalization
Surgery and its outcome
Anesthesia
Invasive procedures
Radiation

Situational (Personal, Environmental)
Related to loss of control and unpredictable outcome secondary to:

Pain   Divorce
New environment   Success
New persons   Failure
Lack of knowledge   Language barrier
Change or loss of
 significant other

Related to potential loss of income

Maturational

Preschool
Related to:

Separation from parents, peers

Being alone

Strangers, animals, snakes

Bodily harm

Age-related fears (dark, strangers, ghosts, monsters)

School Age (6 to 12 years)
Related to:

Being lost

Bad dreams

Being in trouble (12 years)

Weapons (8 years)

Thunder, lightning (6 to 8 years)

Adolescent
Related to uncertainty of:

Appearance

Peer support

Scholastic success

Related to vulnerability to violence
Related to separation from support system

Adult
Related to uncertainty of:

Marriage

Pregnancy

Parenthood

Job security

Effects of aging

Older Adult
Related to:

Anticipated dependence

Prolonged suffering

Vulnerability to crime

Financial insecurity

Abandonment

NOC Anxiety Control, Fear Control

Goals

The adult will relate an increase in psychological and physiologic comfort.

Indicators

- Show decreases in visceral response (pulse, respirations).
- Differentiate real from imagined situations.

- Describe effective and ineffective coping patterns.
- Identify his or her own coping responses.

The child will exhibit or relate an increase in psychological and physiologic comfort.

- Discuss fears.
- Exhibit less crying.

NIC Anxiety Reduction, Coping Enhancement, Presence Counseling, Relaxation Therapy

Generic Interventions

Orient to environment using simple explanations.

Speak slowly and calmly.

Allow personal space.

Use simple, direct statements (avoid detail).

Encourage expression of feelings (helplessness, anger).

Encourage responses that reflect reality. Discuss which aspects can be changed and which cannot.

Provide an emotionally nonthreatening atmosphere. Set up a consistent daily schedule.

When intensity of feelings has decreased, bring behavioral cues into the person's awareness.

Teach relaxation techniques:

Slow, rhythmic breathing

Progressive relaxation of muscle groups

Self-coaching

Thought-stopping

Guided imagery

❖ Pediatric Interventions

Accept the child's fear and provide an explanation, if possible, or some form of control; share with the child that these fears are okay.

Fear of imaginary animals, intruders ("I don't see a lion in your room, but I will leave the light on for you, and if you need me again, please call.")

Fear of parent being late (Establish a contingency plan, e.g., "If you come home from school and Mommy is not here, go to Mrs. S. next door.")

◈ Pediatric Interventions (cont'd)

Fear of vanishing down a toilet or bathtub drain. Wait
until the child is out of the tub before releasing drain.
Wait until the child is off the toilet before flushing.
Leave toys in bathtub, and demonstrate how they do
not go down the drain.

Fear of dark. Give child a night light.

Fear of dogs, cats:
- Allow child to watch a child and a dog playing from
  a distance.
- Do not force child to touch the animal.

Discuss with parents the normalcy of fears in children;
explain the necessity of acceptance and the negative outcomes of punishment or of forcing the child to overcome
the fear.

Provide the child with opportunity to observe how other
children cope successfully with feared object.

▨ Maternal Interventions

Explore fears and emotional responses to pregnancy
(Reeder, Martin, & Koniak-Griffin, 1997).

First trimester
- Uncertainty about future role as mother
- Uncertainty about timing of pregnancy

Third trimester
- Fears about own well-being and "performance" during
  labor
- Fears about well-being of the fetus

Deficient Fluid Volume

DEFINITION

Deficient Fluid Volume: The state in which an individual who is not NPO experiences or is at risk of experiencing dehydration.

⊚ AUTHOR'S NOTE

This diagnosis represents situations in which nurses can prescribe definitive treatment to prevent fluid depletion or to reduce or eliminate related factors, such as insufficient oral intake. Situations that represent hypovolemia caused by hemorrhage or NPO status should be considered collaborative problems, not nursing diagnoses. Nurses monitor to detect these situations and collaborate with doctors for treatment. These situations can be labeled *Potential Complication: Hemorrhage* or *Potential Complication: Hypovolemia.*

DEFINING CHARACTERISTICS
Major (Must be Present, One or More)

Insufficient oral fluid intake
Negative balance of intake and output
Weight loss
Dry skin/mucous membranes

Minor (May be Present)

Increased serum sodium
Decreased urine output or excessive urine output
Concentrated urine or urinary frequency
Thirst, nausea, or anorexia

RELATED FACTORS
Pathophysiologic
Related to excessive urinary output

Uncontrolled diabetes
Diabetes insipidus (inadequate antidiuretic hormone)

Related to increased capillary permeability and evaporative loss from burn wound
Related to losses secondary to:
Fever or increased metabolic rate
Abnormal drainage (e.g., wound, excessive menses)
Peritonitis
Diarrhea

Situational (Personal, Environmental)

Related to vomiting/nausea
Related to decreased motivation to drink liquids secondary to depression or fatigue
Related to fad diets/fasting
Related to high-solute tube feedings
Related to difficulty swallowing or feeding self secondary to oral pain or fatigue
Related to extreme heat/sun, dryness
Related to excessive loss through indwelling catheters or drains
Related to insufficient fluids for exercise effort or weather conditions
Related to excessive use of laxatives, enemas, diuretics, or alcohol

Maturational
Infant/Child
Related to increased vulnerability secondary to decreased fluid reserve and decreased ability to concentrate urine

Older Adult
Related to increased vulnerability secondary to decreased fluid reserve and decreased sensation of thirst

NOC Electrolyte and Acid–Base Balance, Fluid Balance, Hydration

Goals

The person will maintain a urine specific gravity within a normal range.

Indicators

- Increase intake of fluids to a specified amount according to age and metabolic needs.
- Identify risk factors for fluid deficit, and relate the need for increased fluid intake as indicated.
- Demonstrate no signs and symptoms of dehydration.

NIC	Fluid/Electrolyte Management, Fluid Monitoring

Generic Interventions

Assess likes and dislikes; provide favorite fluids within dietary restrictions.

Plan an intake goal for every 8 hours (e.g., 1000 mL during day, 800 mL during evening, 300 mL at night).

Assess the person's understanding of the reasons for maintaining adequate hydration and methods for reaching goal of fluid intake.

Have the person maintain a written record (log) of fluid intake, urinary output, and daily weight (if necessary).

Monitor intake; ensure at least 1500 mL of oral fluids is taken every 24 hours.

Monitor output; ensure an output of at least 1000 to 1500 mL every 24 hours. Monitor for a decrease in urine specific gravity.

Weigh daily in same type of clothing at same time. A 2% to 4% weight loss indicates mild dehydration; a 5% to 9% weight loss indicates moderate dehydration.

Monitor levels of serum electrolytes, blood urea nitrogen, urine and serum osmolality, creatinine, hematocrit, and hemoglobin.

Teach that coffee, tea, and grapefruit juice are diuretics and can contribute to fluid loss.

Consider the additional fluid losses associated with vomiting, diarrhea, fever, tubes, drains.

For wound drainage:

Keep careful records of the amount and type of drainage.

Weigh dressings, if necessary, to estimate fluid loss.

Cover wounds to minimize fluid loss.

❖ Pediatric Interventions

Monitor weight, body temperature, moisture in oral cavity, wet diapers, and urine volume and concentration.

Offer:

Appealing forms of fluids (popsicles, frozen juice bars, snow cones, water, milk, Jell-O with vegetable coloring added; let child help make it)

Unusual containers (colorful cups, straws)

A game or activity (have child take a drink when it is child's turn in a game)

● Geriatric Interventions

Teach to drink 8 to 10 glasses of fluid daily, not including caffeine drinks unless contraindicated (e.g., renal or cardiac insufficiency).

Advise at least four glasses of water: caution on caffeine and sugar drinks.

Explain not to rely on thirst as an indicator of a need for fluids.

Teach to monitor hydration by color of urine.

Evaluate if person is restricting intake to avoid incontinence.

DEFINITION

Excess Fluid Volume: The state in which an individual experiences or is at risk of experiencing intracellular or interstitial fluid overload.

⊗ AUTHOR'S NOTE

This diagnosis represents situations in which nurses can prescribe definitive treatment to reduce or eliminate factors that contribute to edema or can teach preventive actions. Situations that represent vascular fluid overload should be considered collaborative problems, not nursing diagnoses. They can be labeled *Potential Complication: Congestive Heart Failure* or *Potential Complication: Hypervolemia.*

DEFINING CHARACTERISTICS
Major (Must be Present, One or More)
Edema (peripheral, sacral)
Taut, shiny skin

Minor (May be Present)
Intake greater than output
Shortness of breath
Weight gain

RELATED FACTORS
Pathophysiologic
Related to compromised regulatory mechanisms secondary to acute or chronic renal failure
Related to portal hypertension, lower plasma colloidal osmotic pressure, and sodium retention secondary to liver disease, cirrhosis, cancer, or ascites
Related to impaired venous return secondary to:
Varicose veins
Peripheral vascular disease

Thrombus
Chronic phlebitis
Immobility

Treatment-Related

Related to sodium and water retention secondary to corticosteroid therapy

Situational (Personal, Environmental)

Related to excessive sodium intake/fluid intake
Related to low protein intake (e.g., fad diets, malnutrition)
Related to dependent venous pooling/venostasis secondary to immobility, tight cast or bandage, or standing or sitting for long periods
Related to venous compression by pregnant uterus
Related to inadequate lymphatic drainage secondary to mastectomy

Maturational

Older Adult
Related to impaired venous return secondary to increased peripheral resistance and decreased efficiency of valves

NOC Electrolyte Balance, Hydration

Goals

The person will exhibit decreased edema (specify site).

Indicators

- Relate causative factors.
- Relate methods of preventing edema.

NIC Electrolyte Management, Fluid Management, Fluid Monitoring, Skin Surveillance

Generic Interventions

For Edema:

Monitor skin for signs of pressure ulcers.
Gently wash between skin folds, and dry carefully.

Avoid tape when possible.
Change position at least every 2 hours.

**Assess for Evidence of Dependent
Venous Pooling or Venostasis.**

**Keep Edematous Extremity Elevated
Above the Level of the Heart
Whenever Possible (Unless
Contraindicated by Heart Failure).**

**Assess Dietary Intake and Habits that
May Contribute to Fluid Retention
(e.g., Salt Intake).**

Teach the Person to:

Read labels for sodium content.
Avoid convenience foods, canned foods, and frozen foods.
Cook without salt, to use spices to add flavor (lemon, basil,
    tarragon, mint).
Use vinegar in place of salt for flavor (e.g., 2 to 3 teaspoons
    of vinegar to 4 to 6 quarts, according to taste).

**Instruct the Person to Avoid Panty
Girdles/Garters, Knee-Highs, and Leg
Crossing and to Practice Keeping
Legs Elevated When Possible.**

**For Inadequate Lymphatic Drainage
in Arm:**

Keep extremity elevated on pillows.
Take blood pressures in unaffected arm.
Do not give injections or start intravenous fluids in
    affected arm.
Protect affected arm from injury.
Teach the person to avoid using strong detergents, carry-
    ing heavy bags, holding a cigarette, injuring cuticles or
    hangnails, reaching into a hot oven, wearing jewelry or a
    wristwatch, or using Ace bandages.
Caution the person to see a physician if the arm becomes
    red, swollen, or unusually hard.

Protect Edematous Skin from Injury.

Maternal Interventions

Explain the cause of fluid retention (e.g., increased estrogen production, posture that affects blood flow and renal function).

Explain the importance of lying on side at night and during the day (several times).

Teach women to:
  Elevate feet often.
  Drink at least 2000 mL of fluids (three to four servings).
  Eat enough protein and avoid highly salted foods.

Assess for early signs of pregnancy-induced hypertension:
  Weight gain of over 2 lb in 1 week
  Finger edema

Fluid Volume Imbalance, Risk for

DEFINITION

Risk for Fluid Volume Imbalance: A state in which an individual is at risk to experience a decrease, increase, or rapid shift from one to the other of intravascular, interstitial, and/or intracellular fluid.

> ○ **AUTHOR'S NOTE**
>
> This diagnosis can represent a multitude of clinical conditions, such as edema, hemorrhage, dehydration, and compartmental syndrome. If the nurse is monitoring an individual for fluid volume imbalance, labeling the specific imbalance as a collaborative problem, such as hypovolemia, compartmental syndrome, increased intracranial

⊗ **AUTHOR'S NOTE (continued)**

pressure, gastrointestinal bleeding, or postpartum hemorrhage, would clinically be more useful. For example, most intraoperative clients are monitored for hypovolemia; if the procedure is neurosurgery, cranial pressure would also be monitored. If the procedure is orthopedic, compartmental syndrome would be addressed. Refer to Section Two for specific collaborative problems and interventions.

RISK FACTORS
Need to be developed (NANDA, 2001)

Goals
Refer to *Deficient Fluid Volume.*

Generic Interventions
Refer to *Deficient Fluid Volume.*

Grieving*
Grieving, Anticipatory
Grieving, Dysfunctional

Grieving

DEFINITION

Grieving: A state in which an individual or family experiences a natural human response involving psychosocial and physiologic reactions to an actual or perceived loss (person, object, function, status, relationship).

> ### ⊕ AUTHOR'S NOTE
>
> *Grieving, Anticipatory Grieving,* and *Dysfunctional Grieving* represent three types of responses of individuals or families experiencing a loss. *Grieving* describes normal grieving after a loss and participation in grief work. *Anticipatory Grieving* describes someone engaged in grief work before an expected loss. *Dysfunctional Grieving* is a maladaptive process that occurs when grief work is suppressed or absent or when there is a prolonged exaggerated response. For all three diagnoses, the nursing goal is to promote grief work. In addition, for *Dysfunctional Grieving,* the nurse will direct interventions to reduce excessive, prolonged problematic responses.

DEFINING CHARACTERISTICS
Major (Must be Present)

The person reports an actual or perceived loss (person, object, function, status, relationship).

---

*This diagnosis is not currently on the NANDA list but has been included for clarity or usefulness.

Minor (May be Present)

Denial
Guilt
Anger
Despair
Feelings of worthlessness
Suicidal thoughts
Crying
Sorrow

Delusions
Phobias
Anergia
Inability to concentrate
Visual, auditory, and tactile
  hallucinations about the
  object or person
Longing/searching behaviors

RELATED FACTORS

Many situations can contribute to feelings of loss. Some common situations are listed below.

Pathophysiologic

Related to loss of function or independence secondary to:

Neurologic
Cardiovascular
Sensory
Musculoskeletal

Digestive
Renal
Trauma

Treatment-Related

Related to losses associated with, for example, long-term dialysis, surgery (mastectomy, colostomy, hysterectomy)

Situational (Personal, Environmental)

Related to negative effects and losses (e.g., chronic pain, terminal illness, death)
Related to losses in lifestyle associated with:

Childbirth
Marriage
Separation
Divorce

Child leaving home
  (e.g., college or marriage)
Retirement

Related to loss of normalcy secondary to, for example, handicap, scars, illness

Maturational

Related to losses attributed to aging, friends, occupation, function, home
Related to loss of hopes, dreams

NOC Coping, Family Coping, Grief Resolution

Goals

The individual will express his or her grief.

Indicators

- Describe the meaning of the death or loss to him or her.
- Share his or her grief with significant others (children, spouses).

> **NIC** Family Support, Grief Work Facilitation, Coping Enhancement, Anticipatory Guidance, Emotional Support

Generic Interventions

Promote a Trusting Relationship.

Support the Person and the Family's Grief Reactions.

Explain Grief Reactions.
Shock and disbelief
Developing awareness
Restitution
Somatic manifestations

Assess for Experiences with Loss.

Recognize and Reinforce the Strengths of Each Family Member.

Encourage the Family Members to Evaluate Their Feelings and Support One Another.

Allow Each Member Privacy to Share Grief.

Promote Grief Work with Each Response.
Denial
Explain the use of denial by one family member to the other members.
Do not push the client to move past denial without emotional readiness.

Isolation

Reinforce the person's self-worth by allowing privacy.
Encourage client/family to increase social activities
gradually (e.g., support groups, church groups).

Depression

Identify the level of depression, and develop the approach
accordingly.
Use empathic sharing; acknowledge grief ("It must be very
difficult.")

Anger

Explain to family that anger is an attempt to control one's
environment more closely because of inability to control
loss.
Encourage verbalization of the anger.

Guilt

Encourage the client to identify positive
contributions/aspects of the relationship.
Avoid arguing and participating in the person's system of
"shoulds" and "should nots."

Fear

Focus on the present, and maintain a safe and secure
environment.

Rejection

Explain this response to family members.

Hysteria

Reduce environmental stresses (e.g., limit personnel).
Provide the person with a safe, private area to display
grief.
Determine whether family has special requests regarding
viewing the deceased (Vanezis, 1999).
  Respect their requests.
  Prepare them for any body changes.
  Remove all equipment; change soiled linen.
  Support their request (e.g., holding, washing, touching,
  kissing).

Identify Factors that Can Impede Successful Completion of the Mourning Process (Varcorolis, 2002):

High dependence on deceased
Unresolved conflicts

Age of deceased
Inadequate support system
Number of previous losses
Physical and psychological health of person grieving

**Teach the Person and the Family
Signs of Resolution. Refer to
Dysfunctional Grieving.**

Identify Agencies that May Be Helpful.

❖ Pediatric Interventions

Encourage parents and staff to be truthful, and offer explanations that can be understood.
Encourage parents or significant others to nurture children during the grieving process.
Explore with the child his or her concept of death in the context of maturational level.
Correct misconceptions about death, illness, and rituals (funerals).
Prepare the child for grief responses of others.
If the child plans to attend the funeral or visit the funeral home, a thorough explanation of the setting, rituals, and expected behaviors of mourners is necessary beforehand. (The family can plan the visit of the child to be short and to occur before the other mourners arrive.)
Allow child to share fears.
Allow child to remain with significant others while they grieve at home.
Provide accurate explanations for sibling illness or death.

🏠 Maternal Interventions

**Assist Parents of a Deceased Infant
(Newborn, Stillbirth, Miscarriage)
with Grief Work (Mina, 1985):**
Use baby's name when discussing loss.
Allow parents to share their hopes and dreams.
Provide access to hospital chaplain or own religious leader.
Encourage parents to see and hold their infant to validate the reality of the loss.

Maternal Interventions (cont'd)

Prepare a memory packet (wrapped in clean baby blanket) (photograph, identification bracelet, footprints with birth certificate, lock of hair, crib card, fetal monitor strip, infant's blanket).

Encourage parents to share the experience with siblings at home (refer to pertinent literature for consumers).

Provide for follow-up support and referral services after discharge (e.g., social service, support group).

Assist Others to Comfort Grieving Parents:

Stress the importance of openly acknowledging the death.

If the baby or fetus was named, use the name in discussions.

Send sympathy cards.

Grieving, Anticipatory

DEFINITION

Anticipatory Grieving: The state in which an individual or group experiences reactions in response to an expected significant loss.

DEFINING CHARACTERISTICS
Major (Must be Present)

Expressed distress at potential loss

Minor (May be Present)

Denial   Change in sleep patterns
Guilt   Change in social patterns

Anger
Sorrow
Change in eating habits

Change in communication
  patterns
Decreased libido

RELATED FACTORS
See *Grieving*.

NOC Refer to Grieving

Goals

The person will express his or her grief.

Indicators

- Participate in decision-making for the future.
- Share his or her concerns with significant others.

NIC Refer to Grieving

Generic Interventions

Encourage the person to share concerns, fears, effects on
  lifestyle.
Promote the integrity of the person and family by acknowl-
  edging strengths and normalcy of reactions.
Prepare the person and family for grief reactions.
Promote family cohesiveness.
Provide for the concept of hope by:
    Supplying accurate information
    Resisting the temptation to give false hope
    Discussing concerns willingly
Promote grief work with each response.

Denial

Initially support and then strive to increase the development of awareness (when individual indicates readiness
  for awareness).

Isolation

Listen and spend designated time consistently with the
  person and family.
Offer the person and family opportunity to explore their
  emotions.

Depression
Begin with simple problem-solving, and move toward
  acceptance.
Enhance self-worth through positive reinforcement.

Anger
Allow crying to release this energy.
Encourage concerned support from significant others and
  professional support.

Guilt
Allow crying.
Promote more direct expression of feelings.
Explore methods to resolve guilt.

Fear
Help the person and family recognize the feeling.
Explore the person's and family's attitudes about loss,
  death, etc.
Explore the person's and family's methods of coping.

Rejection
Allow verbal expression of this feeling state to diminish
  the emotional strain.
Recognize that expression of anger may create a rejection
  of self to significant others.
Caution against the use of sedatives and tranquilizers,
  which may prevent or delay emotional expressions of loss.
Teach signs of pathologic responses and referrals needed.
Discuss options available during terminal stage:
  Home care
  Institution
  Hospice
Discuss benefits of home care of terminal family member
  (Vickers, 2000):
  Unlimited access to the person
  Keeps family together
  More opportunities for support and assistance from
    extended family and friends
  Dying person is less isolated
Discuss the problems of home care and fears:
  24-hour responsibility
  Unprepared for experience
  Feelings of inadequacy
  Lack of family cohesiveness
Encourage to continue usual schedule or activities (work
  and play).

Grieving, Dysfunctional

DEFINITION

Dysfunctional Grieving: The state in which an individual or group experiences prolonged unresolved grief and engages in detrimental activities.

⊚ AUTHOR'S NOTE

How one responds to loss is highly individual. Responses to acute loss should not be labeled dysfunctional regardless of the severity. *Dysfunctional Grieving* is characterized by its sustained or prolonged detrimental response. The validation of *Dysfunctional Grieving* cannot occur until several months to 1 year after the loss. In many clinical settings, the diagnosis of *Risk for Dysfunctional Grieving* for individuals at risk for unsuccessful reintegration after a loss may be more useful.

DEFINING CHARACTERISTICS
Major (Must be Present, One or More)

Unsuccessful adaptation to loss
Prolonged denial, depression
Delayed emotional reaction
Inability to assume normal patterns of living

Minor (May be Present)

Social isolation or withdrawal
Failure to develop new relationships/interests
Failure to restructure life after loss

RELATED FACTORS
Situational (Personal, Environmental)
Related to:

- Unavailable (or lack of) support system
- Negation of the loss by others
- History of a difficult relationship with the lost person or object

- Multiple past or present losses
- History of ineffective coping strategies
- Unexpected death
- Expectations to "be strong"
- History of unresolved losses
- Thwarted grieving response secondary to role, work responsibilities

NOC See Grieving

Goals

The individual will verbalize an intent to seek professional assistance.

Indicators

- Acknowledge the loss.
- Acknowledge an unresolved grief process.

NIC See also Grieving, Referral, Support Group

Generic Interventions

Teach the normal tasks of mourning (Worden, 1991), and help the person recognize at which task he or she is:
  Acknowledging the loss
  Experiencing the pain
  Adjusting to the loss
  Reinvesting and goal-setting
Encourage person to share perceptions of the situation.
  Review relationship with the lost concept, person.
  Empathically point out misrepresentations.
  Discuss the appropriateness of guilt, anger, or sorrow.
  Encourage expressions of anger or rage.
If denial persists, see *Ineffective Denial.*
Help identify activities that have been ignored or abandoned since loss. Encourage the selection of one to resume.
Encourage participation in large motor activities (e.g., brisk walks, exercise bicycle).
Emphasize past successful coping.
Discuss community resources available for sharing experiences with others.
Refer for counseling if indicated.

Growth and Development, Delayed

DEFINITION

Delayed Growth and Development: The state in which an individual has or is at risk for an impaired ability to perform tasks of his or her age group or impaired growth.

> ⓧ **AUTHOR'S NOTE**
>
> The focus of this diagnosis will be children and adolescents. When an adult has not accomplished a developmental task, the nurse should assess for the altered functioning that has resulted from the failure to meet a developmental task, for example, *Impaired Social Interactions* or *Ineffective Coping.*

DEFINING CHARACTERISTICS
Major (Must be Present, One or More)

Inability to perform or difficulty performing skills or behaviors typical of age group; for example, motor, personal/social, language/cognition *and/or*

Altered physical growth: Weight lagging behind height by two standard deviations; pattern of height and weight percentiles indicating a drop in pattern

Minor (May be Present)

Inability to perform self-care or self-control activities appropriate for age

Flat affect, listlessness, decreased responses, slow social responses, limited signs of satisfaction to caregiver, limited eye contact, difficulty feeding, decreased appetite,

lethargic, irritable, negative mood, regression in self-
toileting, regression in self-feeding
Infants: watchfulness, interrupted sleep pattern

RELATED FACTORS
Pathophysiologic
**Related to compromised physical ability and depen-
dence secondary to:**

Congenital heart defects	Congestive heart failure
Cerebral damage	Cerebral palsy
Congenital defects	
Malabsorption syndrome	Cystic fibrosis
Gastroesophageal reflux	
Congenital anomalies of extremities	
Muscular dystrophy	
Acute illness	
Prolonged pain	
Repeated acute illness, chronic illness	
Inadequate caloric or nutritional intake	

Treatment-Related
**Related to separation from significant others, school;
or inadequate sensory stimulation secondary to:**
Prolonged, painful treatments
Repeated or prolonged hospitalization
Traction or casts
Prolonged bed rest
Isolation due to disease processes
Confinement for ongoing treatment

Situational (Personal, Environmental)
Related to:
Parental stressor secondary to lack of knowledge
Change in usual environment
Separation from significant others (parents, primary
  caregiver)
School-related stressors
Loss of significant other
Loss of control over environment (established rituals,
  activities, established hours of contact with family)

**Related to inadequate, inappropriate parental sup-
port (neglect, abuse)**

Related to inadequate sensory stimulation (neglect, isolation)

Maturational
Infant–Toddler: Birth to 3 Years
Related to limited opportunities to meet social, play, or educational needs secondary to:
Separation from parents/significant others
Restriction of activity secondary to (specify)
Inadequate parental support
Inability to trust significant other
Inability to communicate (deafness)
Multiple caregivers

Preschool Age: 4 to 6 Years
Related to limited opportunities to meet social, play, or educational needs secondary to:
Loss of ability to communicate
Lack of stimulation
Lack of significant other

Related to loss of significant other (death, divorce)
Related to loss of peer group
Related to removal from home environment

School Age: 6 to 11 Years
Related to loss of significant other
Related to loss of peer group
Related to strange environment

Adolescent: 12 to 18 Years
Related to loss of independence and autonomy secondary to (specify)
Related to disruption of peer relationships
Related to disruption in body image
Related to loss of significant other

NIC Child Development (Specify Age)

Goals

The child/adolescent will continue to demonstrate appropriate behavior.

Indicators (specify for age)

- Self-care
- Social skills
- Language
- Cognitive skills
- Motor skills

NIC Development Enhancement, Parenting Promotion, Infant/Child Care

Generic Interventions

Teach parents the age-related developmental tasks (Table I.1).

Carefully assess child's level of development in all areas of functioning by using specific assessment tools (e.g., Brazelton Assessment Table, Denver Developmental Screening Tool).

Provide opportunities for an ill child to meet age-related developmental tasks.

Birth to 1 Year

Provide increased stimulation using variety of colored toys in crib (e.g., mobiles, musical toys, stuffed toys of varied textures, frequent periods of holding and speaking to infant).

Hold while feeding; feed slowly and in relaxed environment.

Provide periods of rest prior to feeding.

Observe mother and child during interaction, especially during feeding.

Investigate crying promptly and consistently.

Assign consistent caregiver.

Encourage parental visits/calls and involvement in care if possible.

Provide buccal experience if infant desires (*i.e.,* thumb, pacifier).

Allow hands and feet to be free if possible.

1 to 3½ Years

Assign consistent caregiver.

Encourage self-care activities (i.e., self-feeding, self-dressing, bathing).

(text continues on p. 193)

Table I.1 Age-Related Developmental Needs

Developmental Tasks/Needs			
Birth to 1 Year	**1–3$\frac{1}{2}$ Years**	**3$\frac{1}{2}$–5 Years**	
Personal/Social Learns to trust and anticipate satisfaction Sends cues to mother/caregiver Begins understanding self as separate from others (body image)	**Personal/Social** Establishes self-control, decision-making, self-independence (autonomy) Extremely curious, prefers to do things independently Demonstrates independence through negativism Very egocentric: believes he or she controls the world Learns about words through senses	**Personal/Social** Attempts to establish self as like parents but independent Explores environment on own initiative Boasts, brags, has feelings of indestructibility Family is primary group Peers increasingly important Assumes sex roles Aggressive	
Motor Responds to sound Social smile Reaches for objects Begins to sit, creep, pull up, and stand with support Attempts to walk	**Motor** Begins to walk and run well Drinks from cup, feeds self	**Motor** Locomotion skills increase, and coordinates easier	

(table continues on p. 190)

Table I.1 Age-Related Developmental Needs (continued)

Developmental Tasks/Needs		
Birth to 1 Year	**1–3½ Years**	**3½–5 Years**
Language/Cognition Learns to signal wants/needs with sounds, crying Begins to vocalize with meaning (two-syllable words: dada, mama) Comprehends some verbal/nonverbal messages (no, yes, bye-bye) Learns about words through senses	Develops fine motor control Climbs Begins self-toileting **Language/Cognition** Has poor time sense Increasingly verbal (4–5-word sentences by age 3½) Talks to self/others Misconceptions about cause/effect	Rides tricycle/bicycle Throws ball, but has difficulty catching **Language/Cognition** Egocentric Language skills flourish Generates many questions: how, why, what? Simple problem-solving; uses fantasy to understand, problem-solve
Fears Loud noises Falling	**Fears** Loss/separation from parents Darkness Machines/equipment Intrusive procedures Unknown Inanimate, unfamiliar objects	**Fears** Mutilation Castration

Developmental Tasks/Needs

5–11 Years	11–15 Years
Personal/Social Learns to include values and skills of school, neighborhood, peers Peer relationships important Focuses more on reality, less on fantasy Family is main base of security and identity Sensitive to reactions of others Seeks approval, recognition Enthusiastic, noisy, imaginative, desires to explore Likes to complete a task Enjoys helping	**Personal/Social** Family values continue to be significant influence Peer group values have increasing significance Early adolescence: outgoing and enthusiastic Emotions are extreme, mood swings, introspection Sexual identity fully mature Wants privacy/independence Develops interests not shared with family Concern with physical self Explores adult roles
Motor Moves constantly Physical play prevalent (sports, swimming, skating, etc.)	**Motor** Well developed Rapid physical growth Secondary sex characteristics

(table continues on p. 192)

Table I.1 Age-Related Developmental Needs (continued)

Developmental Tasks/Needs	
5–11 Years	**11–15 Years**
Language/Cognition Organized, stable thought Concepts more complicated Focuses on concrete understanding	**Language/Cognition** Plans for future career Able to abstract solutions and problem-solve in future tense
Fears Rejections, failure Immobility Mutilation Death	**Fears** Mutilation Disruption in body image Rejection from peers

Reinforce word development by repeating words child uses, naming objects by saying words, and speaking to child often.

Provide frequent periods of play with peers present and with a variety of toys (puzzles, books with pictures, manipulative toys, trucks, cars, blocks, bright colors).

Explain all procedures as you do them.

Provide safe area where the child can locomote; use walker, provide creeping area, and hold hand while taking steps.

Encourage parental visits/calls and involvement in care if possible.

Provide comfort measures after painful procedures.

3¹/₂ to 5 Years

Encourage self-care: self-grooming, self-dressing, mouth care, hair care.

Provide frequent playtime with others and with variety of toys (e.g., models, musical toys, dolls, puppets, books, mini-slide, wagon, tricycle).

Read stories aloud.

Ask for verbal responses and requests.

Say words for equipment, objects, and people, and ask the child to repeat.

Allow time for individual play and exploration of play environment.

Encourage parental visits/calls and involvement in care if possible.

Monitor television, and use television as means to help child understand time ("After *Sesame Street,* your mother will come.")

5 to 11 Years

Talk with child about care provided.

Request input from child (e.g., diet, clothes, routine).

Allow child to dress in clothes instead of pajamas.

Provide periods of interaction with other children on unit.

Provide craft project that can be completed each day or week.

Continue schoolwork at intervals each day.

Praise positive behaviors.

Read stories, and provide variety of independent games, puzzles, books, video games, painting, or other activity.

Introduce the child by name to persons on unit.

Encourage visits and telephone calls from parents, siblings, and peers.

11 to 15 Years

Speak frequently with the child about feelings, ideas, concerns about condition or care.

Provide opportunity for interaction with others of the same age on unit.

Identify interest or hobby that can be supported on unit in some manner, and support it daily.

Allow hospital routine to be altered to suit child's schedule.

Allow the child to dress in own clothes if possible.

Involve child in decisions about care.

Provide opportunity for involvement in variety of activities (e.g., reading, video games, movies, board games, art, trips outside or to other areas).

Encourage visits and telephone calls from parents, siblings, and peers.

Refer to community programs specific to contributing factors (e.g., social services, family services, counseling).

Development, Risk for Delayed

DEFINITION

Risk for Delayed Development: The state in which an individual is at risk for an impaired ability to perform tasks of his or her age group.

RISK FACTORS

Refer to *Delayed Growth and Development.*

Generic Interventions & Goals

Refer to *Delayed Growth and Development.*

Growth, Risk for Disproportionate

DEFINITION
Risk for Disproportionate Growth: The state in which an individual is at risk for an impaired growth.

RISK FACTORS
Refer to *Delayed Growth and Development.*

Goals

The child/adolescent will continue to demonstrate age-appropriate growth.

Indicators

- Height
- Weight
- Head circumference

Generic Interventions

Refer to *Delayed Growth and Development.*

Adult Failure to Thrive

DEFINITION
Adult Failure to Thrive: The state in which an individual experiences insidious and progressive physical and psycho-social deterioration characterized by limited coping and diminished resilience.

DEFINING CHARACTERISTICS
Major

Declining physical functioning	Weight loss
Declining cognitive functioning	Social withdrawal
Depression	Self-care deficit
	Apathy
	Anorexia

RELATED FACTORS

The cause of failure to thrive in adults, usually the elderly, is unknown. Researchers have identified some factors that may contribute to this condition.

Situational (Personal, Environmental)

Related to diminished coping abilities
Related to limited ability to adapt to effects of aging
Related to loss of social skills and the resultant social isolation
Related to loss of social relatedness
Related to increasing dependency and feelings of helplessness

NOC Psychological Adjustment: Life Change
Will to Live

Goals

The person will participate to increase functioning.

Indicators

- Increase social relatedness.
- Maintain or increase self-care activities.

NIC Coping Enhancement
Hope Instillment

Generic Interventions

Consult with therapist to evaluate for depression and medication therapy as indicated.
Evaluate pattern of socialization (refer to *Risk for Loneliness*).

Provide opportunities to increase social relatedness:
  Music therapy
  Recreation therapy
  Reminiscence therapy
Maintain standards of empathic, respectful care.
Attempt to obtain information that will provide useful and
  meaningful topics for conversations (likes, dislikes; inter-
  ests, hobbies; work history). Interview early in the day.
Encourage significant others and caregivers to speak slowly
  with a low voice pitch and at an average volume (unless
  hearing deficits are present), as one adult to another, with
  eye contact, and as if expecting person to understand.
Provide respect and promote sharing:
  Pay attention to what the person is saying.
  Pick out meaningful comments and continue talking.
  Call the person by name and introduce yourself each
    time contact is made; use touch if welcomed.
Engage in useful and meaningful adult conversations:
  Likes, dislikes
  Interests, work history

Health Maintenance, Ineffective

DEFINITION

Ineffective Health Maintenance: The state in which an individual or group experiences or is at risk of experiencing a disruption in health because of an unhealthy lifestyle or lack of
knowledge about managing a condition.

○ AUTHOR'S NOTE

Ineffective Health Maintenance can describe persons who
desire to change an unhealthy lifestyle (obesity, tobacco
use). *Ineffective Therapeutic Regimen Management* can
be used for those who need teaching for self-management
of a disease or condition.

DEFINING CHARACTERISTICS
(IN THE ABSENCE OF DISEASE)
Major (Must be Present, One or More)

Reports or demonstrates an unhealthy practice or lifestyle, e.g.:

Reckless driving
Substance abuse
Excessive sun exposure
Sedentary lifestyle

Inadequate oral hygiene
Inadequate hygiene
Overeating
High-fat diet

Minor (May be Present)
Reports or demonstrates:

Skin and nails

Malodorous
Skin lesions (pustules,
  rashes, dry or scaly skin)

Sunburn
Unusual color, pallor
Unexplained scars

Respiratory system

Frequent infections
Chronic cough

Dyspnea with exertion

Oral cavity

Frequent sores (on tongue, buccal mucosa)
Loss of teeth at early age
Lesions associated with lack of oral care or substance
  abuse (leukoplakia, fistulas)

Gastrointestinal system and nutrition

Obesity
Anorexia
Cachexia

Chronic anemia
Chronic bowel irregularity
Chronic dyspepsia

Musculoskeletal system

Frequent muscle strain, backaches, neck pain
Diminished flexibility and muscle strength

Genitourinary system

Frequent sexually-transmitted infections
Frequent use of potentially unhealthful over-the-counter
  products (e.g., chemical douches, perfumed vaginal
  products, nasal sprays)

Constitutional

Chronic fatigue, headaches, apathy

Psychoemotional

Emotional fragility
Frequent feelings of being overwhelmed

RELATED FACTORS

A variety of factors can produce altered health maintenance. Some common causes are listed below.

Situational (Personal, Environmental)
Related to:
Lack of motivation
Lack of education or readiness
Lack of access to adequate health care services
Inadequate health teaching
Impaired ability to understand secondary to (specify)

Maturational
Child
Related to lack of education of age-related factors.
Examples include:

Sexuality and sexual development	Substance abuse
	Poor nutrition
Safety hazards	Inactivity

Adolescent
Same as children
Cycle, automobile safety practices
Substance abuse (alcohol, other drugs, tobacco)

Adult
Related to lack of education of age-related factors.
Examples include:

Parenthood	Safety practices
Sexual function	

Older Adult
Related to lack of education of age-related factors.
Examples include:
Effects of aging
Sensory deficits

See Table I.2 for age-related conditions.

NOC Health Promoting Behavior, Health Seeking Behaviors, Knowledge: Health Promotion, Knowledge: Health Resources, Participation: Health Care Decisions, Risk Detection, Treatment

(text continues on p. 207)

Table I.2 Primary and Secondary Prevention for Age-Related Conditions

Developmental Level	Primary Prevention	Secondary Prevention

Infancy (0–1 y)	Parent education
	Infant safety
	Nutrition
	Breastfeeding
	Sensory stimulation
	Infant massage and touch
	Visual stimulation
	  Activity
	  Colors
	Auditory stimulation
	  Verbal
	  Music
	Immunizations
	  DPT, hepatitis B
	  IPV
	  H. influenzae
	  pneumococcal influenza
	Oral hygiene
	Teething biscuits
	Fluoride
	Avoid sugared food and drink
		Complete physical examination every 2–3 mo
		Screening at birth
		  Congenital hip
		  Phenylketonuria (PKU)
		  Sickle cell disease
		  Cystic fibrosis
		  Vision (startle reflex)
		  Hearing (response to and localization of sounds)
		  Tuberculin test at 12 mo
		Developmental assessments
		Screen and intervene for high risk
		  Low birth weight
		  Maternal substance abuse during pregnancy
		  Alcohol: fetal alcohol syndrome
		  Cigarettes: sudden infant death syndrome (SIDS)
		  Drugs: addicted neonate
		  Maternal infections during pregnancy

Preschool (1–5 y)	Parent education	Complete physical examination between 2 and 3 y and preschool (urinalysis, CBC)
	Teething	Tuberculin test at 3 y
	Discipline	Developmental assessments (annual)
	Nutrition	Speech development
	Accident prevention	Hearing
	Normal growth and development	Vision
	Child education	Screen and intervene
	Dental self-care	Lead poisoning
	Dressing	Developmental lag
	Bathing with assistance	Neglect or abuse
	Feeding self-care	Strabismus
	Immunizations	Hemoglobin or hematocrit
	DTap	Vision, hearing deficit
	IPV	Strong family history of arteriosclerotic disease (e.g., MI, CVA, peripheral vascular disease), diabetes, hypertension, gout, or hyperlipidemia—fasting serum cholesterol at age 2 years, then every 3–5 years if normal.
	MMR	
	HIB	
	Influenza (for high risk)	
	Varicella Hepatitis A (high risk)	
	Pneumococcal Hepatitis B	
	Dental/oral hygiene	
	Fluoride treatments	
	Fluoridated water	
	Dietary counsel	

(table continues on p. 202)

Table I.2 Primary and Secondary Prevention for Age-Related Conditions (continued)

Developmental Level	Primary Prevention	Secondary Prevention

School age (6–11 y)	Health education of child
	Food pyramid
	Accident prevention
	Outdoor safety (e.g., helmets)
	Substance abuse counsel
	Anticipatory guidance for physical changes at puberty
	Immunizations
	  Tetanus at 11–12 y
	  DTap } Boosters between
	  OPV } 4 and 6 y
	  MMR
	  Varicella (at age 11–12 if no history of infection)
	  Pneumococcal (high risk)
	Professional dental hygiene every 6–12 mo
	Continue fluoridation
	Complete physical examination (yearly)
		Complete physical examination
		Tuberculin test every 3 y (at ages 6 and 9)
		Developmental measurements
		  Language
		  Vision: Snellen charts at school
		    6–8 y, use "E" chart
		    Over 8 y, use alphabet chart
		  Hearing: audiogram

Adolescence (12–19 y)	Health education Proper nutrition and healthful diets	Complete physical examination (yearly) Blood pressure

Young adult (20–39 y)	Sex education (abstinence, family planning, sexually transmitted diseases) Safe driving skills Adult challenges Seeking employment and career choices Dating and marriage Confrontation with substance abuse Safety in athletics, water Skin care, sunscreens Professional dental hygiene every 6–12 mo Immunization Hepatitis B series (if needed) OPV booster at 12–14 y Health education Weight management with good nutrition as basal metabolic rate changes Lifestyle counseling Stress management skills Injury prevention "Safe sex" Parenting skills	Cholesterol profile Tuberculin test at 12 y, and yearly if high risk RPR, CBC, urinalysis, urine for chlamydia and gonorrhea (male) Female: breast self-examination, monthly Male: testicular self-examination, weekly Female, if sexually active: Pap test and pelvic examination, yearly (*Chlamydia* and cervical gonorrhea cultures with pelvic examination) Screening and interventions if high risk Depression Suicide Substance abuse Pregnancy Family history of alcoholism or domestic violence HIV infection Sexually transmitted infections Complete physical examination at about 20 y, then every 5–6 y Female: breast self-examination monthly Gynecologic exam—same as adolescent 12–19 if high risk otherwise every 2 years Male: testicular self-examination weekly All females: baseline mammography at age 40 then every 1–2 y

(table continues on p. 204)

Developmental Level	Primary Prevention	Secondary Prevention
	Substance abuse Environmental health choices Professional dental hygiene every 6–12 mo Immunization Tetanus at 20 y and every 10 y Female: rubella, if zero negative for antibodies Hepatitis B series if needed	Parents-to-be: high-risk screening for Down syndrome, Tay-Sachs disease Pregnant female: screen for sexually transmitted diseases, rubella titer, Rh factor Annual screening and interventions if high risk Female with previous breast cancer: annual mammography at 35 y and after Female with mother or sister who has had breast cancer, same as above Family history of colorectal cancer or high risk: annual stool guaiac, digital rectal examination, and sigmoidoscopy PPD if exposed to tuberculosis Glaucoma screening at 35 years along with routine physical exams Cholesterol profile every 5 years if normal Cholesterol profile every 1–2 years if borderline
Middle-aged adult (40–59 y)	Health education: continue with young adult, perimenopausal Midlife changes, male and female counseling "Empty-nest syndrome" Anticipatory guidance for retirement	Complete physical examination every 5–6 y with complete laboratory evaluation (serum/urine tests, x-ray, ECG) Dexascan screening for osteoporosis once then as needed

	Grandparenting Professional dental hygiene every 6–12 mo Immunizations Tetanus every 10 years Influenza—annual if high risk (i.e., major chronic disease [COPD, CAD]) Pneumococcal—single dose	Female: breast self-examination monthly, Pap test every 1–3 y Male: testicular self-examination monthly All females: mammography every 1–2 y 50 years and over Eye examination every 1–2 y Pregnant female: perinatal screening by amniocentesis if desired Colonoscopy at 50 and 51 y, then every 4 y if negative Stool guaiac test annually at 50 y and thereafter Screening and intervention if high risk Oral cancer: screen more often if substance abuser, smoker Skin cancer PSA yearly after age 40 for blacks, Hispanics and after 50 for others
Older adult (60–74 y)	Health education: continue with previous counseling Home safety Retirement Loss of spouse Special health needs Nutritional changes	Complete physical examination every 2 y with laboratory assessments Blood pressure annually Female: breast self-examination monthly Male: testicular self-examination monthly Female: annual mammogram, Pap test every 1–3 y, depending on risk

(table continues on p. 206)

Table I.2 Primary and Secondary Prevention for Age-Related Conditions (continued)

Developmental Level	Primary Prevention	Secondary Prevention
	Changes in hearing or vision Professional dental/oral hygiene every 6–12 mo Immunizations Tetanus every 10 y Influenza—annual if high risk Pneumococcal (one time only)	Annual stool guaiac test Colonoscopy every 4 y Complete eye examination yearly Podiatric evaluation with foot care PRN Screen for high risk Depression Suicide Alcohol/drug abuse Elder abuse
Old-age adult (75 y and over)	Health education: continue counsel Anticipatory guidance Dying and death Loss of spouse Increasing dependency on others Professional dental/oral hygiene every 6–12 mo Immunizations Tetanus every 10 y Influenza—annual Pneumococcal—if not already received	Complete physical examination annually Female: mammogram every 1–2 y Sigmoidoscopy every 5 y Complete eye examination yearly Podiatrist PRN

(Source: U.S. Department of Health and Human Services [1994]. *Clinician's handbook of preventive services: Putting prevention into practice.* Washington, DC: U.S. Government Printing Office.)

Goals

The individual or caregiver will verbalize an intent or engage in health maintenance behaviors.

Indicator

Identify barriers to health maintenance.

NIC Health Education, Self-Responsibility Facilitation, Health Screening, Risk Identification, Family Involvement Promotion

Generic Interventions

Assess Knowledge of Primary Prevention:

Safety—accident prevention (e.g., car, machinery, outdoor safety, occupational)

Healthful diet (e.g., "basic four," low fat and salt, high complex carbohydrate, sufficient intake of vitamins, minerals, 2 to 3 quarts of water daily)

Weight control

Avoidance of substance abuse (alcohol, drugs, tobacco)

Avoidance of sexually transmitted diseases

Dental/oral hygiene (daily, dentist)

Immunizations

Regular exercise pattern

Stress management

Lifestyle counseling (e.g., safe sex, family planning, parenting skills, financial planning)

Teach Importance of Secondary Prevention (Refer to Table I.2).

Determine Knowledge Needed to Manage Condition:

Causes

Treatments

Medications

Diet

Activity

Risk factors

Signs/symptoms of complications
Restrictions
Follow-up care

**Assess if Needed At-Home Resources
Are Available.**
Caregiver
Finances
Equipment

**Determine If Referrals Are Indicated
(e.g., Social Services, Housekeeping,
Home Health).**

Health Seeking Behaviors (Specify)

DEFINITION
Health Seeking Behaviors: The state in which an individual
in stable health actively seeks ways to alter personal health
habits and/or the environment to move toward a higher level
of wellness.*

> ⊚ **AUTHOR'S NOTE**
>
> This diagnosis can be used to describe the individual/
> family who desires health teaching related to the promo-
> tion and maintenance of health (e.g., preventive behavior,
> age-related screening, optimal nutrition). This diagnosis
> should be used to describe an asymptomatic person. How-

*Stable health is defined as a condition in which the client's
well-being is maximized; signs and symptoms of disease, if present, are controlled; and disabilities follow a predictable, non-
acute course.

⚙ **AUTHOR'S NOTE (continued)**

ever, it can be used for a person with a chronic disease to help that person attain a higher level of wellness. For example, a woman with lupus erythematosus can have the diagnosis *Health Seeking Behaviors related to initiation of a regular exercise program.*

DEFINING CHARACTERISTICS
Major (Must be Present)
Expressed or observed desire to seek information for health promotion

Minor (May be Present)
Expressed or observed desire for increased control of health

Expression of concern about current environmental conditions on health status

Stated or observed unfamiliarity with community wellness resources

Demonstrated or observed lack of knowledge in health-promotion behaviors

RELATED FACTORS
Situational (Personal, Environmental)
Related to anticipated role changes; for example, marriage, parenthood, "empty nest syndrome," retirement

Related to lack of knowledge of:

Preventive behavior (disease)

Screening practices for age and risk

Optimal nutrition and weight control

Regular exercise program

Constructive stress management

Supportive social networks

Maturational
See Table I.2.

NOC Adherence Behavior, Health Behaviors, Health Promoting Behaviors, Well Being

Goals

The person will agree with self-responsibility for wellness (physical, dental, safety, nutritional, family).

Indicators

- Describe screening that is appropriate for age and risk factors.
- Perform self-screening for cancer.
- Participate in a regular physical exercise program.
- State an intent to use positive coping mechanisms and constructive stress management.
- Eat a balance diet to maintain or achieve a BMI <26.

> **NIC** Health Education, Risk Identification, Values Clarification, Behavior Modification, Coping Enhancement, Knowledge: Health Resources

Generic Interventions

Determine the Person's or Family's Knowledge or Perception of:

Life cycle challenges (e.g., marriage, parenting, aging, finances).

Need to maintain responsible relationships with health care providers.

Ability to attain a higher level of health through anticipatory planning for life cycle events (e.g., financial planning).

Need to provide and nurture reciprocity in social support.

Determine the Person's or Family's Past Patterns of Health Care.

Expectations

Interactions with health care system or providers

Influences of family, cultural group, peer group, mass media

Provide Specific Information Concerning Age-Related Health Promotion (Refer to Table I.2).

Discuss Client's Food Choices, and Assist As He or She Identifies New Goals for Health Promotion.

Assist in the selection of foods to sustain life and facilitate body functioning.

Provide information, when needed, about developmental considerations for dependents.

Discuss the risk of excess use of:

salt	snack foods
fried foods	processed meats
fats	soda, fruit drinks

Discuss the Benefits of a Regular Exercise Program.

Discuss the Elements of Constructive Stress Management:

Assertiveness training
Problem solving
Relaxation techniques

Discuss Strategies for Developing Positive Social Networks.

Promote Self-Actualization in the Client Who Is Seeking to Promote Health.

Demonstrate an interested but nonjudgmental attitude.

View the client–nurse relationship as collaborative; the client remains in control of choices, actions, and evaluations.

Facilitate adoption of new behaviors rather than defining them.

Listen, reflect, and converse to clarify the client's current behavior patterns and desired goals.

Enhance the client's strengths, empower with choices and self-control, and always demonstrate respect for those choices.

DEFINITION

Impaired Home Maintenance: The state in which an individual or family experiences or is at risk to experience difficulty in maintaining a safe, hygienic, growth-producing home environment.

> **⊙ AUTHOR'S NOTE**
>
> This diagnosis can describe situations in which the individual or family needs specific support or instruction to manage home care of a family member or activities of daily living.

DEFINING CHARACTERISTICS
Major (Must be Present, One or More)

Expressions or observations of:
   Difficulty in maintaining home hygiene
   Difficulty in maintaining a safe home
   Inability to keep up home
   Lack of sufficient finances

Minor (May be Present)

Repeated infections   Unwashed cooking and
Accumulated wastes   eating equipment
Overcrowding   Offensive odors
Infestations

RELATED FACTORS
Pathophysiologic
Related to compromised functional ability secondary to chronic debilitating disease

Diabetes mellitus   Arthritis
Chronic obstructive   Multiple sclerosis
   pulmonary disease   Muscular dystrophy

Congestive heart failure
Cancer

Parkinson's disease
Cerebrovascular accident

Situational (Personal, Environmental)

Related to change in functional ability of (specify family member) secondary to:
Injury (fractured limb, spinal cord injury)
Surgery (amputation, ostomy)
Impaired mental status (memory lapses, depression, severe anxiety, panic)
Substance abuse (alcohol, other drugs)

Related to unavailable support system
Related to loss of family member
Related to lack of knowledge
Related to insufficient finances

Maturational

Infant
Related to multiple care requirements secondary to high-risk newborn

Older Adult
Related to multiple care requirements secondary to family member with deficits (cognitive, motor, sensory)

NOC Family Functioning

Goals

The person or caregiver will demonstrate the ability to perform skills necessary for the care of the home.

Indicators

- Identify factors that restrict self-care and home management.
- Express satisfaction with home situation.

NIC Home Maintenance Assistance, Environmental Management: Safety, Environmental Management

Generic Interventions

Determine with the person and family the information needed to be taught and learned.

Determine the type of equipment needed, considering availability, cost, and durability.

Determine the type of assistance needed (e.g., meals, housework, transportation), and assist the individual to obtain them.

Discuss the implications of caring for a chronically ill family member (refer to *Caregiver Role Strain*):
  Amount of time
  Effects on other role responsibilities (spouse, children, job)
  Physical requirements (lifting)

Arrange for a home visit.

Allow the caregiver opportunities to share problems and feelings.

Refer to community agencies as indicated (e.g., nursing, social service, meals).

Hopelessness

DEFINITION

Hopelessness: A sustained subjective emotional state in which an individual sees no alternatives or personal choices available to solve problems or to achieve what is desired and cannot mobilize energy on own behalf to establish goals.

> ⊕ **AUTHOR'S NOTE**
>
> *Hopelessness* differs from *Powerlessness* in that a hopeless person sees no solution to the problem or way to achieve what is desired, even if he or she has control of his

DEFINING CHARACTERISTICS
Major (Must be Present, One or More)

Expresses profound, overwhelming, sustained apathy in response to situations perceived as impossible

Physiologic
Slowed responses to stimuli
Lack of energy
Increased sleep

Emotional
The hopeless person often has difficulty experiencing feelings but may feel:
  Unable to seek good fortune, luck, or God's favor
  Lack of meaning or purpose in life
  "Empty" or "drained"
  A sense of loss and deprivation
  Helpless
  Incompetent
  Entrapped

Person exhibits:
Passiveness, lack of involvement in care
Decreased verbalization
Decreased affect
Lack of ambition, initiative, and interest
"Giving up–given up" complex
Inability to accomplish anything
Slowed thought processes
Lack of responsibility for own decisions and life
Isolating behavior

Cognitive
Decreased problem-solving and decision-making capabilities
Deals with past and future, not here and now
Decreased flexibility in thought processes
Rigidity (e.g., "all or none" thinking)

Lacks imagination and wishing capabilities
Unable to identify and/or accomplish desired objectives
  and goals
Unable to plan, organize, or make decisions
Unable to recognize sources of hope
Suicidal thoughts

Minor (May be Present)

Physiologic
Anorexia
Weight loss

Emotional
Person feels:
  "A lump in the throat"
  Discouraged with self and others
  "At the end of my rope"
  Tense
  Overwhelmed (feels he or she just "can't")
  Loss of gratification from roles and relationships
  Vulnerable

Person exhibits:
Poor eye contact—turns away from speaker; shrugs in
  response to speaker
Decreased motivation
Sighing
Regression
Resignation
Depression

Cognitive
Decreased ability to integrate information received
Loss of time perception for past, present, and future
Decreased ability to recall the past
Confusion
Inability to communicate effectively
Distorted thought perceptions and associations
Unreasonable judgment

RELATED FACTORS
Pathophysiologic

Any chronic and/or terminal illness can cause or contribute
to hopelessness (e.g., heart disease, kidney disease, cancer,
AIDS).

Related to impaired ability to cope secondary to (e.g.):
Failing or deteriorating physiologic condition
New and unexpected signs or symptoms of previous disease
  process
Prolonged pain, discomfort, weakness
Impaired functional abilities (walking, elimination, eating)

Treatment-Related
Related to:
Prolonged treatments (e.g., chemotherapy, radiation) that
  cause discomfort (pain, nausea, vomiting)
Treatments that alter body image (e.g., surgery,
  chemotherapy)
Prolonged diagnostic studies
Prolonged dependence on equipment for life support
  (e.g., dialysis, ventilator)
Prolonged dependence on equipment for monitoring bodily
  functions (telemetry)

Situational (Personal, Environmental)
Related to:
Prolonged activity restriction (e.g., fractures, spinal cord
  injury)
Prolonged isolation (e.g., infectious diseases, reverse isola-
  tion for suppressed immune system)
Abandonment of or separation from significant others
  (parents, spouse, children, others)
Inability to achieve goals that one values in life (marriage,
  education, children)
Inability to participate in activities one desires (walking,
  sports)
Loss of something or someone valued (spouse, children,
  friend, financial resources)
Prolonged caretaking responsibilities (spouse, child, parent)
Exposure to long-term physiologic or psychological stress
Loss of belief in transcendent values/God
Ongoing, repetitive losses related to AIDS (individual,
  community)

Maturational
Child
Related to:
Loss of caregivers
Loss of trust in significant other (parents, sibling)

Rejection or abandonment by caregivers
Loss of autonomy related to illness (e.g., fracture)
Loss of bodily functions
Inability to achieve developmental tasks (trust, autonomy, initiative, industry)
Rejection by family

Adolescent
Related to:
Loss of significant other (peer, family)
Loss of bodily functions
Change in body image
Inability to achieve developmental task (role identity)

Adult
Related to:
Impaired bodily functions, loss of body part
Impaired relationships (separation, divorce)
Loss of job, career
Loss of significant others (death of children, spouse)
Inability to achieve developmental tasks (intimacy, commitment, productivity)

Older Adult
Related to:
Sensory deficits
Motor deficits
Cognitive deficits
Loss of independence
Loss of significant others, things
Inability to achieve developmental tasks (integrity)

NOC Decision-Making, Depression Control, Hope, Quality of Life

Goals

Short-Term
The person will express feelings of optimism about the present.

Indicators
- Share suffering openly and constructively with others.
- Reminisce and review life positively.

- Consider own values and the meaning of life.
- Express confidence in a desired outcome and goals.
- Express confidence in self and others.
- Practice energy conservation.

Long-Term
The person will express positive expectations about the future, expressing purpose and meaning in life.

Indicators

Demonstrate an increase in energy level, as evidenced by activities (e.g., self-care, exercise, hobbies).
Demonstrate initiative, self-direction, and autonomy in decision-making and problem-solving.
Make statement similar to the following:
- "I am looking forward to . . ."
- "When things are not so good, it helps me to think of . . ."
- "I have enough time to do what I want."
- "There are more good times ahead."
- "I expect to succeed in . . ."
- "I expect to get more out of the good things in life."
- "My past experiences have helped me be prepared for my future."
- "In the future, I'll be happier."
- "I have faith in the future."

Develop, improve, and maintain positive relationships with others.
Participate in a significant role.
Express spiritual beliefs.
Redefine the future and set realistic goals.
Exhibit peace and comfort with situation.

NIC Hope Instillation, Values Clarification, Decision-Making Support, Spiritual Support, Support System Enhancement

Generic Interventions

Convey empathy to promote verbalization of doubts, fears, and concerns.
Determine risk for suicide (Refer to Risk for Suicide).
Encourage verbalization of why and how hope is significant in client's life.

Encourage expressions of how hope is uncertain and areas in which hope has failed.

Teach how to deal with the hopeless aspects by separating them from the hopeful aspects.

Assess and mobilize the person's internal resources (autonomy, independence, rationale, cognitive thinking, flexibility, spirituality).

Assist with identification of sources of hope (e.g., relationships, faith, things to accomplish).

Create an environment in which spiritual expression is encouraged.

Assist with development of realistic short- and long-term goals (progress from simple to more complex; may use a "goals poster" to indicate type and time for achieving specific goals).

Teach how to anticipate pleasurable experiences (e.g., walking, reading favorite book, writing letter).

Assess and mobilize person's external resources (significant others, health care team, support groups, God or higher powers).

Help person to recognize that he or she is loved, cared about, and important in the lives of others regardless of failing health.

Encourage sharing of concerns with others who have had a similar problem or disease and have had positive experiences from coping effectively with it.

Assess belief support system (values, religious activities, relationship with God, meaning and purpose of prayer; refer to *Spiritual Distress*).

Allow time and opportunities to reflect on the meaning of suffering, death, and dying.

Initiate referrals as indicated (e.g., counseling, spiritual leader).

❖ Pediatric Interventions (Adolescent)

Provide truthful explanations.

Engage in activities.

If appropriate, discuss knowledge of survivors.

Focus on future.

Discuss topics interesting to the child.

Use humor if appropriate.

DEFINITION

Disorganized Infant Behavior: The state in which the neonate has an alteration in integration and modulation of the physiologic and behavioral systems of adaptation (autonomic, motor, state, organizational, self-regulatory, and attention-interactional).

> ### ⓧ AUTHOR'S NOTE
>
> This diagnosis describes an infant who has difficulty regulating and adapting to external stimuli. This difficulty is the result of immature neurobehavioral development and increased environmental stimuli associated with neonatal units. When an infant is overstimulated or stressed, she or he uses energy to adapt, which depletes the supply of energy needed for physiologic growth. The goal of nursing care is to assist the infant with energy conservation by reducing environmental stimuli, allowing the infant sufficient time to adapt to handling, and providing sensory input when appropriate to the infant's physiologic and neurobehavioral status.

DEFINING CHARACTERISTICS
(Vandenberg, 1990; Wong, 2003)

Autonomic System

Cardiac
Increased rate

Respiration
Pauses, tachypnea, gasping

Color changes
Paling around nostrils, perioral duskiness, mottled, cyanotic, gray, flushed, ruddy

Visceral
Hiccups, gagging, grunting, spitting up
Straining as if actually producing a bowel movement

Motor

Seizures	Sneezing
Tremoring/startling	Yawning
Twitching	Sighing
Coughing	

Motor System

Fluctuating tone

Flaccidity of:

Trunk	Face
Extremities	

Hypertonicity:

Leg extensions	Arching
Salutes	Finger splays
Airplaning	Tongue extensions
Sitting on air	Fisting

Hyperflexions:

Trunk	Fetal tuck
Extremities	

Frantic diffuse activity

State System (Range)

Difficulty maintaining state control

Difficulty in transitions from one state to another

Sleeping:

Twitches	Whimpers
Sound	Grimacing
Jerky moves	Fussy in sleep
Irregular respirations	

Awake:

Eye-floating	Panicked, worried,
Glassy-eyed	or dull look
Strained, fussy	Weak cry
Staring	Irritability
Gaze aversion	Abrupt state changes

Attention-Interaction System

Attempts at engaging behaviors elicit stress

Impaired ability to orient, attend, engage in reciprocal social interactions

Difficult to console

Self-Regulatory System

Limited or absent use of self-regulatory behaviors to maintain or regain control

Postural changes
Foot, leg bracing
Sucking fists
Finger folding
Hand to mouth
Stressed with more than one mode of stimuli

RELATED FACTORS
Pathophysiologic
Related to immature or impaired central nervous system secondary to:
Prematurity
Prenatal exposure to drugs
Congenital anomalies
Hypoglycemia
Infection
Hyperbilirubinemia
Decreased oxygen saturation

Related to nutritional deficits secondary to: reflux emesis, colic, swallowing problems, or feeding intolerances
Related to excess stimulation secondary to: pain, hunger, oral hypersensitivity, or temperature variation

Treatment-Related
Related to excess stimulation secondary to, for example, invasive procedures, chest physical therapy, restraints, lights (e.g., bililights), tubes, tape, medication administration, movement, feeding, noise (e.g., prolonged, alarms)
Related to inability to see caregivers secondary to eye patches

Situational (Personal, Environmental)
Related to multiple caregivers
Related to imbalance of task touch and consoling touch
Related to decreased ability to self-regulate secondary to sudden movement, noise, fatigue, or insufficient sleep

---

NOC Neurological Status, Preterm Infant Organization, Sleep, Comfort Level

Goal

The infant will demonstrate increased signs of stability.

Indicators

- Smooth, stable respirations; pink, stable color; consistent tone, improved posture; calm; focused alertness; well-modulated sleep; responsive to auditory, visual, and social stimuli
- Self-regulatory skills such as sucking, hand to mouth, hand holding, position changes

The parent(s)/caregiver(s) will describe techniques to reduce environmental stress in agency and/or at home.

- Describe situations that stress the infant.
- Describe signs/symptoms of stress in the infant.

> **NIC** Environmental Management, Neurological Monitoring, Sleep Enhancement, Newborn Care, Parent Education: Newborn, Positioning

Generic Interventions

Assess for Causative/ Contributing Factors:

Pain
Fatigue
Disorganized sleep-wake pattern
Feeding problems
Excessive stimulation person, environmental

Reduce or Eliminate Contributing Factors if Possible.

Pain

Determine the baseline behavioral manifestations of the infant and document.

Observe for responses different from baseline that have been associated with neonatal pain responses (Bozzette, 1993):

Facial responses (open mouth, brow bulge, grimace, chin quiver, nasolabial furrow, taut tongue)

Motor responses (flinch, muscle rigidity, clenched hands, withdrawal)

If unsure whether behavior indicates pain but pain is sus-
pected, consult with physician for an analgesic trial.
Evaluate the infant's response.
Aggressively manage obvious pain stimuli (e.g., postsurgi-
cal, lack of feeding, painful procedures, hyperglycemia;
Acute Pain Management Guideline Panel, 1992).
Consult with physician for an analgesic.
Provide analgesic before painful procedures.
Consider topical analgesia for frequent painful procedures
(e.g., heelstick, venipuncture).
When administering analgesics (Acute Pain Management
Guideline Panel, 1992):
Reduce initial dose, and monitor respiratory response
cautiously.
Determine optimal dose and interval.
Monitor when pain breaks through.
Determine if the infant appears comfortable after the dose.
When indicated, wean infant from the drug slowly over a
period of days. Assess response to withdrawal. Consult
with physician to manage withdrawal symptoms if
indicated.

Fatigue/disorganized sleep-wake patterns
Evaluate the need and, if needed, the frequency of each
intervention.
Organize care plan for every-4-hour interventions.

Feeding problems (Flandermeyer, 1993)
Reduce the stress of feeding:
Initiate contact slowly.
Touch the infant's back lightly.
Swaddle the infant with hands crossing midline.
When this is tolerated, pick the infant up, facing out
toward room to eliminate visual stimulation.
Prevent auditory stimulation (e.g., do not talk).
Give bottle; provide jaw support if needed.
After the infant is settled, use soothing techniques, hand
holding, vertical rocking.
Allow the infant's behavioral cues to set the pace and tone
of the interaction.
Position to facilitate feeding.

**Provide Comfort Measures When
Infant Is in a Nonarousal State
(Blackburn, 1993).**
Tactile stimulation (e.g., kangaroo care, massage)

Music, intrauterine sounds (Callins, 1991); play music, and
evaluate response
Swaddling, rocking

Reduce Environmental Stimuli:
Noise (Thomas, 1989)
Do not tap on incubator.
Place a folded blanket on top of incubator if it is the only
work surface available.
Slowly open and close portholes.
Pad incubator doors to reduce banging.
Remove water from ventilator tubing.
Speak softly at the bedside and only when necessary.
Slowly drop the head of the mattress.
Position the infant's bed away from sources of noise
(e.g., telephone, intercom, unit equipment).
Evaluate the effectiveness of a quiet hour each shift. Col-
lect data before and after to evaluate effects on staff,
infants, and parents (Blackburn, 1993).

Lights
Use full-spectrum light instead of white light at bedside.
Cover cribs, incubators, and radiant warmers completely
during sleep periods; partially during awake times.
Shade the infant's eyes with a blanket tent or cutout box.
Avoid usual stimuli on cribs (e.g., toys)

Position the Infant in Postures that Permit Flexion, and Minimize Flailing, Arching, and Squirming.
Avoid oversized diapers
Use prone-lying positions

Reduce the Stress Associated with Handling:
When moving or lifting the infant, contain the infant with
your hands by wrapping or placing rolled blankets
around his or her body.
Maintain containment during procedures and caregiving
activities.
Handle slowly and gently.
Initiate all interactions and treatments with one sense
stimulus at a time (e.g., touch), then slowly progress to
visual, auditory, movement.

Assess for cues for readiness, impending disorganization, or stability; respond to cues.

Allow to be protected and undisturbed for 2- to 3-hour intervals.

Use suctioning or postural drainage as needed instead of routinely.

Reduce Disorganized Neurobehavior During Transport (Transfer) (Little et al., 1994).

Have a plan for transport with assigned roles for each team member.

Establish behavior cues of stress for this infant with primary nurse before transport.

Swaddle the infant or place in a nest made of blankets.

Ensure the transport equipment is ready (e.g., ventilator). Warm mattress, or use sheepskin.

Carefully and smoothly move the infant. Avoid talking if possible.

If stress behaviors manifest, stop and allow the infant to return to a stable state.

Reposition every 2–3 hours or sooner if infant behavior suggests discomfort.

Enhance Parent Participation:

Encourage parents to share their feelings, fears, and expectations. Gently correct misconceptions.

Teach the behavioral cues and signs of stress in their infant.

Assist parents to interact with their infant as appropriate to status and maturity.

Initiate Health Teaching and Referrals As Indicated.

Home Care. Provide parents with teaching related to (Johnson-Crowley, 1993):

Teach caregivers to continually observe the changing capabilities to determine the appropriate positioning and bedding options (Wong 2003).

Health concerns

Feeding, hygiene

Safety, temperature

Illness, infection

Growth, development

State modulation
Appropriate stimulation
Sleep-wake patterns

Parent–infant interaction
Behavior cues
Signs of stress

Infant's environment
Animate, inanimate stimulation
Role of father and siblings
Playing with infant

Parental coping and support
Refer for follow-up home visits.

Infant Behavior, Risk for Disorganized

DEFINITION

Risk for Disorganized Infant Behavior: The state in which the neonate is at risk for an alteration in integration and modulation of the physiologic and behavioral systems of adaptation (autonomic, motor, state, organizational, self-regulatory, and attentional-interactional).

RISK FACTORS

Refer to Related Factors.

RELATED FACTORS

Refer to *Disorganized Infant Behavior.*

Interventions

Refer to *Disorganized Infant Behavior.*

Infant Behavior, Readiness for Enhanced Organized

DEFINITION

Readiness for Enhanced Organized Infant Behavior: A pattern of modulation of the physiologic and behavioral systems of functioning of an infant (autonomic, motor, state, organizational, self-regulatory, and attentional-interactional) that is satisfactory but can be improved, resulting in higher levels of integration in response to environmental stimuli.

ⓩ AUTHOR'S NOTE

This diagnosis describes an infant who is responding to the environment with stable and predictable autonomic, motor, and state cues. The focus of interventions is to promote continued stable development and to reduce excess environmental stimuli that may stress the infant.

Because this is a wellness diagnosis, the use of related factors is not needed. The diagnostic statement can be written as *Readiness for Enhanced Organized Infant Behavior as evidenced by ability to regulate autonomic, motor, and state systems to environmental stimuli.*

DEFINING CHARACTERISTICS
(Blackburn & Vandenberg, 1993)
Autonomic System

Able to regulate color and respiration
Reduction of tremors, twitches
Reduction of visceral signals (e.g., smooth)
Digestive functioning, feeding tolerance

Motor System

Smooth, well-modulated posture and tone
Synchronous smooth movements with:
  Hand/foot clasping
  Grasping

Hand-to-mouth activity
Suck/suck searching
Hand-holding
Tucking

State System

Well-differentiated range of states
Clear, robust sleep states
Active self-quieting/consoling
Focused, shiny-eyed alertness with intent or animated
   facial expressions
"Ooh" face
Cooing
Attentional smiling

RELATED FACTORS

Because this is a diagnosis of effective functioning, the use
of related factors is not warranted.

NOC Child Development, Specify Age, Sleep, Comfort Level

Goals

The infant will continue age-appropriate growth and development.

Indicators

• Not experience excessive environmental stimuli.
• Demonstrate continued organized sleep states and calm
  alert states.

The parent(s) will describe developmental needs of the
infant.

• Demonstrate handling that promotes stability.
• Describe signs of stress or exhaustion.
• Demonstrate (Reeder, Martin, & Koniak-Griffin, 1997):
      Gentle, soothing touch
      Melodic tone of voice, coos
      Mutual gazing
      Rhythmic movements
• Acknowledge all of baby's vocalizations.
• Recognize soothing qualities of actions.

NIC Developmental Care, Infant Care, Sleep Enhancement, Environmental Management: Comfort, Parent Education: Infant, Attachment Promotion, Caregiver Support, Calming Technique

🔹 Pediatric Interventions

Explain Developmental Needs of Infants.

Stimulation (visual, auditory, vestibular, tactile, olfactory, gustatory)

Periods of alertness

Sleep requirements

Explain the Effects of Excess Environmental Stress on the Infant:

Provide a list of signs of stress for the infant.

Teach to terminate stimulation if the infant shows signs.

When providing developmental intervention(s):

Offer only when the infant is alert.

If possible, show parents examples of their infant when alert and not alert.

Begin with one stimulus at a time (touch, voice).

Provide intervention for a short time.

Increase interventions according to the infant's cues.

Provide frequent, short-duration interventions instead of infrequent, long-term ones.

Explain Role Model, and Observe Parent Engaging in Developmental Interventions.

Visual (Reeder et al., 1997)

Eye-to-eye contact

Face-to-face experiences

Provide with high-contrast colors, geometric shapes (e.g., black-and-white shapes on paper mobile)

Auditory

Use high-pitched vocalization.

Play classical music softly.

Avoid loud talking.

Call the infant by name.

Avoid monotone speech patterns.

◆ Pediatric Interventions (cont'd)

Tactile
Use firm, gentle touch as initial approach.
Use skin-to-skin contact in a warm room.
For a massage, stroke skin very slowly and gently in head-to-toe direction. Begin at trunk.
Provide alternative textures (e.g., sheepskin, velvet, satin).
Avoid stroking if responses are disorganized.

Vestibular (Movement)
Rock in chair; provide head support.
Place in sling and rock.
Slowly change position during handling.

Olfactory
Wear a light perfume.

Gustatory
Allow non-nutritive sucking (e.g., pacifier, hand in mouth).

Promote Adjustment and Stability to Caregiving Activities (Blackburn & Vandenberg, 1993).

Waking
Enter room slowly.
Turn on light; open curtains slowly.
Avoid waking if asleep.

Changing
Keep room warm.
Gently change position; contain limbs during movement.
Stop changing if the infant is irritable.

Feeding
Time feedings with alert states.
Hold the infant close and, if needed, swaddle in blanket.

Bathing
Ventral openness may be stressful.
Cover body parts not being bathed.

🔷 Pediatric Interventions (cont'd)

Proceed slowly; allow for rest.
Offer a pacifier or hand to suck.
Eliminate unnecessary noise.
Use soft, soothing voice.

**Explain the Need to Reduce
Environmental Stimuli When Taking
the Infant Outside Home:**

Shelter eyes from light.
Swaddle the infant so hands can reach mouth.
Protect from loud noises.

**Praise Parents on their Interaction
Patterns. Point Out the Infant's
Engaging Responses.**

**Initiate Health Teaching and
Referrals If Needed:**

Explain that developmental interventions will change
as the child develops. Refer to *Delayed Growth and
Development* for specific age-related developmental
needs.
Provide parents with resources for assistance at home
(e.g., community resources).

Infection, Risk for

DEFINITION
Risk for Infection: The state in which an individual is at risk to be invaded by an opportunistic or pathogenic agent (virus, fungus, bacterium, protozoan, or other parasite) from endogenous or exogenous sources.

> ### ⦿ AUTHOR'S NOTE
>
> *Risk for Infection* describes a situation when host defenses are compromised, making the host more susceptible to environmental pathogens. Nursing interventions focus on minimizing introduction of organisms or increasing resistance to infection (e.g., improving nutritional status).

RISK FACTORS
Presence of risk factors (see Related Factors)

RELATED FACTORS
A variety of health problems and situations can create favorable conditions that encourage the development of infections. Some common factors are listed below.

Pathophysiologic
Related to compromised host defenses secondary to:

Cancer

Renal failure

Hematologic disorders

Diabetes mellitus

Alcoholism

Immunodeficiency

AIDS

Hepatic disorders

Respiratory disorders

Immunosuppression

Altered or insufficient
  leukocytes

Periodontal disease   Altered integumentary
Arthritis   system

Related to compromised circulation secondary to:
Lymphedema
Obesity
Peripheral vascular disease

Treatment-Related
Related to a site for organism invasion secondary to:
Surgery   Presence of invasive lines
Dialysis   Intubation
Total parenteral nutrition Enteral feedings

Related to compromised host defenses secondary to:
Radiation therapy
Organ transplant
Medication therapy (specify; e.g., chemotherapy, immuno-
  suppressants)

Situational (Personal, Environmental)
Related to compromised host defenses secondary to:
Prolonged immobility   Stress
Increased length of   Smoking
  hospital stay   History of infections
Malnutrition

Related to a site for organism invasion secondary to:
Trauma (accidental, intentional)
Postpartum period
Bites (animal, insect, human)
Thermal injuries
Warm, moist, dark environment (skin folds, casts)

**Related to contact with contagious agents (nosocomial
or community-acquired)**

Maturational
Newborn
**Related to increased vulnerability of infant second-
ary to:**
Lack of maternal antibodies (dependent on maternal
  exposure)
Lack of normal flora
Open wounds (umbilical, circumcision)
Immature immune system

Infant/Child
Related to increased vulnerability secondary to lack of immunization

Older Adult
Related to increased vulnerability of elderly secondary to: debilitated condition, decreased immune response, or multiple chronic diseases

NOC	Infection Status, Wound Healing, Primary Intention, Immune Status

Goals

The person will report risk factors associated with infection and precautions needed.

Indicators

- Demonstrate meticulous hand washing technique by the time of discharge.
- Describe methods of transmission of infection.
- Describe the influence of nutrition on prevention of infection.

NIC	Infection Control, Wound Care, Incision Site Care, Health Education

Generic Interventions

Identify Individuals at Risk for Nosocomial Infections.

Assess for predictors that increase the risk of infection.
Infection (preoperatively)
Abdominal or thoracic surgery
Surgery longer than 2 hours
Genitourinary procedure
Instrumentation (ventilator, suction, catheters, nebulizers, tracheostomy, invasive monitoring)
Anesthesia

Assess for confounding factors.
Age younger than 1 year or older than 65 years
Obesity

Underlying disease conditions (chronic obstructive pulmonary disease, diabetes, cardiovascular, blood dyscrasias)

Substance abuse

Medications (steroids, chemotherapy, antibiotic therapy)

Nutritional status (intake less than minimum daily requirements)

Smoker

Reduce the Entry of Organisms into Individuals.

Meticulous hand washing

Aseptic technique

Isolation measures

No unnecessary diagnostic or therapeutic procedures

Reduction of airborne microorganisms

Protect the Immune-Deficient Individual from Infection:

Instruct individual to ask all visitors and personnel to wash their hands before approaching him or her.

Limit visitors when appropriate.

Restrict invasive devices (intravenous line, laboratory specimens) to those that are necessary.

Teach individual and family members signs and symptoms of infection.

Reduce Individual's Susceptibility to Infection:

Encourage and maintain caloric and protein intake in diet (see *Imbalanced Nutrition*).

Monitor use or overuse of antimicrobial therapy.

Administer prescribed antimicrobial therapy within 15 minutes of scheduled time.

Minimize length of stay in hospital.

Observe for Clinical Manifestations of Infection (e.g., Fever, Cloudy Urine, Purulent Drainage).

Instruct Individual and Family Regarding the Causes, Risks, and Communicability of the Infection.

Report Communicable Diseases As Appropriate to Public Health Department.

❖ Pediatric Interventions

Monitor for signs of infection (e.g., lethargy, feeding difficulties, vomiting, temperature instability, subtle color
changes).

Provide umbilical cord care. Teach cord care and signs of
infection (e.g., increased redness, purulent drainage).

Teach signs of infection of circumcised area (e.g., bleeding,
increased redness, or unusual swelling).

🗝 Maternal Interventions

Explain the increased vulnerability to infection during
pregnancy.

Teach how to prevent urinary tract infections during
pregnancy:
  Drink at least eight 8-oz glasses of water.
  Void frequently.
  Void before and after intercourse (Reeder et al., 1997).

Teach how to prevent infection postpartum:
  Wipe from front to back.
  Clean perineal area after voiding or defecating (e.g., sitz
    bath, squirt bottle).
  Change perineal pads after each voiding.
  Teach proper breast care.

Identify risk factors for postpartum infections:
  Anemia
  Poor nutrition
  Lack of prenatal care
  Obesity
  Intercourse after membrane rupture
  Immunosuppression
  Prolonged labor
  Prolonged membrane rupture
  Intrauterine fetal monitoring (in high-risk mothers)
  Hemorrhage

Instruct on signs and symptoms of infection (e.g., fever,
purulent drainage), and report promptly.

🎯 Geriatric Considerations

Explain that the usual signs of infection may not be present (e.g., fever, chills).

Assess for anorexia, weakness, change in mental status, or hypothermia.

Monitor skin and urinary system for signs of fungal, viral, or mycobacterial pathogens.

Infection Transmission, Risk for*

DEFINITION
Risk for Infection Transmission: The state in which an individual is at risk for transferring an opportunistic or pathogenic agent to others.

RISK FACTORS
Presence of risk factors (see Related Factors)

RELATED FACTORS
Pathophysiologic
Related to:
Colonization with highly antibiotic-resistant organism
Airborne transmission exposure
Contact transmission exposure (direct, indirect, contact droplet)

Treatment-Related
Related to contaminated wound

---

*This diagnosis is not currently on the NANDA list but has been included for clarity or usefulness.

Related to devices with contaminated drainage (urinary and chest tubes, suction equipment, endotracheal tubes)

Situational (Personal, Environmental)

Related to:

Disaster with hazardous infectious material

Unsanitary living conditions (sewage, personal hygiene)

Areas considered high risk for vector-borne diseases
  (malaria, rabies, bubonic plague, natural disasters)

Areas considered high risk for vehicle-borne diseases
  (hepatitis A, shigella, *Salmonella*)

Lack of knowledge of sources or prevention of infection

Intravenous drug use

Multiple sexual partners

Unprotected sexual intercourse

Natural disaster (e.g., flood, hurricane)

Maturational

Newborn

Related to birth outside a hospital setting in an uncontrolled environment

Related to exposure during prenatal or perinatal period to communicable disease via mother

---

NOC Infection Status, Risk Control, Risk Detection

Goals

The person will describe the mode of transmission of disease by the time of discharge.

Indicators

• Relate the need to be isolated until noninfectious.
• Demonstrate meticulous hand washing during hospitalization.

NIC Teaching: Disease Process, Infection Protection,
Infection Protection

Generic Interventions

Identify susceptible host individuals based on focus assessment for risk factors and history of exposure.

Identify the mode of transmission based on infecting agent:
Airborne
Contact
- Direct
- Indirect
- Contact droplet

Vehicle-borne (e.g., food, water, blood, body fluids)
Vector-borne (insects, animals)

Initiate appropriate isolation precautions. Consult with infection control practitioner.

Secure appropriate room assignment, depending on the type of infection and hygienic practices of the infected person.

Adhere to the Universal Infection Precautions.

In the case of acute exposure to HIV (e.g., sexual assault, needlestick, break in barrier with an HIV-infected person), immediately refer to health care facility (e.g., emergency room, occupational health) to evaluate the immediate initiation of postexposure prophylaxis of antiviral therapy (Sharbaugh, 1999).

Refer to infection control practitioner for follow-up with the health department concerning family exposure and cause of exposure, and assist in appropriate isolation of the client.

Teach client regarding the chain of infection and patient responsibility in the hospital and at home.

Injury, Risk for
Aspiration, Risk for
Falls, Risk for
Poisoning, Risk for
Suffocation, Risk for
Trauma, Risk for

Injury, Risk for

DEFINITION

Risk for Injury: The state in which an individual is at risk for harm because of a perceptual or physiologic deficit, a lack of awareness of hazards, or maturational age.

> ⟳ **AUTHOR'S NOTE**
>
> This diagnosis has five subcategories: *Risk for Aspiration, Falls, Poisoning, Suffocation,* and *Trauma.* Should the nurse choose to isolate interventions only for prevention of poisoning, then the diagnosis *Risk for Poisoning* would be useful.

RISK FACTORS
Presence of risk factors (see Related Factors for specific factors)

RELATED FACTORS
Pathophysiologic
Related to altered cerebral function secondary to, for example, tissue hypoxia, vertigo, syncope
Related to altered mobility secondary to:

Unsteady gait	Cerebrovascular accident
Amputation	Parkinsonism
Arthritis	Loss of limb

Related to impaired sensory function (e.g., vision, hearing, thermal/touch, smell)
Related to fatigue
Related to orthostatic hypotension
Related to vestibular disorders
Related to carotid sinus syncope
Related to lack of awareness of environmental hazards secondary to, for example, confusion, hypoglycemia, depression, electrolyte imbalance
Related to tonic-clonic movements secondary to seizures

Treatment-Related
Related to effects of (specify) on mobility or sensorium:
Medications

Sedatives	Diuretics
Vasodilators	Phenothiazines
Antihypertensives	Psychotropics
Hypoglycemics	

Related to casts/crutches, canes, walkers

Situational (Personal, Environmental)
Related to decrease in or loss of short-term memory
Related to faulty judgment secondary to, for example, dehydration (e.g., summer), stress, alcohol
Related to prolonged bed rest
Related to vasovagal reflex
Related to household hazards (specify):

Unsafe walkways	Stairs
Unsafe toys	Slippery floors
Inadequate lighting	Faulty electric wires
Bathrooms (tubs, low toilets)	Improperly stored poisons

Related to automotive hazards
Related to fire hazards
Related to unfamiliar setting (hospital, nursing home)
Related to improper footwear
Related to inattentive caregiver
Related to improper use of aids (crutches, canes, walkers, wheelchairs)
Related to history of accidents

Maturational
Infant/Child
Related to lack of awareness of hazards

Older Adult
Related to faulty judgment secondary to:
Sensory deficits
Medication
Cognitive deficits

NOC Risk Control, Safety Status: Falls Occurrence, Safety Behavior: Home Physical Environment, Safety Behavior: Personal

Goals

The person will relate fewer injuries and less fear of injury.

Indicators

- Identify factors that increase the risk for injury.
- Relate an intent to use safety measures to prevent injury (e.g., remove throw rugs or anchor them).
- Relate an intent to practice selected prevention measures (e.g., wear sunglasses to reduce glare).
- Increase daily activity, if feasible.

NIC Fall Prevention, Environmental Management: Safety, Health Education, Surveillance: Safety, Risk Identification

Generic Interventions

Orient each new admission to surroundings, explain the call system, and assess the person's ability to use it.
Closely supervise the person during the first few nights to assess safety.
Use night light.
Encourage the person to request assistance during the night.
Keep bed at lowest level during the night.
Teach proper use of crutches, canes, walkers, prosthesis.
Instruct the person to wear shoes that fit properly and that have nonskid soles.
Assess for the presence of side effects of drugs that may cause vertigo.
Teach the person to:
    Eliminate throw rugs, litter, and highly polished floors.

Provide nonslip surfaces in bathtub or shower by applying commercially available traction tapes.

Provide handgrips in bathroom.

Provide railings in hallways and on stairs.

Remove protruding objects (e.g., coat hooks, shelves,
light fixtures) from stairway walls.

Institute safety precautions for confused persons
(Schoenfelder, 2000).

Observe frequently.

Ask roommate, if capable, to alert nurses of a problem.

Use low bed, with side rails up.

Use mattress on floor.

Place bedside table or commode chair in front of patient
when sitting in a chair.

Consider an alarm system.

Place person in room near traffic (e.g., nurses' station).

Provide a distraction: music, companion, simple craft,
pet therapy.

🐾 Pediatric Interventions

Teach parents to expect frequent changes in infants' and
children's ability and to take precautions (e.g., infant who
suddenly rolls over for the first time might be on a changing table unattended).

Discuss with parents the necessity of constant monitoring
of small children.

Provide parents with information to assist them in selecting a babysitter.

Determine previous experiences and knowledge of emergency measures.

Observe the interaction of the sitter with the child.

Teach parents to expect children to mimic them and to
teach their children what they can do with or without
supervision (seat belts, helmets, safe driving).

Explain and expect compliance with certain rules (depending on age) concerning:

Streets

Playground equipment

Water (pools, bathtubs)

Bicycles

❖ Pediatric Interventions (cont'd)

Fire
Animals
Strangers
Instruct how to "child-proof" the home.
Explain why children should not ride in front (air bags).
Refer to local fire department for assistance in staging
  home fire drills.
Encourage parents to learn basic life-saving skills (CPR,
  Heimlich maneuver).
Teach children how to dial 911.
Teach parents to assist their children in handling peer
  pressure that involves risk-taking behavior.

⊙ Geriatric Interventions

Assess for orthostatic hypotension. Compare brachial blood
  pressure (supine, standing).
Discuss physiology of orthostatic hypotension with client.
Teach techniques to reduce orthostatic hypotension.
  Change positions slowly.
  Move from lying to an upright position in stages.
  During day, rest in a recliner rather than in bed.
  Avoid prolonged standing.
Teach to avoid dehydration and vasodilation (e.g., hot tubs).
Teach exercises to increase strength and flexibility.
Perform ankle-strengthening exercises daily (Schoenfelder,
  2000).
  Stand behind a straight chair, with feet slightly apart.
  Slowly raise both heels until body weight is on balls
    of feet; hold for count of 3 (e.g., "1 Mississippi,
    2 Mississippi, 3 Mississippi").
  Do 5 to 10 repetitions; increase repetitions as strength
    increases.
Walk at least two or three times a week.
  Use ankle exercises as a warm-up before walking.
  Begin walking with someone at side if needed for
    10 minutes.
  Increase time and speed according to capabilities.

DEFINITION
Risk for Aspiration: The state in which a person is at risk for entry of secretions, solids, or fluids into the tracheobronchial passages.

RISK FACTORS
Presence of favorable conditions for aspiration (see Related Factors).

RELATED FACTORS
Pathophysiologic
Related to reduced level of consciousness secondary to:

Anesthesia	Coma
Head injury	Presenile dementia
Cerebrovascular accident	Seizures

Related to depressed cough and gag reflexes
Related to increased intragastric pressure secondary to:

Lithotomy position	Obesity
Enlarged uterus	Ascites

Related to impaired swallowing or decreased laryngeal and glottic reflexes secondary to:

Achalasia	Catatonia
Scleroderma	Myasthenia gravis
Esophageal strictures	Guillain-Barré syndrome
Cerebrovascular accident	Multiple sclerosis
Parkinson's disease	Muscular dystrophy
Debilitating conditions	

Related to tracheoesophageal fistula
Related to impaired protective reflexes secondary to:
Facial/oral/neck surgery or trauma
Paraplegia or hemiplegia

Treatment-Related
Related to depressed laryngeal and glottic reflexes secondary to:

Presence of tracheostomy/endotracheal tube
Sedation
Tube feedings

Related to impaired ability to cough secondary to:
Wired jaw
Imposed prone position

Situational (Personal, Environmental)

Related to inability/impaired ability to elevate upper body

Related to eating when intoxicated

Maturational

Premature
Related to impaired sucking/swallowing reflexes

Neonate
Related to decreased muscle tone of inferior esophageal sphincter

Older Adult
Related to poor dentition

NOC   Aspiration Control

Goals

The person will not experience aspiration.

Indicators

- Relate measures to prevent aspiration.
- Name foods or fluids that are high risk for aspiration.

NIC   Aspirations: Precautions, Airway Management, Positioning, Airway Suctioning

Generic Interventions

Reduce the Risk of Aspiration.

For individuals with decreased strength, decreased sensorium, or autonomic disorders:
  Maintain a side-lying position if not contraindicated by injury.

Assess for position of the tongue, ensuring that it has not dropped backward, occluding the airway.

Keep the head of the bed elevated if not contraindicated.

Clear secretions from mouth and throat with a tissue or gentle suction.

Reassess frequently for presence of obstructive material in mouth and throat.

For persons with tracheostomies or endotracheal tubes:

Inflate cuff (during continuous mechanical ventilation, during and after eating, during and 1 hour after tube feeding, during intermittent positive-pressure breathing treatments).

Suction every 1 to 2 hours and as needed.

For persons with gastrointestinal tubes and feedings:

Verify that feeding tube has not moved upward since insertion.

Aspirate for residual contents before each feeding for tubes positioned gastrically.

Elevate head of bed for 30 to 45 minutes during feeding period and 1 hour after to prevent reflux by reverse gravity.

Administer feeding if residual contents are less than 150 mL (intermittent), *or*

Administer feeding if residual is not greater than 150 mL at 10% to 20% of hourly rate (continuous).

Regulate gastric feedings using an intermittent schedule, allowing periods of stomach emptying between feeding intervals.

Ensure emergency management of obstructions is known.

❖ Pediatric Interventions

Position infant in side-lying position or supine, not prone.

Teach parents:

Not to prop bottle

To keep small objects (e.g., coins) out of reach

To remove all plastic bags

To inspect toys for removable parts or long strings

Teach what foods to avoid for young children (e.g., fruits with pits, nuts, gum, whole grapes, hot dogs, popcorn kernels).

Teach emergency management of airway obstruction:

Back blows and chest thrusts (infants)

Heimlich maneuver (children)

Risk for Falls

DEFINITION
Risk for Falls: The state in which an individual has increased susceptibility to falling.

RISK FACTORS
Presence of risk factors (see Related Factors under *Risk for Injury*).

> ⊗ **AUTHOR'S NOTE**
>
> This nursing diagnosis can be used to specify an individual at risk for falls. If the person is at risk for various types of injuries (e.g., as a cognitively impaired person), the broader diagnosis *Risk for Injury* is more useful.

Goals

The person will relate fewer falls and less fear of falling.

Indicators

- Identify factors that increase the risk for injury.
- Relate an intent to use safety measures to prevent injury (e.g., remove throw rugs or anchor them).
- Relate an intent to practice selected prevention measures (e.g., wear sunglasses to reduce glare).
- Increase daily activity, if feasible.

Generic Interventions

Refer to *Risk for Injury*.

Poisoning, Risk for

DEFINITION
Risk for Poisoning: The state in which an individual is at risk of accidental exposure to or ingestion of drugs or dangerous substances.

RISK FACTORS
Presence of risk factors (see Related Factors under *Risk for Injury*).

Suffocation, Risk for

DEFINITION
Risk for Suffocation: The state in which an individual is at risk for smothering and asphyxiation

RISK FACTORS
Presence of risk factors (see Related Factors under *Risk for Injury*)

Trauma, Risk for

DEFINITION

Risk for Trauma: The state in which an individual is at risk of accidental tissue injury (e.g., wound, burns, fracture).

RISK FACTORS

Presence of risk factors (see Related Factors under *Risk for Injury*)

Injury, Risk for Perioperative Positioning

DEFINITION

Risk for Perioperative Positioning Injury: The state in which an individual is at risk for harm as a result of positioning requirements for surgery and loss of usual protective responses secondary to anesthesia.

> ∞ **AUTHOR'S NOTE**
>
> This diagnosis focuses on identifying the vulnerability for tissue, nerve, and joint injury resulting from required positions for surgery. The addition of the term "perioperative positioning" to the *Risk for Injury* diagnosis adds etiology to the label.
>
> If a client has no preexisting risk factors that make him or her more vulnerable to injury, this diagnosis could be used with no related factors because they are evident. If

> ⓧ **AUTHOR'S NOTE (continued)**
>
> related factors are desired, the statement could read, for
> example, *Risk for Perioperative Positioning Injury related
> to position requirements for surgery and loss of usual sen-
> sory protective measures secondary to anesthesia.* When a
> client has preexisting risk factors, the statement should
> include them: for example, *Risk for Perioperative Posi-
> tioning Injury related to compromised tissue perfusion sec-
> ondary to peripheral arterial disease.*

RISK FACTORS

Presence of risk factors (see Related Factors).

RELATED FACTORS
Pathophysiologic
Related to increased vulnerability secondary to:

Chronic disease	Radiation therapy
Renal, hepatic dysfunction	Cancer
Osteoporosis	Infection
Compromised immune system	Thin body frame

Related to compromised tissue perfusion secondary to:

Diabetes mellitus	Cardiovascular disease
Peripheral vascular disease	Anemia
Hypothermia	History of thrombosis
Ascites	Dehydration
Edema	

Related to vulnerability of stoma during positioning
**Related to preexisting contractures or physical impair-
ments secondary to: for example, rheumatoid arthritis,
polio**

Treatment-Related
***Related to position requirements and loss of usual
sensory protective responses secondary to anesthesia**

---

*This risk factor is always present and may be deleted from the
diagnostic statement.

Related to surgical procedures of 2 hours or longer
Related to vulnerability of implants or prostheses (e.g., pacemakers) during positioning

Situational (Personal, Environmental)

Related to compromised circulation secondary to:

Obesity   Pregnancy
Tobacco use

Maturational

Related to increased vulnerability to tissue injury secondary to decreased circulatory volume (infant, elder)

NOC Circulation Status, Neurological Status, Tissue Perfusion: Peripheral

Goals

The person will have no neuromuscular damage or injury related to the surgical position.

Indicators

- Padding is used as indicated for procedure.
- Limbs are secured when at risk.
- Limbs are flexed when indicated.

NIC Positioning: Intraoperative, Surveillance, Pressure Management

Generic Interventions

Determine if client has preexisting risk factors (refer to Risk Factors). Communicate findings to the surgical team.

Prior to positioning, assess and document the following:
  Range-of-motion ability
  Physical abnormalities
  External/internal prostheses or implants
  Neurovascular status
  Circulatory status

Move the person from the stretcher to the operating room bed according to protocol. Lift; do not pull or drag. Do not leave unattended.

Discuss the surgical position desired with the surgeon.
Advise if any preexisting factors exist. Determine
if the position will be arranged before or after
anesthesia.

Always ask the anesthesiologist's or nurse anesthetist's
permission before moving or repositioning an anes-
thetized person.

Reduce vulnerability to tissue injury.
Align neck and spine at all times.
Gently manipulate joints. Do not abduct more than
90 degrees.
Do not let limbs extend off the operating room bed.
Reposition slowly and gently.
Use a draw sheet above the elbows to tuck in arms at
side, or abduct arm on an arm board with padding.

Protect eyes and ears from pressure. Ensure that ears are
not bent. Use eye shields if needed.

Depending on the surgical position, pad areas vulnerable
to injury. Refer to unit protocols.

If feasible, ask client if he or she feels pain, burning, pressure, or any discomforts after positioning.

Continually assess that team members are not leaning on
the client, especially on the limbs.

Ensure that the head is lifted slightly every 30 minutes.

When repositioning or returning the person to a supine
position after certain surgical positions (e.g., Trendelenburg, lithotomy, reverse Trendelenburg, jack-knife,
lateral), slowly change position to prevent severe
hypotension.

Assess client's skin condition when surgery is completed,
and document findings. Inform postanesthesia nurses
whether preexisting risk factors are present that increase
vulnerability postoperatively.

Deficient Knowledge

DEFINITION
Deficient Knowledge: The state in which an individual or group experiences a deficiency in cognitive knowledge or psychomotor skills concerning the condition or treatment plan.

> **⨂ AUTHOR'S NOTE**
>
> *Deficient Knowledge* does not represent a human response, alteration, or pattern of dysfunction; rather, it is an etiologic or contributing factor (Jenny, 1987). Lack of knowledge can contribute to a variety of responses (e.g., anxiety, self-care deficits). All nursing diagnoses have related client/family teaching as a part of nursing interventions (e.g., *Impaired Bowel Elimination, Impaired Verbal Communication*). When the teaching relates directly to a specific nursing diagnosis, incorporate the teaching into the plan. When specific teaching is indicated before a procedure, the diagnosis *Anxiety related to unfamiliar environment or procedure* can be used. When information is given to assist a person or family with self-care at home, the diagnosis *Ineffective Therapeutic Regimen Management* may be indicated.

DEFINING CHARACTERISTICS
Major (Must be Present, One or More)
Verbalizes a deficiency in knowledge or skill or requests information

Expresses an inaccurate perception of health status

Does not correctly perform a desired or prescribed health behavior

Minor (May be Present)
Lack of integration of treatment plan into daily activities

Exhibits or expresses psychological alteration (e.g., anxiety, depression) resulting from misinformation or lack of information

Latex Allergy

DEFINITION
Latex Allergy: The state in which an individual experiences an immunoglobin E–mediated allergic response to latex.

DEFINING CHARACTERISTICS
Major
Positive skin test to natural rubber latex (NRL) extract

Minor

Allergic conjunctivitis	Rhinitis
Urticaria	Asthma

RELATED FACTORS
Biopathophysiologic
Related to hypersensitivity response to the protein component of NRL

NOC Immune Hypersensitivity Control

Goals
The person will report no exposure to latex.

Indicators
- Describe products of NRL.
- Describe strategies to avoid exposure.

NIC Allergy Management, Latex Precautions, Environmental Risk Protection

Generic Interventions

Explain the importance of completely avoiding direct contact with all NRL products.

Advise that a person with a history of mild skin reaction to latex is at risk for anaphylaxis.

Instruct the patient to wear a medical alert bracelet stating "Latex Allergy" and to carry autoinjectable epinephrine.

Instruct to warn all health care providers (e.g., dental, medical, surgical) of the allergy.

Use nonlatex alternative supplies:

  Clear disposable amber bags

  Silicone baby nipples

  2×2 gauze pads with silk tape in place of adhesive bandages

  Clear plastic or Silastic catheters

  Vinyl or neoprene gloves

  Silk or plastic tape, not plastic or adhesive

Protect from exposure to latex.

  Cover skin with cloth before applying blood pressure cuff.

  Do not allow rubber stethoscope tubing to touch person.

  Do not inject through rubber parts (e.g., heparin locks); use syringe and stopcock.

  Change needles after each puncture of rubber stopper.

  Cover rubber parts with tape.

Teach what products are commonly made of latex:

Health care equipment:

NRL gloves, powdered or unpowdered, including those labeled "hypoallergenic"

Blood pressure cuffs

Stethoscopes

Tourniquets

Electrode pads

Airways, endotracheal tubes

Syringe plunges, bulb syringes

Masks for anesthesia

Rubber aprons

Catheters, wound drains

Injection ports

Tops of multidose vials

Adhesive tape

Ostomy pouches

Wheelchair cushions

Briefs with elastic
Pads for crutches

Office/household products:
Erasers
Rubber bands
Dishwashing gloves
Balloons
Condoms, diaphragms
Baby bottle nipples, pacifiers
Rubber balls and toys
Racquet handles, cycle grips
Tires
Hot water bottles
Carpeting
Shoe soles
Elastic in underwear
Rubber cement

Latex Allergy, Risk for

DEFINITION

Risk for Latex Allergy: The state in which an individual is at
risk for experiencing an immunoglobin E–mediated allergic
response to latex.

RISK FACTORS
Biopathophysiologic
Related to history of atopic eczema
Related to history of allergic rhinitis
Related to history of asthma

Treatment-Related
Related to frequent urinary catheterizations
Related to frequent rectal disimpaction removal
Related to frequent surgical procedures

Situational (Personal, Environmental)

Related to history of food allergy to banana, kiwi, avocado, tomato, raw potato, peach, chestnuts, mango, papaya, passion fruit

Food handler

History of allergy to gloves, condoms, etc.

Frequent occupational exposure to natural rubber latex, such as:

Health care workers

Food handlers

Workers making NRL
  products

Housekeepers

Greenhouse workers

Loneliness, Risk for

DEFINITION

Risk for Loneliness: The state in which an individual is at risk for experiencing discomfort associated with a desire or need for contact with others.

> ⊚ **AUTHOR'S NOTE**
>
> *Risk for Loneliness* was added to the NANDA list in 1994. *Social Isolation* is also on the NANDA list. *Social Isolation* is a conceptually incorrect diagnosis because it does not represent a response but instead is the cause. *Loneliness* and *Risk for Loneliness* better describe the negative state of aloneness.
>
> Loneliness is a subjective state that exists whenever a person says it does and is perceived as imposed by others. Loneliness is *not* the result of voluntary solitude that is necessary for personal renewal, nor is it the creative aloneness of the artist or the initial aloneness one may experience as a result of seeking individualism and independence (e.g., moving to a new city, going away to college).

RISK FACTORS
See Related Factors.

RELATED FACTORS
Pathophysiologic
Related to fear of rejection secondary to:
Obesity
Cancer (disfiguring surgery of head or neck, superstitions
  of others)
Physical handicaps (paraplegia, amputation, arthritis,
  hemiplegia)
Emotional handicaps (extreme anxiety, depression, para-
  noia, phobias)
Incontinence (embarrassment, odor)
Communicable diseases (AIDS, hepatitis)
Psychiatric illness (schizophrenia, bipolar affective disorder,
  personality disorders)

**Related to difficulty accessing social events second-
ary to:**
Debilitating diseases
Physical disabilities

Treatment-Related
Related to therapeutic isolation

Situational (Personal, Environmental)
Related to insufficient planning for retirement
Related to death of a significant other
Related to divorce
Related to disfiguring appearance
**Related to fear of rejection secondary to: for example,
obesity, extreme poverty, hospitalization or terminal
illness (dying process), or unemployment**
**Related to moving to another culture (e.g., unfamiliar
language)**
**Related to history of unsatisfying social experiences
secondary to: drug abuse, alcohol abuse, immature
behavior, unacceptable social behavior, or delusional
thinking**
Related to loss of usual means of transportation
**Related to change in usual residence secondary to
long-term care or relocation**

Maturational

Child
Related to protective isolation or a communicable disease

Older Adult
Related to loss of usual social contacts secondary to retirement, relocation, death of (specify), or loss of driving ability

NOC Loneliness, Social Development

Goals

The person will report decreased feelings of loneliness.

Indicators

- Identify the reasons for feelings of isolation.
- Discuss ways of increasing meaningful relationships.

NIC Socialization Enhancement, Spiritual Support, Behavior Modification: Social Skills, Presence, Anticipatory Guidance

Generic Interventions

The nursing interventions for a variety of contributing factors that might be associated with a diagnosis of *Risk for Loneliness* are very similar.

Identify Causative and Contributing Factors.

Reduce or Eliminate Causative and Contributing Factors:
Promote social interaction.
Support the individual who has experienced a loss as he or she works through grief (see *Grieving*).
Validate the normalcy of grieving.
Encourage the person to talk about feelings of loneliness and the reasons they exist.
Mobilize the person's support system of neighbors and friends.
Discuss the importance of quality socialization rather than a great number of interactions.

Refer to social skills teaching (see *Social Interaction, Impaired*).

Offer feedback on how the person presents himself or herself to others (see *Social Interactions, Impaired*).

Decrease barriers to social contact.

Determine available transportation in the community (public, church-related, volunteer).

Determine if person must be taught how to use alternate transportation (e.g., drive a car).

Identify activities that help keep people busy, especially during times of high risk of loneliness (see *Deficient Diversional Activity*).

Assist with the development of alternate means of communication for persons with compromised sensory ability (e.g., amplifier on phone; see *Impaired Communication*).

Assist with the management of aesthetic problems (e.g., consult enterostomal therapist if odor is a problem).

Assist the person in locating stores that sell clothing especially made for those who have had disfiguring surgery (e.g., mastectomy).

Refer to *Impaired Urinary Elimination* for specific interventions to control incontinence.

For individuals with poor or offensive social skills.

Engage in one-to-one social dialogue. Explain the difference between casual and meaningful conversation.

Discuss the characteristics of meaningful conversation:

Initiating interactions

Being spontaneous

Being alert

Showing interest

Giving and receiving compliments

Showing interest in others, in activities

Requesting help when needed

Using increased eye contact

Using appropriate speech tone and nonverbal behavior

Allow person opportunities to observe others engaged in meaningful conversation.

Observe the person socializing, and discuss the interactions after. Offer praise. Gently discuss alternative approaches. Role-play skills.

Initiate Referrals as Indicated:
Community-based groups that contact the socially isolated
Self-help groups for clients isolated due to specific medical
  problems (Reach to Recovery, United Ostomy Association)
Wheelchair groups
Psychiatric consumer rights associations

⊙ Geriatric Interventions
**Discuss the Anticipated Effects of
Retirement on the Person's Life.
Assist with Planning (Stanley &
Beare, 2000):**
Plan to ensure adequate income.
Decrease time at work the last 2 to 3 years (e.g., shorter
  days, longer vacations).
Cultivate friends outside of work
Develop routines at home to replace work structure.
Rely on others rather than spouse for leisure activities.
Cultivate leisure activities that are realistic (energy,
  cost).
Prepare self for ambivalent feelings and short-term nega-
  tive impact on self-esteem.

**Identify Strategies to Expand the
World of the Isolated:**
Senior centers and church groups
Foster grandparent program
Day care centers for the elderly
Retirement communities
House sharing, group homes
College classes open to older persons
Pets
Telephone contact
Psychiatric day hospital or activity program

**Identify Community Sources
for Socialization.**

**Refer to Transportation Services
if Needed.**

Therapeutic Regimen Management, Effective Individual

DEFINITION

Effective Individual Therapeutic Regimen Management: A pattern in which the individual integrates into daily living a program for treatment of illness and its sequelae that is satisfactory for meeting health goals.

ⓧ AUTHOR'S NOTE

Effective Individual Therapeutic Regimen Management describes an individual who is successfully managing an illness or condition. The concept of enhanced is appropriate. The nurse can assist the person to enhance his or her management. The focus would be one of anticipatory guidance (e.g., teaching the person what events could negatively impact his or her management and how to reduce the negative impact).

This diagnosis does not need related factors. Writing related factors would only repeat the characteristics of persons who manage their conditions well (e.g., motivated, knowledgeable).

DEFINING CHARACTERISTICS

Appropriate choices of daily activities for meeting the goals of a treatment or prevention program

Illness symptoms within a normal range of expectation

Verbalization of desire to manage the treatment of illness and prevention of sequelae

Verbalization of intent to reduce risk factors for progression or illness and sequelae

RELATED FACTORS

Refer to Author's Note for an explanation.

NOC Compliance Behavior, Knowledge: Treatment Regimen, Participation: Health Care Decisions, Risk Control

Goals

The person will describe strategies to address progression or complication of his or her condition if it should arise.

Indicators

- Discuss situations that can challenge his or her continued successful management.
- Describe or demonstrate self-care techniques needed.

> **NIC** Behavior Modification, Mutual Goal Setting, Teaching: Individual, Decision-Making Support, Health System Guidance, Anticipatory Guidance

Generic Interventions

Discuss Possible Changes in Person's Condition that May Affect the Usual Management.

Exacerbation
Complications
Side effects of medication

Advise Early Contact with Care Provider to Discuss Possible Changes in Management Regimen.

Discuss How Increased Levels of Stress Can Negatively Affect Previous Successful Management and Possibly Decrease Resistance to Colds or Influenza.

Explore with the Person His or Her Evaluation of the Level of Stress with Which He or She Usually Lives.

Usual level of stress
Signs of overload

Discuss that Stress Comes with Favorable and Unfavorable Life

Events (e.g., Marriage, Divorce, Birth, Death, Vacations, Work).

When Faced with Upcoming Additional Stresses, Plan to:

Reduce stress in other aspects of life, if possible.
Increase adherence to healthy habits:
  Sleep 7 to 8 hours.
  Eat breakfast.
  Exercise daily (at least a 30-minute brisk walk).
  Eliminate or minimize alcohol intake.
  Increase intake of complex carbohydrates/fiber.
  Decrease intake of fat.
  Decrease caffeine intake.
Increase spiritually related activities:
  Meditation
  Listening to relaxing music
  Nature walks (e.g., woods, near water, mountains).
  Reading poetry

Initiate Health Teaching and Referrals Regarding Stress-Reduction Techniques.

Therapeutic Regimen Management, Ineffective

Therapeutic Regimen Management, Ineffective Family

Therapeutic Regimen Management, Ineffective Community

Therapeutic Regimen Management, Ineffective

DEFINITION

Ineffective Therapeutic Regimen Management: A pattern in which the individual experiences or is at risk to experience difficulty integrating into daily living a program for treatment of illness and the sequelae of illness and reduction of risk situations (e.g., unsafe, pollution).

☞ AUTHOR'S NOTE

Ineffective Therapeutic Regimen Management is a useful diagnosis for nurses in most settings. Individuals and families experiencing a variety of health problems, acute or chronic, are usually faced with treatment programs that require changes in previous functioning or lifestyle. These regimens are activities or habits of medication therapy, treatments, diet, exercise, stress management, problem-solving, symptom management, and other strategies that improve health and well-being.

This diagnosis describes individuals or families who are experiencing difficulty in achieving positive outcomes. The nurse is the primary professional who, with the client, determines what choices are available and how success can be achieved. The primary nursing interventions are exploring available options with the client and family and teaching the client how to implement the selected option.

When an individual is faced with a complex regimen to follow or has compromised functioning that impedes

---

> ⊕ **AUTHOR'S NOTE (continued)**
>
> successful management, the diagnosis *Risk for Ineffective Therapeutic Regimen Management* is appropriate. In addition to teaching the client how to manage the regimen, the nurse must also assist him or her to identify the adjustments needed because of a functional deficit. *Risk for Ineffective Therapeutic Regimen Management* is a useful diagnosis for discharge teaching.

DEFINING CHARACTERISTICS
Major (Must be Present, One or More)
Verbalized desire to manage the treatment of illness and prevention of sequelae

Verbalized difficulty with regulation/integration of one or more prescribed regimens for treatment of illness and its effects or for prevention of complications

Minor (May be Present)
Acceleration (expected or unexpected) of illness symptoms

Verbalization that client did not take action to include treatment regimens in daily routines

Verbalization that client did not take action to reduce risk factors for progression of illness and sequelae

RELATED FACTORS
Treatment-Related
Related to:
Complexity of therapeutic regimen
Financial cost of regimen
Complexity of health care system
Side effects of therapy
Unfamiliar treatments or techniques

Situational (Personal, Environmental)
Related to:
Decisional conflicts
Insufficient knowledge
Family conflicts
Mistrust of regimen
Mistrust of health care personnel
Health belief conflicts

Questions about seriousness of problem
Questions about susceptibility
Questions about benefits of regimen
Insufficient social support
Insufficient confidence
Previous unsuccessful experiences

Related to barriers to comprehension secondary to:

Cognitive deficits	Fatigue
Hearing impairments	Motivation
Anxiety	Memory problems

Maturational
Child, Adolescent
Related to fear of being different

 NOC Compliance Behavior, Knowledge: Treatment Regimen, Participation: Health Care Decisions, Treatment Behavior: Illness or Dying

Goals

The person/family will relate an intent to practice health behaviors needed or desired for recovery from illness and prevention of recurrence or complications.

Indicators

- Relate less anxiety related to fear of the unknown, fear of loss of control, or misconceptions.
- Describe disease process, causes, and factors contributing to symptoms, and the regimen for disease or symptom control.

Generic Interventions

Identify Causative or Contributing Factors that Impede Effective Management:

Lack of trust
Insufficient confidence (self-efficacy)
Insufficient knowledge
Insufficient resources

Build Trust and Strength
(Zerwich, 1992).

Gain entrance to family system. Do not take over.

Avoid impression of pressuring.

Listen to discover concerns, not to impose expectations.

Attempt to discover a match between expressed needs and services the nurse can provide.

Discover and affirm strengths.

Accept persons where they are.

Demonstrate persistence, but proceed slowly.

Demonstrate honesty, consistency, stability.

Maintain preestablished contacts in person or by phone.

Promote Confidence and Positive
Self-Efficacy (Bandura, 1982).

Explore past successful management of problems.

Tell stories of other successes.

If appropriate, encourage opportunities to witness others successfully coping in a similar situation.

Encourage participation in self-help groups.

If high autonomic response (e.g., rapid pulse, diaphoresis) is reducing feeling of confidence, teach short-term anxiety interrupters (Grainger, 1990).

  Look up.

  Control breathing.

  Lower shoulders.

  Slow thoughts.

  Alter voice.

  Give self-directions (out loud, if possible).

  Exercise.

  "Scruff your face"—change facial expression.

  Change perspective (imagine watching the situation from a distance).

Identify Factors that
Influence Learning.

Perception of seriousness

Susceptibility to complications

Prognosis

Perception of control of progression

Level of anxiety

Financial status

Support system

Past experiences

Physical status
Emotional status
Cognitive ability

Promote a Positive Attitude and Active Participation of the Person and Family.

Solicit expressions of feelings, concerns, and questions from person and family.
Encourage person/family to seek information and make informed decisions.
Explain responsibilities of person/family and how these can be assumed.

Explain and Discuss:

Disease process
Treatment regimen (medications, diet, procedures, exercises, equipment use)
Rationale of regimen
Expectations (client, family) of regimen
Side effects of regimen
Lifestyle changes needed
Methods to monitor condition
Follow-up care needed
Signs or symptoms of complications
Resources, support available
Home environment alterations needed

Explain that Changes in Lifestyle and Needed Learning Will Take Time to Integrate.

Provide printed material.
Explain whom to contact with questions.

Identify Referrals or Community Services Needed for Follow-Up.

Geriatric Interventions

To Promote Learning:
Avoid times of day when fatigued.
Reduce distractions.

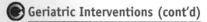

🜨 Geriatric Interventions (cont'd)

Relate information to prior experiences.
Use visual cues.
Provide outlines prior to class.

Allow Person to Self-Pace the Learning.

Create a List of Cues to Organize Activities.

Therapeutic Regimen Management, Ineffective Family

DEFINITION

Ineffective Family Therapeutic Regimen Management: A pattern in which the family experiences or is at risk to experience difficulty integrating into daily living a program for treatment of illness and the sequelae of illness and reduction of risk situations (e.g., safety, pollution).

> ☺ AUTHOR'S NOTE
>
> Refer to *Ineffective Therapeutic Regimen Management.*

DEFINING CHARACTERISTICS
Major

Inappropriate family activities for meeting the goals of a treatment or prevention program

Minor

Acceleration (expected or unexpected) of illness symptoms of a family member

Lack of attention to illness and its sequelae

Verbalization of desire to manage the treatment of illness and prevention of sequelae

Verbalization of difficulty with regulation/integration of one or more prescribed regimens for treatment of illness and its effects or prevention of complications

Verbalization that family did not take action to reduce risk factors for progression of illness and sequelae

RELATED FACTORS

Refer to *Ineffective Therapeutic Regimen Management.*

Generic Interventions

Refer to *Ineffective Therapeutic Regimen Management.*

Therapeutic Regimen Management, Ineffective Community

DEFINITION

Ineffective Community Therapeutic Regimen Management: A pattern in which the community experiences or is at high risk to experience difficulty integrating a program for prevention/treatment of illness and the sequelae of illness and reduction of risk situations (e.g., safety, pollution).

◯◯ AUTHOR'S NOTE

This diagnosis describes a community that has evidence that a population is underserved because of insufficient availability of, access to, or knowledge of health care re-

⊗ **AUTHOR'S NOTE (continued)**

sources. The community nurse, using the results of a community assessment, can identify at-risk groups and overall community needs. In addition, the nurse will assess health systems, transportation, social services, and access.

DEFINING CHARACTERISTICS
Major
Verbalized difficulty in meeting health needs in communities
Acceleration (expected or unexpected) of illness(es)
Morbidity, mortality rates above the norm

RELATED FACTORS
Situational (Environmental)
Related to availability of community programs for (specify):

Prevention of diseases   Screening for diseases
Immunizations   Dental care
Accident prevention   Fire safety
Smoking cessation   Substance abuse
Alcohol abuse   Child abuse

Related to problem accessing program secondary to, for example, inadequate communication, limited hours, no transportation, insufficient funds
Related to complexity of population's needs
Related to lack of awareness of availability
Related to presence of environmental or occupational health hazards
Related to multiple needs of vulnerable groups (specify):
Homeless
Pregnant teenagers
Persons living below poverty level
Home-bound individuals

Related to unavailable or insufficient health care agencies

Goals

The community will promote the use of community resources for health problems.

Indicators

- Identify community resources that are needed.
- Participate in program development as needed.

Generic Interventions

Create a Survey to Determine:

Health problem identification
Awareness of health services
Use of health services
Interest in health-promotion programs
Recommendation for funding sources

Survey Samples of the Target Population:

Mail survey
One-to-one survey at community center, sports field, supermarket
Group survey (e.g., church groups, clubs)
Survey of key community leaders

Design the Survey for Easy Reading and Answering (e.g., Circle the Number that Best Describes Your Answer: 1—No Concern; 2—Medium; 3—High).

How concerned are you about, e.g.:
Hypertension
Stress
Alcohol misuse

Violence
Nutrition
HIV

Organize the Response Data.

Analyze the Findings.

What are the overall health problems reported?
What are the health concerns of:
  Elderly population
  Households with children up to age 20 years
  Single-parent households
  Respondents younger than 45 years
  Individuals below the poverty level

Evaluate Community Resources.

What resources are available for the health problems
  identified?
Are there use or access problems with the services?
How does the population know of services?
Identify problems that do not have community services
  available.

**If Services Are Available but Are
Underused, Evaluate:**

Hours of operation (convenient?)
Location of services (access, esthetics)
Efficiency and atmosphere
Advertising strategies

**If Services Are Unavailable, Pursue
Program Development.**

Examine and evaluate similar programs in other
  communities:
  Basic information
  Purpose, goals
  Services available
  Funding
  Cost to participants
  Availability of services
  Accessibility of services
  Satisfaction (citizen, employees)
Meet with appropriate persons to discuss findings (survey,
  on-site visits).

Address the following:
   Presence of community support
   Available expertise and technology in community
   Financial support
Identify appropriate community sources of assistance
   (e.g., hospital departments, schools of nursing, private
   foundations).
Plan the program (refer to *Readiness for Enhanced
   Community Coping* for interventions for community
   planning).

**Evaluate Vulnerable Population's
Access to Health Care and Knowledge
of Risk Factors.**

Rural families, elderly
Migrant workers
New immigrants
Homeless
Individuals and groups below the poverty level

**Make a Priority of Ensuring that Basic
Needs for Food, Shelter, Clothing, and
Safety Are Met before Attempting to
Address Higher Health Needs.**

**Provide Information Regarding
Illness Prevention, Health Promotion,
and Health Services to
Vulnerable Populations.**

Mobility, Impaired Physical
Bed Mobility, Impaired
Walking, Impaired
Wheelchair Mobility, Impaired
Wheelchair Transfer Ability, Impaired

Mobility, Impaired Physical

DEFINITION

Impaired Physical Mobility: The state in which an individual experiences or is at risk of experiencing limitation of physical movement but is not immobile.

> ### ⊗ AUTHOR'S NOTE
>
> *Impaired Physical Mobility* describes an individual with limited use of arm(s) or leg(s) or limited muscle strength. *Impaired Physical Mobility* should not be used to describe complete immobility; instead, *Disuse Syndrome* is more applicable. Limitation of physical movement can also be the etiology of other nursing diagnoses, such as *Self-Care Deficit* or *Risk for Injury*.
>
> Nursing interventions for *Impaired Physical Mobility* focus on strengthening and restoring function and preventing deterioration.

DEFINING CHARACTERISTICS
(Levin et al., 1989)
Major (80% to 100%)

Compromised ability to move purposefully within the environment (e.g., bed mobility, transfers, ambulation)
Range-of-motion (ROM) limitations

Minor (50% to 80%)

Imposed restriction of movement

Reluctance to move

RELATED FACTORS
Pathophysiologic
Related to decreased strength and endurance secondary to:

Neuromuscular impairment

Autoimmune alterations (e.g., multiple sclerosis, arthritis)

Nervous system diseases (e.g., parkinsonism, myasthenia gravis)

Muscular dystrophy

Partial or total paralysis (e.g., spinal cord injury, stroke)

Central nervous system tumor

Increased intracranial pressure

Sensory deficits

Musculoskeletal impairment

Fractures

Connective tissue disease (systemic lupus erythematosus)

Related to edema (increased synovial fluid)

Treatment-Related
Related to external devices (casts or splints, braces, intravenous tubing).

Related to insufficient strength and endurance for ambulation with (specify; e.g., prosthesis, crutches, walker)

Situational (Personal, Environmental)
Related to fatigue, decreased motivation, or pain

Maturational
Children

Related to abnormal gait secondary to:

Congenital skeletal deficiencies

Osteomyelitis

Congenital hip dysplasia

Legg-Calvé-Perthes disease

Older Adults

Related to decreased motor agility or muscle weakness

NOC Ambulation: Walking, Joint Movement: Active, Mobility Level

Goals

The person will report an increase in strength and endurance of limbs.

Indicators

- Demonstrate the use of adaptive devices to increase mobility.
- Use safety measures to minimize potential for injury.
- Describe rationale for interventions.
- Demonstrate measures to increase mobility.

NIC Exercise Therapy: Joint Mobility, Exercise Promotion: Strength Training, Exercise Therapy: Ambulation, Positioning, Teaching: Prescribed Activity: Exercise, Teaching: Assistance Device, Teaching: Safety

Generic Interventions

Refer to *Disuse Syndrome* for Interventions to Prevent the Complications of Immobility.

Teach to Perform active ROM Exercises on Unaffected Limbs at Least Four Times a Day.

Perform passive ROM exercises on affected limbs.
   Perform slowly.
   Support the extremity above and below the joint.
Gradually progress from active ROM to functional activities.

Position in Alignment to Prevent Complications.

Use a foot board.
Avoid prolonged periods of sitting or lying in the same position.
Change position of the shoulder joints every 2 to 4 hours.
Use a small pillow or no pillow when in Fowler's position.
Support the hand and wrist in natural alignment.
If the client is supine or prone, place a rolled towel or small pillow under the lumbar curvature or under the end of the rib cage.

Place a trochanter roll or sandbags alongside the hips and upper thighs.

If the client is in the lateral position, place pillow(s) to support the leg from groin to foot and a pillow to flex the shoulder and elbow slightly; if needed, support the lower foot in dorsal flexion with a sandbag.

Use hand and wrist splints.

Provide Progressive Mobilization.*

Assist slowly to sitting position.

Allow to dangle legs over the side of the bed for a few minutes before standing.

Limit the time to 15 minutes, three times a day, the first few times out of bed.

Increase time out of bed, as tolerated, by 15-minute increments.

Progress to ambulation, with or without assistive devices.

If client is unable to walk, assist out of bed to a wheelchair or chair.

Encourage ambulation for short, frequent walks (at least three times daily), with assistance if unsteady.

Increase lengths of walks progressively each day.

Observe and Teach the Use of:

Crutches

No pressure should be exerted on axilla; hand strength should be used.

Type of gait varies with diagnosis.

Measure crutches 2 to 3 inches below axilla and tips 6 inches away from feet.

Walkers

Use arm strength to support weakness in lower limbs.

Gait varies with individual's problems.

Wheelchairs

Practice transfers.

Practice maneuvering around barriers.

Prostheses

Stump wrapping before application of the prosthesis.

Application of the prosthesis.

---

*This may require a primary care professional's order.

Principles of stump care.

Importance of cleaning the stump, keeping it dry, and applying the prosthesis only when the stump is dry.

Slings

Assess for correct application; sling should be loose around neck and should support elbow and wrist above level of the heart.

Remove slings for ROM.

Ace bandages

Observe for correct position.

Apply with even pressure, wrapping distally to proximally.

Observe for bunching.

Observe for signs of skin irritation (redness, ulceration) or tightness (compression).

Rewrap twice per day or as needed unless contraindicated (e.g., if bandage is postoperative compression dressing, check physician's orders).

Teach Safety Precautions.

Protect areas of decreased sensation from extremes of heat and cold.

Practice falling and how to recover from falls while transferring or ambulating.

For decreased perception of lower extremity (post-CVA "neglect"), instruct the individual to check where limb is placed when changing positions or going through doorways; check to make sure that both shoes are tied, that affected leg is dressed with trousers, and that pants are not dragging.

Instruct individuals who are confined to wheelchair to shift position and lift up buttocks every 15 minutes to relieve pressure; maneuver curbs, ramps, inclines, and around obstacles; and lock wheelchair before transferring.

Encourage Use of Affected Arm When Possible.

Encourage the person to use affected arm for self-care activities (e.g., feeding, dressing, brushing hair).

For post-CVA neglect of upper limb, see also *Unilateral Neglect*.

Instruct the person to use unaffected arm to exercise the affected arm.

Use appropriate adaptive equipment to enhance the use of
arms:

Universal cuff for feeding in individuals who have poor
control in both arms, hands.

Large-handled or padded silverware to assist individuals
with poor fine-motor skills.

Dishware with high edges to prevent food from
slipping.

Suction-cup aids to hold dishes in place and prevent slid-
ing of plate.

Use a warm bath to alleviate early morning stiffness
and improve mobility.

Have Person Demonstrate:

Strengthening exercises
ROM exercises
Care of adaptive devices
Safety precautions

Impaired Bed Mobility

DEFINITION

Impaired Bed Mobility: The state in which an individual
experiences, or is at risk of experiencing, limitation of movement in bed.

⊚ AUTHOR'S NOTE

Impaired Bed Mobility is a clinically useful diagnosis
when an individual is a candidate for rehabilitation to
improve strength, range of motion, and movement. The
nurse could consult with a physical therapist for a specific plan for the individual. This diagnosis would be
inappropriate for an unconscious or terminally ill person.

DEFINING CHARACTERISTICS

Impaired ability to turn from side to side
Impaired ability to move from supine to sitting or from sitting to supine
Impaired ability to "scoot" or reposition self in bed
Impaired ability to move from supine to prone or from prone to supine
Impaired ability to move from supine to long sitting or from long sitting to supine

RELATED FACTORS

Refer to *Impaired Physical Mobility*.

Goals

Refer to *Impaired Physical Mobility*.

Generic Interventions

Refer to *Impaired Physical Mobility*.

Impaired Walking

DEFINITION

Impaired Walking: The state in which an individual experiences or is at risk of experiencing limitation in walking.

DEFINING CHARACTERISTICS

Impaired ability to climb stairs
Impaired ability to walk required distances
Impaired ability to walk on an incline
Impaired ability to walk on uneven surfaces
Impaired ability to navigate curbs

RELATED FACTORS

Refer to *Impaired Physical Mobility.*

Goals

The person will increase walking distances (specify distance goal).

Indicators

- Demonstrate safe mobility.
- Use mobility aids correctly.

Generic Interventions

Explain that Safe Ambulation Is a Complete Movement Involving the Musculoskeletal, Neurologic, and Cardiovascular Systems and Cognitive Factors Such As Mentation and Orientation.

If the Person Is Deconditioned, a Progressive Program of Exercise Is Needed; Consult with Physical Therapist for an Evaluation and Plan.

Ascertain that Ambulatory Aids Are Being Used Correctly and Safely (e.g., Cane, Walker, Crutches).

Wears well-fitting, firm shoes

Can ambulate on inclines, uneven surfaces, and up and down stairs

Is aware of hazards (e.g., wet floors, throw rugs)

Provide Progressive Mobilization If Indicated:

Assist slowly to a sitting position.

Allow to dangle legs over the side of the bed for a few minutes before standing.

Limit the time to 15 minutes, three times a day, the first few times out of bed.

Increase time out of bed, as tolerated, by 15-minute increments.

Progress to ambulation, with or without assistive devices.

If client is unable to walk, assist out of bed to a wheelchair or chair.

Encourage ambulation for short, frequent walks (at least three times daily), with assistance if unsteady.

Increase lengths of walks progressively each day.

Evaluate Response to Ambulation.
Refer to *Activity Intolerance,* **if needed.**

Impaired Wheelchair Mobility

DEFINITION

Impaired Wheelchair Mobility: The state in which an individual experiences or is at risk of experiencing difficulty with wheelchair mobility and safety.

DEFINING CHARACTERISTICS

Impaired ability to operate manual or power wheelchair on even or uneven surface

Impaired ability to operate manual or power wheelchair on an incline

Impaired ability to operate wheelchair on curbs

RELATED FACTORS

Refer to *Impaired Physical Mobility.*

Goals

The person will report satisfactory, safe wheelchair mobility.

Indicators

- Demonstrate safe use of wheelchair.
- Demonstrate safe transfer to wheelchair.

Generic Interventions

Determine Factors that Are Interfering with Proper Wheelchair Use.
Knowledge
Strength
Mentation

Consult with Physical Therapist if Strengthening Exercises Are Indicated.

Teach Transfer Techniques.
Weight-bearing
Non–weight-bearing

Have Person Demonstrate Technique and Evaluate Effectiveness and Safety.

Impaired Wheelchair Transfer Ability

DEFINITION

Impaired Wheelchair Transfer Ability: The state in which an individual experiences or is at risk of experiencing difficulty with transfer to and from the wheelchair.

DEFINING CHARACTERISTICS

Impaired ability to transfer from bed to chair and from chair to bed

Impaired ability to transfer on or off a toilet or commode

Impaired ability to transfer in and out of tub or shower

Impaired ability to transfer between uneven levels

Impaired ability to transfer from chair to car or from car to chair

Impaired ability to transfer from chair to floor or from floor to chair

Impaired ability to transfer from standing to floor or from floor to standing

RELATED FACTORS

Refer to *Impaired Physical Mobility*.

NOC Transfer Performance

Goals

The person will demonstrate transfer to and from wheelchair.

Indicators

- Identify when assistance is needed.
- Demonstrate ability to transfer in varied situations (e.g., toilet, bed, car, chair, uneven levels).

NIC (See also Impaired Physical Mobility), Positioning: Wheelchair

Generic Interventions

Explain that safe ambulation is a complete movement involving the musculoskeletal, neurologic, and cardiovascular systems and cognitive factors such as mentation and orientation.

If the person is deconditioned, a progressive program of exercise is needed; consult with physical therapist for an evaluation and plan.

Explain that one should always transfer toward the unaffected side.

Determine whether an assisted device is needed (e.g., walking belt with handles, mechanical lift, transfer sheets).

Consult with physical therapist to determine how much assistance is needed:

   Requires no assistance

   Requires only verbal cuing

   Support by clinician's hand if additional help is needed

   Requires physical assistance

   Needs mechanical device to execute transfer (e.g., lifts)

Advise that ability may fluctuate and to request assistance to prevent injury.

Noncompliance

DEFINITION

Noncompliance: The state in which an individual or group desires to comply, but factors are present that deter adherence to agreed-upon health-related advice given by health professionals.

> ### ⊛ AUTHOR'S NOTE
>
> *Noncompliance* describes the individual who desires to comply, but the presence of certain factors prevents him or her from doing so. The nurse must attempt to reduce or eliminate these factors for the interventions to be successful. However, the nurse is cautioned against using the diagnosis of *Noncompliance* to describe an individual who has made an informed, autonomous decision not to participate. Behaviors may be acts of omission or commission and may be intentional or unintentional (Brandt et al., 1997).

DEFINING CHARACTERISTICS

Major (Must be Present)

Verbalization of difficulty with compliance or confusion about therapy *or*

Minor (May be Present)

Missed appointments
Partially used or unused medications
Persistence of symptoms
Progression of disease process
Occurrence of undesired outcomes (postoperative morbidity, pregnancy, obesity, addiction, regression during rehabilitation)

RELATED FACTORS
Pathophysiologic
Related to impaired ability to perform tasks because of disability secondary to (e.g., poor memory, motor and sensory deficits)

Related to increasing amount of disease-related symptoms despite adherence to advised regimen

Treatment-Related
Related to:
Side effects of therapy
Previous unsuccessful experiences with advised regimen
Impersonal aspects of referral process
Nontherapeutic environment
Cost of therapy
Complex unsupervised or prolonged therapy
Financial cost of therapy

Situational (Personal, Environmental)
Related to barriers to access secondary to:
Mobility problems
Financial issues
Lack of child care
Transportation problems
Inclement weather

Related to concurrent illness of family member
Related to nonsupportive family, peers, community
Related to barriers to care secondary to homelessness
Related to barriers to comprehension secondary to:

Cognitive deficits	Visual deficits
Hearing deficits	Poor memory
Anxiety	Fatigue
Decreased attention span	Motivation

Related to perception of seriousness and susceptibility

NOC Adherence Behavior, Compliance Behavior, Symptom Control, Treatment Behavior: Illness/Dying

Goals

The person will report a desire to change or initiate change.

Indicators

- Describe reasons for suggested regimen.
- Identify barriers to adhering to regimen.

> **NIC**   Health Education, Self-Modification Assistance, Self-Responsibility Facilitation, Coping Enhancement, Decision Making Support, Health System Guidance, Mutual Goal Setting, Teaching: Disease Process

Generic Interventions

Using Open-Ended Questions, Encourage Person to Talk about Experiences with Health Care (e.g., Hospitalizations, Family Deaths, Diagnostic Tests, Blood Tests, X-Ray Tests).

Ask Client Directly, "What Are Your Concerns About:

taking this drug?"
following this diet?"
having a blood test?"
going through the cystoscopy?"
having your gallbladder removed?"
using a diaphragm?"
paying for the operation?"

Explore the Person's Understanding of the Problem and His or Her Expectations of Treatment and of Outcomes. Determine If Beliefs Are Realistic and Correct.

Assess Problematic Factors of Prescribed Therapy (e.g., Time, Cost, Complexity, Convenience, Adverse Effects).

Assess Person for Recent Changes in Lifestyle (Personal, Work, Family, Health, Financial).

Assist to Reduce Side Effects, If Possible.

For gastric irritation, suggest that drug be taken with milk
or food; it may be advisable to eat yogurt (unless contraindicated).

For drowsiness, take medication at bedtime or late in
afternoon; consult physician for dose reduction.

**Discuss the Risks and Benefits of
Adhering to the Prescribed Regimen.**

**Affirm Client's Right to Refuse All or
Part of the Prescribed Regimen.**

**Nutrition, Imbalanced:
   Less than Body Requirements**
Impaired Dentition
Impaired Swallowing
Ineffective Infant Feeding Pattern

**Nutrition, Imbalanced:
Less Than Body Requirements**

DEFINITION

Imbalanced Nutrition: Less Than Body Requirements: The
state in which an individual, who is not NPO, experiences or
is at risk for inadequate intake or metabolism of nutrients
for metabolic needs with or without weight loss.

> ∞ **AUTHOR'S NOTE**
>
> This diagnosis describes individuals who can ingest food
> but have an intake of less-than-adequate amounts. This

⊚ **AUTHOR'S NOTE (continued)**

diagnosis should not be used to describe individuals who are NPO or cannot ingest food. These situations should be described by the collaborative problems of

Potential Complication:
  Electrolyte imbalances
  Negative nitrogen balance

Nurses monitor to detect complications of an NPO state and confer with physicians for parenteral therapy. Some nursing diagnoses that may relate to an individual who is NPO are *Risk for Impaired Oral Mucous Membrane* and *Impaired Comfort*.

DEFINING CHARACTERISTICS
Major (Must be Present, One or More)
One who is not NPO reports or has: inadequate food intake less than recommended daily allowance with or without weight loss *or*
Actual or potential metabolic needs in excess of intake

Minor (May be Present)
Weight 10% to 20% or more below ideal for height and frame
Triceps skinfold, midarm circumference, and midarm muscle circumference less than 60% standard measurement
Muscle weakness and tenderness
Mental irritability or confusion
Decreased serum prealbumin
Decreased serum transferrin or iron-binding capacity

RELATED FACTORS
Pathophysiologic
Related to increased caloric requirements and difficulty in ingesting sufficient calories secondary to burns (postacute phase), infection, chemical dependence, cancer, or trauma
Related to dysphagia secondary to:

CVA	Parkinson's disease
Amyotrophic lateral sclerosis	Neuromuscular disorders
Cerebral palsy	Muscular dystrophy
	AIDS

Related to decreased absorption of nutrients secondary to Crohn's disease, cystic fibrosis, or lactose intolerance

Related to decreased desire to eat secondary to altered level of consciousness

Related to self-induced vomiting, physical exercise in excess of caloric intake, or refusal to eat secondary to anorexia nervosa

Related to reluctance to eat for fear of poisoning secondary to paranoid behavior

Related to anorexia, excessive physical agitation secondary to bipolar disorder

Related to anorexia and diarrhea secondary to protozoal infection

Related to vomiting, anorexia, and impaired digestion secondary to pancreatitis

Related to anorexia, impaired protein and fat metabolism, and impaired storage of vitamins secondary to cirrhosis

Treatment-Related

Related to increased protein and vitamin requirements for wound healing and decreased intake secondary to: surgery, medications (cancer chemotherapy), surgical reconstruction of the mouth, wired jaw, or radiation therapy

Related to inadequate absorption as a side effect of (specify):

Colchicine	Neomycin
Pyrimethamine	Para-aminosalicylic acid
Antacid	

Related to decreased oral intake, mouth discomfort, nausea, vomiting secondary to: radiation therapy, chemotherapy, or tonsillectomy

Situational (Personal, Environmental)

Related to decreased desire to eat secondary to: anorexia, depression, stress, social isolation, nausea and vomiting, or allergies

Related to inability to procure food (physical limitations, financial or transportation problems)

Related to inability to chew (damaged or missing teeth, ill-fitting dentures)
Related to diarrhea secondary to (specify)

Maturational

Infant/Child
Related to inadequate intake secondary to: lack of emotional/sensory stimulation or lack of knowledge of caregiver
Related to malabsorption, dietary restrictions, and anorexia secondary to celiac disease, lactose intolerance, or cystic fibrosis
Related to sucking difficulties (infant) and dysphagia secondary to: cerebral palsy or cleft lip and palate
Related to inadequate sucking, fatigue, and dyspnea secondary to: congenital heart disease or prematurity

Older Adult
Related to effects of declining metabolic rate, estrogen levels, and bone mineral density (women)
Related to degeneration of periodontal membrane with loose teeth

---

NOC Nutritional Status, Teaching: Nutrition

Goals

The person will ingest daily nutritional requirements in accordance with his or her activity level and metabolic needs.

Indicators

- Relate importance of good nutrition.
- Identify deficiencies in daily intake.
- Relate methods to increase appetite.

NIC Nutrition Management, Nutrition Monitoring

Generic Interventions

Determine daily caloric requirements that are realistic and adequate. Consult with dietitian.

Weigh daily; monitor laboratory results.

Explain the importance of adequate nutrition. Negotiate with client intake goals for each meal and snacks.

Teach client to use spices to help improve the taste and aroma of food (lemon juice, mint, cloves, basil, thyme, cinnamon, rosemary, bacon bits).

Encourage client to eat with others (meals served in dining room or group area or at local meeting place, such as community center, by church groups).

Plan care so that unpleasant or painful procedures do not take place before meals.

Provide pleasant, relaxed atmosphere for eating (no bedpans in sight; do not rush); try a "surprise" (e.g., flowers with meal).

Arrange plan of care to decrease or eliminate nauseating odors or procedures near mealtimes.

Teach or assist client to rest before meals.

Teach client to avoid cooking odors—frying foods, brewing coffee—if possible (take a walk; select foods that can be eaten cold).

Maintain good oral hygiene (brush teeth, rinse mouth) before and after ingestion of food.

Offer frequent small feedings (six per day plus snacks) to reduce the feeling of a distended stomach.

Arrange to have highest protein/calorie nutrients served at the time client feels most like eating (e.g., if chemotherapy is in early morning, serve in late afternoon).

Instruct person with decreased appetite to:

Eat dry foods (toast, crackers) on arising.

Eat salty foods if permissible.

Avoid overly sweet, rich, greasy, or fried foods.

Try clear, cool beverages.

Sip slowly through straw.

Take whatever can be tolerated.

Eat small portions low in fat, and eat more frequently.

Try commercial supplements available in many forms (liquids, powder, pudding).

If person has an eating disorder (Townsend, 1994):

Establish intake goals with client, physician, and nutritionist.

Discuss the benefits of compliance and the consequences of nonadherence.

If intake is refused, notify physician.

Sit with person during meals. Limit meal times to 30 minutes.

Observe for at least 1 hour after meals. Accompany to bathroom.

Weigh on arising and after first voiding.

Provide reinforcement for improvement, but do not focus discussions on food or eating.

As person improves, explore issues of body image, weight gain, and control.

For a hyperactive person (Townsend, 1994):

Provide high-protein, high-calorie finger foods and drinks.

Offer frequent snacks. Avoid empty calories (e.g., soda).

Walk or pace with person as finger foods are eaten.

🅒 Geriatric Interventions

Evaluate Ability to Process and Prepare Food.

Finances
Transportation
Mobility
Manual dexterity

Explain Community Resources Available.

Meals on Wheels
Senior centers
Supermarkets that deliver

For Women Older Than 50 Years, Advise to:

Increase calcium intake to 1200 mg/d (1500 mg/d if not taking hormone replacement therapy).

Reduce calorie intake to 1700 to 1800.

Balance intake and exercise.

Include beta-carotene and vitamin C and E supplements daily.

Impaired Dentition

DEFINITION

Impaired Dentition: The state in which an individual experiences a disruption in tooth development/eruption patterns or structural integrity of individual teeth.

ⓧ AUTHOR'S NOTE

Impaired Dentition describes a multitude of problems with teeth. It is unclear how this diagnosis would be used by nurses or any health care professional. If the client has caries, abscesses, or misaligned or malformed teeth, the nurse would refer him or her to a dental professional. If the tooth problem is affecting comfort or nutrition, *Impaired Comfort* or *Imbalanced Nutrition* would be the appropriate nursing diagnosis.

DEFINING CHARACTERISTICS

Excessive plaque
Crown or root caries
Halitosis
Tooth enamel discoloration
Toothache
Loose teeth
Excessive calculus
Incomplete eruption for age (may be primary or permanent teeth)
Malocclusion or tooth misalignment
Premature loss of primary teeth
Worn-down or abraded teeth
Tooth fracture(s)
Missing teeth or complete absence
Erosion of enamel
Asymmetric facial expression

DEFINITION

Impaired Swallowing: The state in which an individual has decreased ability to voluntarily pass fluids or solid foods from the mouth to the stomach.

DEFINING CHARACTERISTICS
(Jeng et al., 2001)
Major (Must be Present)

Observed evidence of difficulty swallowing *or*
Stasis of food in oral cavity
Choking
Coughing after fluid/food intake

Minor (May be Present)

Slurred speech
Nasal-sounding voice
Drooling

RELATED FACTORS
Pathophysiologic
Related to decreased/absent gag reflex, mastication difficulties, or decreased sensations secondary to:
Cerebrovascular accident
Right or left hemispheric damage to the brain
Damage to the 5th, 7th, 9th, 10th, or 11th cranial nerves

Cerebral palsy
Muscular dystrophy
Amyotrophic lateral
  sclerosis
Parkinsonism
Myasthenia gravis
Guillain-Barré syndrome
Poliomyelitis

Related to tracheoesophageal tumors, edema
Related to irritated oropharyngeal cavity
Related to decreased saliva

Treatment-Related
Related to surgical reconstruction of the mouth, throat, jaw, and/or nose

Related to mechanical obstruction secondary to tracheostomy tube
Related to esophagitis secondary to radiotherapy
Related to decreased consciousness secondary to anesthesia
Related to increased viscosity and diminished quantity of saliva (e.g., secondary to medications, radiation)

Situational (Personal, Environmental)
Related to fatigue
Related to limited awareness, distractibility

Maturational
Infant/Children
Related to decreased sensations or difficulty with mastication
Refer to *Ineffective Infant Feeding Pattern.*

NOC Aspiration Control, Swallowing Status

Goals
The person will report improved ability to swallow.

Indicators
- Describe causative factors when known.
- Describe rationale and procedures for treatment.

NIC Aspiration Precautions, Swallowing Therapy, Surveillance, Referral, Positioning

Generic Interventions
Reduce the Possibility of Aspiration.
Before beginning feeding, assess that person is adequately alert and responsive, is able to control mouth, has cough/gag reflex, and can swallow own saliva.
Have suction equipment available and functioning properly.
Position correctly.

Sit upright (60 to 90 degrees) in chair or dangle feet at
side of bed if possible (prop pillows if necessary).

Assume position 10 to 15 minutes before eating, and
maintain position for 10 to 15 minutes after finishing
eating.

Flex head forward on the midline about 45 degrees to
keep esophagus patent.

Keep individual focused on task by giving directions until
he or she has finished swallowing each mouthful.

Start with small amounts, and progress slowly as person
learns to handle each step:

Ice chips

Part of eyedropper filled with water

Use juice in place of water

¼, ½, 1 teaspoon semisolid

Pureed food or commercial baby foods

One-half cracker

Soft diet/regular diet

**Assist with Moving the Bolus of Food
from the Anterior to the Posterior of
Mouth. Place Food in the Posterior
Mouth Where Swallowing Can
Be Ensured.**

Prevent/Decrease Thick Secretions.

**Progress to Ice Chips, Water, and Then
Food When Danger of Aspiration
is Decreased.**

**For Individuals with Impaired
Cognition or Awareness:**

Concentrate on solids rather than liquids, because liquids
are generally less well tolerated.

Keep extraneous stimuli at minimum while eating (e.g., no
television or radio, no verbal stimuli unless directed at
task).

Have person concentrate on task of swallowing.

Have person sit up in chair with neck slightly flexed.

Instruct person to hold breath while swallowing.

Observe for swallowing and check mouth for emptying.

Avoid overloading mouth, because this decreases swallowing effectiveness.

Give solids and liquids separately.
Reinforce behaviors with simple one-word commands.

**Feed Slowly, Making Certain Previous
Bite Has Been Swallowed.**

Consult with Speech Pathologist.

**Teach Family Emergency
Interventions for Obstruction
(e.g., Heimlich Maneuver).**

Ineffective Infant Feeding Pattern

DEFINITION

Ineffective Infant Feeding Pattern: A state in which an infant
(birth to 9 months) demonstrates an impaired ability to suck
or coordinate the suck-swallow response, resulting in inadequate oral nutrition for metabolic needs.

ⓧ **AUTHOR'S NOTE**

This diagnosis represents a specific type of nutritional
problem of infants grouped under the more general diagnosis *Imbalanced Nutrition: Less Than Body Requirements.* The nursing role is to provide or assist caregivers
to provide appropriate calories to gain weight. Specific
feeding techniques and energy expenditure reduction are
used to achieve oral feedings for all nutrition. Some infants with sucking or such swallow-response difficulties
can meet nutritional needs unless additional factors that
increase caloric needs are present (e.g., infection).

DEFINING CHARACTERISTICS
Major (Must be Present, One or More)
Inability to initiate or sustain an effective suck; inability to
  coordinate sucking, swallowing, and breathing
Actual metabolic needs in excess of oral intake with weight
  loss or need for enteral feeding supplement

Minor (May be Present)
Inconsistent oral intake (volume, time interval, duration)
Oral motor developmental delay
Tachypnea with increased respiratory effort
Regurgitation or vomiting after feeding

RELATED FACTORS
Pathophysiologic
Related to increased caloric need secondary to:

Body temperature instability	Wound healing
Growth needs	Infection
Tachypnea with increased respiratory effort	Major organ system disease or failure

Related to muscle weakness/hypotonia secondary to:

Malnutrition	Congenital defects
Prematurity	Major organ system disease or failure
Acute/chronic illness	
Lethargy	Neurologic impairment/delay

Treatment-Related
**Related to hypermetabolic state and increased caloric
needs secondary to: surgery or painful procedures**
**Related to muscle weakness and lethargy secondary
to sleep deprivation or medications (muscle relaxants,
e.g., antiseizure medications, paralyzing agents in past,
sedatives, narcotics)**
Related to oral hypersensitivity
Related to previous prolonged NPO state

Situational (Personal, Environmental)
Related to inconsistent caregivers (feeders)
**Related to lack of knowledge of or commitment
of caregiver (feeder) to special feeding needs or
regimen**
**Related to presence of noxious facial or absence of
oral stimuli**

NOC Muscle Function, Nutritional Status, Swallowing Status

Goals

The infant will ingest adequate nutrition for growth appropriate to age and need.

Indicators

- The parent will demonstrate increasing skill.
- The parent will identify techniques that increase effective feeding.

NIC Non-nutritive Swallowing, Swallowing Therapy, Aspiration Precautions, Bottle Feeding, Parent Education: Infant

❖ Pediatric Interventions

Assess the Infant's Feeding Pattern and Nutritional Needs.

Assess volume, duration, and effort during feeding; respiratory rate and effort; signs of fatigue.

Assess past caloric intake, weight gain, trends in intake and output, renal function, fluid retention.

Collaborate with Clinical Dietitian to Set Calorie, Volume, and Weight Gain Goals.

Collaborate with Parent(s) about Effective Techniques Used with This Infant.

Provide Specific Interventions to Promote Effective Oral Feeding.

Non-nutritive sucking

Nutritive sucking for identified amount of time

Consistency in approach to feeding

Specific interventions for oral motor delays (position, equipment, jaw/mouth manipulation)

Control of adverse environmental stimuli and noxious stimuli to face and mouth

❖ Pediatric Interventions (cont'd)

Promote Sleep and Reduce Unnecessary Energy Expenditure.

If Needed, Plan for Enteral Feeding Includes Guidelines for Increasing Oral Feeding and Decreasing Enteral Feeding as the Infant Eats More Effectively by Mouth.

Establish Partnership with Parent(s) in All Stages of Plan.

Provide Ongoing Information to Parent(s) about Special Needs, and Assist Them in Establishing Needed Resources (Equipment, Nursing Care, Other Caregivers).

Nutrition, Imbalanced: More Than Body Requirements

DEFINITION

Imbalanced Nutrition: More Than Body Requirements: The state in which an individual experiences or is at risk of experiencing weight gain related to an intake in excess of metabolic requirements.

∞ AUTHOR'S NOTE

Obesity is a complex condition with sociocultural, psychological, and metabolic implications. This diagnosis, when used to describe obesity or overweight con-

> ⊕ **AUTHOR'S NOTE (continued)**
>
> ditions, focuses on them as nutritional problems. The focus of treatment is behavioral modification and lifestyle changes. It is recommended that *Ineffective Health Maintenance related to intake in excess of metabolic requirements* be used in place of this diagnosis. In addition, *Ineffective Coping related to increased food consumption secondary to response to external stressors* may be used. When weight gain is the result of physiologic conditions (e.g., altered taste); pharmacologic interventions, such as corticosteroid therapy; or history of excessive weight gain during pregnancy, this diagnosis can be clinically useful.

DEFINING CHARACTERISTICS
Major (Must be Present, One or More)
Overweight (weight 10% over ideal for height and frame) *or*
Obese (weight 20% or more over ideal for height and frame)
Triceps skinfold greater than 15 mm in men and 25 mm in women

Minor (May be Present)
Reported undesirable eating patterns
Intake in excess of metabolic requirements
Sedentary activity patterns

RELATED FACTORS
Pathophysiologic
Related to altered satiety patterns secondary to (specify)
Related to decreased sense of taste and smell

Treatment-Related
Related to altered satiety secondary to:
Medications (corticosteroids, antihistamines)
Radiation (decreased sense of taste and smell)

Situational (Personal, Environmental)
Related to risk of gaining more than 25 to 30 lb when pregnant
Related to lack of basic nutritional knowledge
Related to sedentary activity patterns

Maturational

Adult/Older Adult
Related to decreased activity patterns and decreased metabolic needs

NOC Nutritional Status, Weight Control

Goals

The person will describe why he or she is at risk for weight gain.

Indicators

- Describe reasons for increased intake with taste or olfactory deficits.
- Discuss nutritional needs during pregnancy.
- Discuss effects of exercise on weight control.

NIC Nutrition Management, Weight Management, Teaching: Individual, Behavioral Modification, Exercise Promotion

Generic Interventions

Increase Individual's Awareness of Amount/Type of Food Consumed.

Instruct person to keep a diet diary for 1 week:
    What, when, where, and why eaten
    Whether doing anything else (e.g., watching television, preparing dinner)
    Emotions just before eating
    Others present (spouse, children)
Review diet diary with individual to point out patterns (e.g., time, place, people, emotions, foods) that affect intake.
Review high- and low-calorie food items.

Assist Person to Set Realistic Goals (e.g., Decreasing Oral Intake by 500 Calories Will Result in a 1- to 2-Lb Loss Each Week).

Teach Behavior Modification Techniques.

Eat only at a specific spot at home (e.g., kitchen table).
Do not eat while doing other activities, such as reading or watching television; eat only when sitting.

Drink an 8-oz glass of water immediately before eating.

Use small plates (portions look bigger).

Prepare small portions, just enough for a meal, and discard leftovers.

Never eat from another person's plate.

Eat slowly, and chew thoroughly.

Put down utensils and wait 15 seconds between bites.

Eat low-calorie snacks that need to be chewed to satisfy oral need (carrots, celery, apples).

Decrease liquid calories; drink diet sodas or water.

Plan a Daily Walking Program, and Gradually Increase Rate and Length of Walk.

Start out at 5 to 10 blocks for 0.5 to 1 mile per day; increase 1 block or 0.1 mile per week.

Progress slowly.

Avoid straining or pushing too hard and becoming overly fatigued.

Stop immediately if any of the following signs occur:
  Tightness or pain in chest
  Severe breathlessness
  Lightheadedness
  Dizziness
  Loss of muscle control
  Nausea

Establish a regular time of day for physical activity; the goal is three to five times a week for a duration of 15 to 45 minutes and with a heart rate of 80% of stress test or gross calculation (170 beats/min for ages 20 to 29 years; decrease 10 beats/min for each additional decade of life; e.g., 160 beats/min for ages 30 to 39 years, 150 beats/min for ages 40 to 49 years).

Advise that intermittent physical activity that accumulates to 30 or more minutes daily is beneficial.

Suggest taking every opportunity to increase activity (e.g., walk down stairs instead of using elevator, park car further from store).

Refer to Support Groups (e.g., Weight Watchers, Overeaters Anonymous, TOPS, Trim Clubs, the Diet Workshop, Inc.).

Nutrition, Imbalanced: Potential for More Than Body Requirements

DEFINITION

Imbalanced Nutrition: Potential for More Than Body Requirements: The state in which an individual is at risk of experiencing an intake of nutrients that exceeds metabolic needs.

> #### ⊛ AUTHOR'S NOTE
>
> This diagnosis is similar to *Risk for Imbalanced Nutrition: More Than Body Requirements*. It describes an individual who has a family history of obesity, who is demonstrating a pattern of higher weight, or who has had a history of excessive weight gain (e.g., previous pregnancy). Until clinical research differentiates this diagnosis from other accepted diagnoses, use *Ineffective Health Maintenance* (Actual or Risk) or *Risk for Imbalanced Nutrition: More Than Body Requirements* to direct teaching to assist families and individuals to identify unhealthy dietary patterns.

DEFINING CHARACTERISTICS

Reported or observed obesity in one or both parents
Rapid transition across growth percentiles in infants or children
Reported use of solid food as major food source before 5 months of age
Observed use of food as a reward or comfort measure
Reported or observed higher baseline weight at beginning of each pregnancy
Dysfunctional eating patterns

Parenting, Impaired

DEFINITION

Impaired Parenting: The state in which one or more care-givers demonstrate real or potential inability to provide a constructive environment that nurtures the growth and development of his, her, or their child (children).

> ⚛ **AUTHOR'S NOTE**
>
> A family's ability to function is at a high risk of develop-ing problems when the child or parent has a condition that increases the stress of the family unit. The term *parent* refers to any individual defined as the primary care-giver for a child.

DEFINING CHARACTERISTICS
Major (Must be Present, One or More)

Inappropriate or non-nurturing parenting behaviors
Lack of parental attachment behavior

Minor (May be Present)

Frequent verbalization of dissatisfaction or disappoint-ment with infant or child
Verbalization of frustration of role
Verbalization of perceived or actual inadequacy
Diminished or inappropriate visual, tactile, or auditory stimulation of infant

311

Evidence of abuse or neglect of child
Growth and developmental delays in infant or child

RELATED FACTORS
Individuals or families who may be at risk for developing or
experiencing parenting difficulties

Parent
Single
Adolescent
Abusive
Psychiatric disorder
Alcoholic

Addicted to drugs
Terminally ill
Acutely disabled
Accident victim

Child
Of unwanted pregnancy
With undesired
  characteristics
Mentally handicapped
Terminally ill

Of undesired gender
Physically handicapped
With hyperactive
  characteristics

Situational (Personal, Environmental)
**Related to interruption of bonding process secondary
to: illness (child, parent), incarceration, or relocation**
Related to separation from nuclear family
Related to inconsistent caregivers or techniques
Related to lack of knowledge
Related to lack of available role model
Related to relationship problems (specify):
Marital discord
Separation
Live-in partner

Divorce
Stepparents
Relocation

**Related to ineffective adaptation to stressors asso-
ciated with illness, new baby, elder care, economic
problems, or substance abuse**

Maturational
Adolescent
**Related to the conflict of meeting own needs over
child's**
**Related to history of ineffective relationships with own
parents**
**Related to parental history of abusive relationship
with parents**

Related to unrealistic expectations of child by parent
Related to unrealistic expectations of self by parent
Related to unrealistic expectations of parent by child
Related to unmet psychosocial needs of child by parent

 Child Development (Specify), Family Coping, Family
Environment: Internal, Family Functioning, Parent-Infant
Attachment

Goals

The parent/primary caregiver will acknowledge a problem
with parenting skills.

Indicators

- Provide a safe environment for child.
- Describe resources available for assistance with
  improvement of parenting skills.

NIC Parenting Promotion, Developmental Enhancement,
Anticipatory Guidance, Parent Education,
Behavior Management

Generic Interventions

**Encourage Parents to Share Parenting
Difficulties and Usual or
Recent Stressors.**

**If Abuse Is Suspected, Notify
Appropriate Authorities (See *Disabled
Family Coping*).**

**Provide Family with
Information about:**
Age-related development needs
Age-related problematic behavior

**Observe Parents Interacting
with Child.**
Support strengths.
Role model in uncomfortable or problematic areas.
Emphasize child's strengths or unique characteristics.

Allow Parents to Watch Nurse Care for Child. Role-Model Comfort Measures and Sensory Stimulation (Verbal, Toys, Touch).

Encourage Parents to Participate in Care.

Explain All Procedures and the Associated Discomforts.

Encourage Parents to Be Present for Procedures When Possible and to Comfort Child.

Explore Parents' Expectations of Child; Differentiate Realistic from Unrealistic.

Assess Usual Discipline Methods for Appropriateness and Follow-Through.

Explore with Parents the Child's Problem Behavior (Herman-Staab, 1994):

Frequency, duration

Situational context (when, where, triggers)

Consequences of problem behavior (parental attention, discipline, inconsistencies in response)

Behavior desired by parents

Discuss Positive Parenting Techniques (Herman-Staab, 1994).

Convey to child that he or she is loved.

Catch child being good; use good eye contact.

Set aside "special time" when the parent guarantees a time with child without interruptions.

Ignore minor transgressions by having no physical contact, eye contact, or discussion about the behavior.

Practice active listening. Describe what child is saying, reflect back the child's feelings, and do not judge.

Use "I" statements when disapproving of behavior. Focus on the act, not the child, as undesirable.

Discuss Discipline Methods.

For small child—sit in chair 1 minute for each year of age (if child gets up, put back in chair, and reset timer).

For older child—deprive of favorite pastime (e.g., bicycle, television show).

Avoid hitting except for one hand slap for a small child for dangerous touching (e.g., stove, electric plug).

Do not threaten. Clarify punishment, and follow through with it.

Expect child to obey.

Parents should agree jointly and follow through with consistency.

Discuss Resources Available (e.g., Counseling, Community, Social Service, Parenting Classes).

Initiate a Referral to Community Nursing Service If Indicated.

Parent-Infant-Child Attachment, Risk for Impaired

DEFINITION

Risk for Impaired Parent-Infant-Child Attachment: The state in which there is a risk for a disruption of a nurturing, protective, interactive process between a parent/primary caregiver and infant.

⊚ AUTHOR'S NOTE

This new diagnosis describes a parent or caregiver who is at risk for attachment difficulties with his or her infant. Barriers to attachment can be the environment, knowledge, anxiety, and health of the parent or infant. This diagnosis is appropriate as a risk or high-risk diagnosis. If the nurse diagnoses a problem in infant–parent attach-

> ## ⊙ AUTHOR'S NOTE (continued)
> ment, the diagnosis *Risk for Impaired Parenting related to inadequate parent attachment* would be more useful so that the nurse could focus on improving attachment and preventing destructive parenting patterns.

RISK FACTORS
Refer to Related Factors.

RELATED FACTORS
Pathophysiologic
Related to interruption of bonding process secondary to:
Parental illness
Infant illness

Treatment-Related
Related to barriers to holding secondary to: bililights or intensive care monitoring

Situational (Personal, Environmental)
Related to unrealistic expectations (e.g., of child or self)
Related to unwanted pregnancy
Related to disappointment with infant (e.g., gender, appearance)
Related to ineffective adaptation to stressors associated with new baby and other responsibilities secondary to:
Health problems   Substance abuse
Mental illness   Relationship problems
Economic problems

Related to history of ineffective relationship with own parents
Related to lack of knowledge or available role model for parental role
Related to physical disabilities of parent (e.g., blindness, paralysis, deafness)

Maturational

Adolescent
Related to difficulty delaying own gratification for the gratification of the infant

Goals

The parent will demonstrate increased attachment behaviors, such as holding infant close, smiling and talking to infant, and seeking eye contact with infant.

Indicators

* Be supported in his or her need to be involved in infant's care.
* Begin to verbalize positive feelings regarding infant.

Generic Interventions

**Assess Causative or
Contributing Factors.**
Maternal
Unwanted pregnancy
Prolonged or difficult labor and delivery
Postpartum pain or fatigue
Lack of positive support system (mother, spouse, friends)
Lack of positive role model (mother, relative, neighbor)

Parental inadequate coping patterns (one or both parents)
Alcoholic
Drug addict
Marital difficulties (separation, divorce, violence)
Change in lifestyle related to new role
Adolescent parent
Career change (e.g., working woman to mother)
Illness in family

Infant
Premature, defective, ill
Multiple birth

**Eliminate or Reduce Contributing
Factors if Possible.**

Illness, pain, fatigue

Establish with mother what infant-care activities are
feasible.

Provide mother with uninterrupted sleep periods of at least
2 hours during the day and 4 hours during the night.

Provide relief for discomforts.

Lack of experience or lack of positive mothering role model

Explore with mother her feelings and attitudes concerning
her own mother.

Assist her to identify someone who is a positive mother,
and encourage her to seek that person's aid.

Outline the teaching program available to her during hospitalization.

Determine who will assist her at home initially.

Identify community programs and reference material that
can increase her learning about child care after discharge.

Lack of positive support system

Identify parent's support system, and assess its strengths
and weaknesses.

Assess the need for counseling.

Encourage the parents to express feelings about the
experience and about the future.

Be an active listener to the parents.

Observe the parents interacting with the infant.

Provide Opportunities for the Attachment Process.

Promote attachment in the immediate postdelivery phase.

Encourage mother to hold infant following birth (may need
a short recovery period).

Provide skin-to-skin contact if desired; keep room warm
(72° to 76°F), or use a heat panel over the infant.

Provide mother with an opportunity to breastfeed if
desired.

Delay the administration of silver nitrate to allow for eye
contact.

Give family as much time as they need together, with minimum interruption from staff (the "sensitive period" lasts
from 30 to 90 minutes).

Encourage father to hold infant.

Facilitate the attachment process during the post-partum phase.

Check mother regularly for signs of fatigue, especially if she had anesthesia.

Offer flexible rooming-in to the mother; establish with her the amount of care she will assume initially, and support her requests for assistance.

Discuss the future involvement of the father in the infant's care. (If desired, discuss opportunities for father to participate in his child's care at home.)

Provide support to the parents.

Listen to the mother's replay of her labor and delivery experience.

Allow for verbalization of feelings.

Indicate acceptance of feelings.

Point out the infant's strengths and individual characteristics to the parents.

Demonstrate the infant's responses to the parents.

Have a system of follow-up after discharge, especially for families considered at risk (e.g., phone call or a home visit by the community health nurse).

Assess the need for teaching.

Observe the parents interacting with the infant.

Support each parent's strengths.

Assist parents in areas in which they are uncomfortable (role-modeling).

Offer classes in infant care.

Have handouts and audiovisual aids available for parents to view at their own time.

Assess for level of knowledge in the area of growth and development, and provide information as needed.

Help parents understand the infant's cues and temperament.

See References/Bibliography for recommended printed material on parenting and child care.

When immediate separation of the child from the parents is necessary because of prematurity or illness, provide for bonding or attachment experiences, as possible.

Allow parents to see and touch infant prior to transport.

Encourage father to visit the neonatal intensive care unit and bring back verbal reports of infant and pictures if possible.

Encourage earliest visiting for mother as feasible, with frequent phone contact with infant's caregivers if visiting is not possible.

Initiate Referrals as Needed.
Consult with community agencies for follow-up visits if indicated.
Refer parents to pertinent organizations.

Parental Role Conflict

DEFINITION

Parental Role Conflict: The state in which a parent or primary caregiver experiences or perceives a change in role in response to external factors (e.g., illness, hospitalization, divorce, separation). Birth of child with special needs.

ⓧ **AUTHOR'S NOTE**

This diagnosis describes a parent or parents whose previously effective functioning ability is challenged by external factors. In certain situations, such as illness, role confusion and conflict are expected. This diagnosis differs from *Impaired Parenting,* which describes a parent (or parents) who demonstrates or is at high risk of demonstrating inappropriate parenting behaviors or lack of parental attachment. If parents are not assisted in adapting their role to external factors, *Parental Role Conflict* can lead to *Impaired Parenting.* The term *parent* refers to any individual defined as the primary caregiver for a child.

This diagnosis was developed by the Nursing Diagnosis Discussion Group, Rainbow Babies' and Children's Hospital, University Hospitals of Cleveland.

DEFINING CHARACTERISTICS
Major (Must be Present, One or More)

Parent expresses concerns about changes in parental role.

Parent demonstrates disruption in care and/or caretaking routines.

Minor (May be Present)

Parent expresses concerns/feelings of inadequacy to provide for child's physical and emotional needs during hospitalization or in the home.

Parent expresses concern about effect of child's illness on other children.

Parent expresses concerns about care of siblings at home.

Parent expresses concern about perceived loss of control over decisions relating to child.

RELATED FACTORS
Situational (Personal, Environmental)

Related to separation from child secondary to:

Birth of a child with a congenital defect or chronic illness

Hospitalization of a child with an acute or chronic illness

Change in acuity, prognosis, or environment of care (e.g., transfer to or from an intensive care unit)

Related to fear of involvement secondary to invasive or restrictive treatment modalities (e.g., isolation, intubation)

Related to interruption of family life secondary to:

Home care of a child with special needs (e.g., apnea monitoring, postural drainage, hyperalimentation)

Frequent visits to hospital

Addition of new family member (aging relative, newborn)

Related to change in ability to parent secondary to:

Illness of parent	Travel requirements
Work responsibilities	Divorce
Remarriage	Dating
Death	

NOC (See also Parental Role Conflict)

Goals

The parent will demonstrate control over decision-making concerning the child and collaborate with health professionals in making decisions about the health/illness care of the child.

Indicators

- Relate information about the child's health status and treatment plan.
- Participate in caring for the child in the home/hospital setting to the extent he or she desires.
- Verbalize feelings about the child's illness and the hospitalization.
- Identify and use available support systems that allow parent time and energy to cope with ill child's needs.

NIC **(See also Parental Role Conflict)**

Generic Interventions

Discuss what has influenced a change in role (e.g., divorce, remarriage, illness [child, parent], boarding away, family additions [newborn, aging parent]).

Allow parents to share frustrations.

Assist parents to determine the type of role desired and if realistic.

If indicated, refer for counseling for management of stressors and role changes.

For ill or hospitalized child:

Help parents adapt parenting behaviors to allow for continuation of parenting role during hospitalization or illness.

Provide information about hospital routines and policies, such as visiting hours, mealtimes, division routines, medical and nursing routines, rooming-in.

Explain procedures and tests to parents; help them interpret these activities to child; discuss child's age-appropriate range of responses.

Instruct parents to continue limit-setting strategies and demonstrations of caring behaviors (e.g., touching, hugging despite hospitalization and equipment).

Provide information to empower parents to adapt parenting role to the situation of hospitalization or the event of chronic illness of the child.

Foster open communication with parents, allowing time for questions, frequent repetition of information; provide direct and honest answers.

Approach parents with new information; do not make them assume the responsibility for seeking out the information.

When parents cannot be with their child, facilitate information-sharing through telephone calls; allow parents to call primary nurse or nurse caring for child.

Support continued decision-making of parents regarding child's care.

Provide parents opportunity to help formulate plan of care for their child.

Use parents as source of information about child; child's usual behaviors, reactions, and preferences.

Recognize parents as "experts" about their child.

Allow parents the choice to be present during treatments and procedures.

Allow parents to participate in caring for their child to the extent they desire.

Provide for 24-hour rooming-in for at least one parent and extended visiting for other family members.

Collaborate and negotiate with parents about parental tasks they want to continue to do, tasks they want others to assume, tasks they want to share, and tasks they want to learn to do; continually assess changes in their desired involvement in care.

Allow parents to have uninterrupted time with child.

Explore with parents their personal responsibilities (e.g., work schedule, sibling care, household responsibilities, responsibilities to extended family); assist them in establishing a schedule that allows sufficient caretaking time for child or visiting time with hospitalized child, without frustration in meeting other role responsibilities (e.g., if visiting is not possible until evening hours, delay child's bath time, and allow parent to bathe child then).

Support parents' ability to normalize the hospital/home environment for themselves and child.

Encourage parents to bring clothing and toys from home.

Allow parents to prepare home-cooked food or bring food from home if desired.

Encourage opportunities for families to eat meals together.

Encourage opportunities for parents to take child on leaves from the hospital, including visits home, as possible.

Help parents verbalize feelings about child's illness or hospitalization and adaptation of the parenting role to the situation.

Provide for parents' physical and emotional needs.

Assess and facilitate parents' ability to meet self-care needs (e.g., rest, nutrition, activity, privacy).

Allow parents an opportunity to determine the caregiving schedule to correspond with a schedule to meet their own needs.

Assess support systems: parent to parent, family, friends, minister, etc.

Initiate referrals if indicated: chaplain, social service, community agencies (respite care), parent self-help groups.

Peripheral Neurovascular Dysfunction, Risk for

DEFINITION

Risk for Peripheral Neurovascular Dysfunction: A state in which an individual is at risk of experiencing a disruption in circulation, sensation, or motion of an extremity.

> ○ **AUTHOR'S NOTE**
>
> This diagnosis represents a situation that nurses can prevent by identifying who is at risk and implementing measures to reduce or eliminate the causative or contributing factors. If undetected, compromised neurovascular function can lead to compartmental syndrome. Compartmental syndrome requires medical intervention (e.g., fasciotomy and nursing care before and after surgery).

RISK FACTORS
Presence of risk factors (see Related Factors)

RELATED FACTORS
Pathophysiologic
Related to increased volume of (specify extremity) secondary to:
Bleeding (e.g., trauma, fractures)
Coagulation disorder
Venous obstruction/pooling
Arterial obstruction

Related to increased capillary filtration secondary to:
Trauma
Severe burns (thermal, electrical)
Hypothermia
Frostbite
Allergic response (e.g., insect bites)
Venomous bites (e.g., snake)
Nephrotic syndrome

Related to restrictive envelope secondary to:
Circumferential burns of extremities
Excessive pressure

Treatment-Related
Related to increased volume secondary to:
Infiltration of intravenous infusion
Excessive movement
Dislocated prosthesis (knee, hip)
Nonpatent wound drainage system

Related to increased capillary filtration secondary to:
Total knee replacement
Total hip replacement

Related to restrictive envelope secondary to:
Tourniquet
Blood pressure cuff
Cast
Brace
Restraints
Antishock trousers
Excessive traction
Circumferential dressings, Ace wraps
Air splints
Premature or tight closure of fascial defects

NOC Neurological Status

Goals

The individual will report changes in peripheral sensation or movement.

Indicators

- Have palpable peripheral pulses.
- Have warm extremities.
- Have capillary refill less than 3 seconds.

NIC Peripheral Sensation Management, Positioning, Embolus Precautions

Generic Interventions

Assess and Evaluate Neurovascular Status at Least Every Hour for First 24 Hours. Compare with Unaffected Limb if Possible.

Peripheral pulses
Skin color, temperature
Capillary refill time

For Injured Arms:
Assess for ability to:
Hyperextend thumbs, wrist, and four fingers
Abduct (fan out) all fingers
Touch thumb to small finger

Assess sensation with pressure from a sharp point.
Web space between thumb and index finger
Distal fat pad of small finger
Distal surface of the index finger

For Injured Legs:
Assess for ability to:
Dorsiflex (upward movement) ankle and extend toes at
  metatarsal phalangeal joints
Plantarflex (downward movement) ankle and toes

Assess sensation with pressure from a sharp point:
Web space between great toe and second toe
Medial and lateral surfaces of the sole (upper third)

Instruct to Report Unusual, New, or Different Sensations (e.g., Tingling, Numbness, or Decreased Ability to Move Toes or Fingers; Pain with Passive Stretch; Unrelieved Pain).

Reduce Edema or Its Effects on Function.

Remove jewelry from affected limb.

Elevate limbs unless contraindicated.

Advise to move fingers or toes of affected limb two to four times per hour.

Apply ice bags around injured site. Place a cloth between ice bag and skin.

Monitor drainage (characteristics, amount) from wounds or incisional site.

Maintain patency of the wound drainage system.

Notify the Physician If the Following Occur:

Change in sensation
Movement ability
Pale, mottled, or cyanotic skin
Slowed capillary refill more than 3 seconds
Diminished or absent pulse
Increasing pain or pain not controlled by medication
Pain with passive stretching of muscle
Pain increased with elevation

If Previous Signs or Symptoms Occur, Discontinue Elevation and Ice Application.

Promote Circulation in Affected Limb.

Ensure hydration is optimal to maximize circulation.

Monitor traction apparatus and splints for pressure on vessels or nerves.

If wrist or ankle restraints are used, monitor for pressure on vessels or nerves. Remove at least every hour, and perform range-of-motion (ROM) exercises.

Encourage active ROM exercises of unaffected body parts
and ambulation if permissible.

**After Hip or Knee Joint Replacement,
Maintain Correct Positioning to
Prevent Prosthetic Dislocation.**

Initiate Health Teaching As Indicated.
**Teach client and family to watch for and report the
following symptoms:**
Severe pain
Numbness or tingling
Swelling
Skin discoloration
Paralysis or reduced movement
Cool, white toes or fingertips
Foul odor, warm spots, soft areas, or cracks in the cast

Emphasize the importance of follow-up evaluations.

Post-trauma Response
Post-trauma Response, Risk for
Rape-Trauma Syndrome

Post-Trauma Response

DEFINITION

Post-trauma Response: The state in which an individual experiences a sustained painful response for more than 1 month
to one or more overwhelming traumatic events that have not
been assimilated.

DEFINING CHARACTERISTICS
Major (Must be Present, One or More)

Reexperiencing the traumatic event, which may be identi-
  fied in cognitive, affective, or sensory-motor activities,
  such as:
  Flashbacks, intrusive thoughts
  Repetitive dreams/nightmares
  Excessive verbalization of the traumatic events
  Survival guilt or guilt about behavior required for
    survival
  Painful emotion, self-blame, shame, or sadness
  Vulnerability or helplessness, anxiety, or panic
  Fear of repetition, death, loss of bodily control
  Anger outburst/rage, startle reaction
  Hyperalertness or hypervigilance

Minor (May be Present)
Psychic/Emotional Numbness

Impaired interpretation of reality, impaired memory
Confusion, dissociation, or amnesia
Vagueness about traumatic event
Narrowed attention or inattention/daze
Feeling of numbness, constricted affect
Feeling detached/alienated
Reduced interest in significant activities

Altered Lifestyle

Submissiveness, passiveness, or dependency
Self-destructiveness (e.g., alcohol/drug abuse, suicide
  attempts, reckless driving, illegal activities)
Thrill-seeking activities
Difficulty with interpersonal relationships
Development of phobia regarding trauma
Avoidance of situations or activities that arouse recollection
  of the trauma
Social isolation/withdrawal, negative self-concept
Sleep disturbances, emotional disturbances
Irritability, poor impulse control, or explosiveness
Loss of faith in people or the world/feeling of meaningless-
  ness in life
Chronic anxiety or chronic depression
Somatic preoccupation/multiple physiologic symptoms

RELATED FACTORS
Situational (Personal, Environmental)
Related to traumatic events of natural origin, including:

Floods	Epidemics (may be of
Earthquakes	human origin)
Volcanic eruptions	Other natural disasters,
Storms	which are overwhelming
Avalanches	to most people

Related to traumatic events of human origin, such as:

Wars	Concentration camp
Airplane crashes	confinement
Serious car accidents	Torture
Large fires	Assault
Bombing	Rape

Related to industrial disasters (nuclear, chemical, or other life-threatening accidents)

NOC Abuse Recovery, Coping, Fear Control

Goals

The person will assimilate the experience into a meaningful whole and go on to pursue his or her life, as evidenced by goal-setting.

Indicators

- Report a lessening of reexperiencing the trauma or numbing symptoms.
- Acknowledge the traumatic event and begin to work with the trauma by talking over the experience and expressing feelings such as fear, anger, and guilt.
- Identify and make connection with support persons/resources.

NIC Counseling, Anxiety Reduction, Emotional Support, Family Support, Support System Enhancement, Coping Enhancement, Active Listening, Presence, Grief Work Facilitation, Referral

Generic Interventions

In a quiet room, explore with the person what happened. If the person is too anxious, discontinue assessment.

Communicate to the person that you are sorry that this happened, that he or she is not to blame, that you are glad he or she is alive, and that he or she is safe here.

Assist the person to decrease extremes of reexperiencing or numbing symptoms.

Provide a safe, therapeutic environment where the person can regain control.

Stay with the person, and offer support during an episode of high anxiety.

Assist the person to control impulsive acting-out behavior by setting limits, promoting ventilation, and redirecting excess energy into physical exercise activity (e.g., going to the gym, walking, jogging).

Reassure the person that these feelings/symptoms are often experienced by individuals who underwent such traumatic events.

Assist the person to acknowledge the traumatic event and begin to work through the trauma by talking about the experience and expressing feelings, such as fear, anger, and guilt.

Assist the person to make connections with support and resources according to his or her needs.

Encourage the person to resume old activities and begin some new ones.

Assist family/significant others to understand what is happening to the victim.

Encourage ventilation of their feelings.

Provide counseling sessions, or link the person with appropriate community resources as necessary.

Explain to the person and significant others:

Flashbacks, nightmares
Avoidance behavior
Detached behavior
Hypervigilance
Exaggerated startle reflex
Angry outbursts

Provide or arrange follow-up treatment where the person/family can continue to work through the trauma and integrate the experience into new ego synthesis.

◆ Pediatric Interventions

Assist Child to Understand and Integrate the Experience in Accordance with His or Her Developmental Stage.

Assist to describe the experience and to express feelings (e.g., fear, guilt, rage) in safe, supportive places, such as play therapy sessions.

Provide accurate information and explanations to child in terms child can understand.

Provide family counseling to promote family members' understanding of child's needs.

Assist Family/Significant Others.

Assist them to understand what is happening to child.

Encourage ventilation of their feelings.

Provide family counseling and/or link them with appropriate community resources, as necessary.

Post-Trauma Response, Risk for

DEFINITION

Risk for Post-trauma Response: A state in which the individual is at risk to experience a sustained painful response to one or more overwhelming traumatic events that have not been assimilated.

RISK FACTORS

Refer to Related Factors in *Post-trauma Response.*

Goals

The person will continue to function appropriately after the traumatic event.

Indicators

- Identify signs or symptoms that necessitate professional consultation.
- Express feelings regarding traumatic event.

Generic Interventions

Refer to *Post-trauma Syndrome.*

Rape-Trauma Syndrome

DEFINITION

Rape-Trauma Syndrome: The state in which an individual experiences a forced, violent sexual assault (vaginal or anal penetration) against his or her will and without his or her consent. The trauma syndrome that develops from this attack or attempted attack includes an acute phase of disorganization of the victim and family's lifestyle and a long-term process of reorganization of lifestyle (Holmstrom & Burgess, 1975).

DEFINING CHARACTERISTICS
Major (Must be Present)

Reports or evidence of sexual assault

Minor (May be Present)

If the victim is a child, parents may experience similar responses.

Acute Phase
Somatic responses
Gastrointestinal irritability (nausea, vomiting, anorexia)
Genitourinary discomfort (pain, pruritus)
Skeletal muscle tension (spasms, pain)

Psychological Responses
Denial
Emotional shock
Anger
Fear of being alone or that the rapist will return (a child
   victim will fear punishment, repercussions, abandon-
   ment, rejection)
Guilt
Panic on seeing assailant or scene of attack

Sexual Responses
Mistrust of men (if victim is a woman)
Change in sexual behavior

Long-Term Phase
Any response of the acute phase may continue if resolution
   does not occur.

Psychological Responses
Phobias
Nightmares or sleep disturbances
Anxiety
Depression

NOC Abuse Protection, Abuse Recovery Coping

Goals

The person will return to precrisis level of functioning.
The child will express feelings concerning the assault and
   the treatment.

Indicators

- Share feelings.
- Describe rationale and treatment procedures.
- Identify members of support system, and use them
   appropriately.

NIC Abuse Protection Support, Coping Enhancement, Rape-Trauma Treatment, Support Groups, Anxiety Reduction, Presence, Emotional Support, Calming Technique, Active Listening, Family Support, Grief Work Facilitation

The parents, spouse, or significant other will return to pre-crisis level of functioning.

Short-Term Goals
- Share feelings.
- Describe rationale and treatment procedures.
- Identify members of support system and use them appropriately.

Long-Term Goals
- Report sleeping well.
- Report return to former eating pattern.
- Report no or occasional somatic reactions.
- Demonstrate calmness and relaxation.

Generic Interventions

Promote Trusting Relationship, and Stay with Person During Acute Stage or Arrange for Other Support.

Communicate.
Victim is safe here.
It was not his or her fault.
You are sorry this happened.
You are glad he or she is alive.

Provide This Analogy: "Every Time You Think You Are Responsible for This Rape, Think Instead that You Were Hit Over the Head with a Shovel (e.g., 'I Would Not Have Been Hit over the Head with a Shovel if I Didn't Wear that Dress, Drink Too Much, Kiss Him, Walk Home ...')." This May Help Effect the Realization that This Was a Crime of Violence and Control, Not Sex.

Explain the Care and Examination She or He Will Experience.

Conduct the examinations in an unhurried manner.

Explain every detail before action.

If this is the person's first pelvic examination, explain the
position and the instruments.

Discuss the possibility of pregnancy and a sexually transmitted disease and treatments available.

Explain the Legal Issues and Police Investigation (Heinrich, 1987).

Explain the need to collect specimens for future possible
court use.

Explain that the choice to report the rape is the
victim's.

If the police interview is permitted:

Negotiate with victim and police for an advantageous
time.

Explain to victim what kind of questions will be
asked.

Remain with the victim during the interview; do not ask
questions or offer answers.

Record Presence and Location of Bruises, Lacerations, Edema, or Abrasion.

Whenever Possible, Provide Crisis Counseling within 1 Hour of Rape-Trauma Event.

Before Person Leaves Hospital, Provide Card with Information about Follow-up Appointments and Names and Telephone Numbers of Local Crisis and Counseling Centers.

Encourage Person to Recognize Positive Responses or Support from Sexual Partner or Members of Opposite Sex.

🔸 Pediatric Interventions

Addressing the child's developmental level, elicit the child's reaction.

Explain what happened. Reinforce that the child did not deserve this.

Use play therapy with puppets or dolls with genitalia.

Evaluate the risk for suicide, especially in adolescent boys.

For adolescents:

Educate the individual and family that rape is a violent crime.

Discourage focusing on "what if . . ." or "I should have. . . ."

Discourage violent, destructive, or irrational retribution toward rapist.

Help family to be supportive of individual.

Refer child and caregivers for counseling.

⚫ Geriatric Interventions

Assess for change in behavior in cognitively impaired (elderly, developmentally delayed) (Burgess, 2000):

Fearful behavior of men

Avoidance behavior with men

Withdrawal behavior

Staying near nurses' station

Lying in fetal position

Powerlessness

DEFINITION
Powerlessness: The state in which an individual or group perceives a lack of personal control over certain events or situations, which affects outlook, goals, and lifestyle.

> ℗ **AUTHOR'S NOTE**
>
> Most individuals are subject to feelings of powerlessness in varying amounts in various situations. This diagnosis can be used to describe individuals who respond to loss of control with apathy, anger, or depression. Prolonged states of powerlessness may lead to hopelessness.

DEFINING CHARACTERISTICS
Major (Must be Present)
Overt or covert expressions of dissatisfaction about inability to control situation (e.g., work, illness, prognosis, care, recovery rate) that is negatively affecting outlook, goals, and lifestyle

Minor (May be Present)
Apathy
Anger
Violent behavior
Anxiety
Unsatisfactory dependence
  on others

Passivity
Resignation
Acting-out behavior
Depression

RELATED FACTORS
Pathophysiologic

Any disease process—acute or chronic—can contribute to powerlessness. Some common sources are the following:

Related to inability to communicate secondary to: e.g.,
Cerebrovascular accident
Guillain-Barré syndrome
Intubation

Related to inability to perform activities of daily living secondary to: e.g., cerebrovascular accident, cervical trauma, myocardial infarction, or pain
Related to inability to perform role responsibilities secondary to: e.g., surgery, trauma, or arthritis
Related to progressive debilitating disease secondary to: for example, multiple sclerosis, terminal cancer, AIDS
Related to substance abuse

Situational (Personal, Environmental)

Related to feeling of loss of control and lifestyle restrictions secondary to (specify)
Related to change from curative status to palliative status
Related to overeating patterns
Related to personal characteristics that highly value control (e.g., internal locus of control)
Related to effects of hospital or institutional limitations
Related to lifestyle of helplessness
Related to fear of disapproval
Related to unmet dependency needs
Related to consistent negative feedback
Related to long-term abusive relationship

Maturational

Parents of Adolescent Children
Related to child-rearing problems

Older Adult
Related to multiple losses secondary to aging (e.g., retirement, sensory deficits, motor deficits, financial status, or significant others)

NOC Depression Control, Health Beliefs, Health Beliefs: Percieved Control, Participation: Health Care Decisions

Goals

The person will verbalize ability to control/influence situations and outcomes.

Indicators

- Identify factors that can be controlled by him or her.
- Make decisions regarding his or her care, treatment, and future when possible.

NIC Mood Management, Teaching: Individual, Decision-Making Support, Self-Responsibility Facilitation, Health System Guidance, Spiritual Support

Generic Interventions

Explore the effects of condition on:
   Occupation
   Leisure activities
   Role responsibilities
   Relationships
Allow to share losses (e.g., independence, roles, income).
Assist not to see self as helpless. Help to identify personal strengths and assets.
Explain all procedures, rules, and options. Allow time to answer questions; ask person to write questions down so as not to forget them.
Keep person informed about condition, treatments, and results.
Anticipate questions/interest, and offer information.
While being realistic, point out positive changes in person's condition.
Provide opportunities for person to control decisions.
Allow person to manipulate surroundings, such as deciding what is to be kept where (shoes under bed, picture on window).
Record person's specific choices on care plan to ensure that others on staff acknowledge preferences ("Dislikes orange juice." "Takes showers." "Plan dressing change at 7:30 prior to shower.").

Provide daily recognition of progress.

For the person with chronic helplessness:

Encourage to take responsibility for self-care.

Assist to set realistic goals.

Help to differentiate areas of life that she or he can and cannot control.

Provide opportunities for person to be successful.

Pediatric Interventions

Explore with child perceptions of the situation.

Use play therapy to help gain mastery of stressful situations.

Encourage personal possessions.

Explain all procedures. Allow child some aspect of control or choices.

Actively encourage child to ask questions.

If possible, elicit information from child rather than parent or caregiver.

Geriatric Interventions

Involve in discussing plans and options early.

Provide time to adjust to changes.

Listen carefully to person's perceptions of the situation.

DEFINITION

Risk for Powerlessness: The state in which an individual or group is at risk to perceive a lack of personal control over certain events or situations that affects outlook, goals, and lifestyle.

RISK FACTORS

Refer to *Powerlessness,* Related Factors.

Goals

The person will continue to make decisions regarding his or her life, health care, and future.

Indicators

- Engage in discussions of options.
- Raise questions regarding choices.

Generic Interventions

Refer to *Powerlessness.*

Protection, Ineffective
Tissue Integrity, Impaired
Skin Integrity, Impaired
Skin Integrity, Impaired, Risk for
Oral Mucous Membrane, Impaired

Protection, Ineffective

DEFINITION

Ineffective Protection: The state in which an individual experiences a decrease in the ability to guard against internal or external threats, such as illness or injury.

⊗ AUTHOR'S NOTE

Ineffective Protection represents a broad diagnostic category under which several specific nursing diagnoses are clustered: *Impaired Tissue Integrity, Impaired Oral Mucous Membrane,* and *Impaired Skin Integrity.* These diagnoses are more clinically useful than *Ineffective Protection.*

The nurse should be cautioned concerning the substitution of *Ineffective Protection* as a new name for compromised immune system, AIDS, disseminated intravascular coagulation, diabetes mellitus, etc. The nurse should focus on the functional abilities of the individual that are or may be compromised because of altered protection, such as *Fatigue, Risk for Infection,* and *Risk for Social Isolation.* The nurse should also focus on the physiologic complications of altered protection that require nursing and medical interventions for management (i.e., collaborative problems, such as Potential Complication: Thrombocytopenia or Potential Complication: Sepsis).

DEFINING CHARACTERISTICS
Major (Must be Present, One or More)
Deficient immunity
Impaired healing
Altered clotting
Maladaptive stress response
Neurosensory alterations

Minor (May be Present)

Chilling	Cough
Perspiration	Itching
Dyspnea	Restlessness
Insomnia	Immobility
Fatigue	Disorientation
Anorexia	Pressure sores
Weakness	

Tissue Integrity, Impaired

DEFINITION
Impaired Tissue Integrity: The state in which an individual experiences or is at risk for altered integumentary, corneal, or mucous membranous tissues of the body.

> ⊗ **AUTHOR'S NOTE**
>
> *Impaired Tissue Integrity* is the broad category under which the more specific nursing diagnoses of *Impaired Skin Integrity* and *Impaired Oral Mucous Membranes* fall. Because tissue is composed of epithelium and connective muscle and nervous tissue, *Impaired Tissue Integrity* correctly describes some pressure ulcers that are deeper than dermal. *Impaired Skin Integrity* should be used to describe potential or actual disruptions of epidermal and dermal tissue only.

> ⓩ **AUTHOR'S NOTE (continued)**
>
> When a pressure ulcer is stage IV, necrotic, or infected, it may be more appropriate to label the diagnosis a collaborative problem as Potential Complication: Stage IV pressure ulcer. This would represent a situation a nurse manages with physician- and nurse-prescribed interventions. When a stage II or III pressure ulcer needs a dressing that requires a physician's order in an acute care setting, the nurse should continue to label the situation a nursing diagnosis because other than hospital regulation, it would be appropriate and legal for a nurse to treat the ulcer independently (e.g., in the community).
>
> If an individual is at risk for damage to corneal tissue, the nurse can use the diagnosis *Risk for Impaired Corneal Tissue Integrity related to,* for example, corneal drying and reduced lacrimal production secondary to unconscious state. If an individual is immobile and multiple systems—respiratory, circulatory, musculoskeletal, and integumentary—are threatened, the nurse can use *Disuse Syndrome* to describe the entire situation.

DEFINING CHARACTERISTICS
Major (Must be Present, One or More)
Disruptions of corneal, integumentary, or mucous membranous tissue or invasion of body structure (incision, dermal ulcer, corneal ulcer, oral lesion)

Minor (May be Present)
Lesions (primary, secondary) Dry mucous membrane
Edema Leukoplakia
Erythema Coated tongue

RELATED FACTORS
Pathophysiologic
Related to inflammation of dermal-epidermal junctions secondary to:
Autoimmune alterations
Lupus erythematosus Scleroderma

Metabolic and endocrine alterations
Diabetes mellitus Jaundice

Hepatitis

Cirrhosis

Renal failure

Cancer

Thyroid dysfunction

Bacterial (impetigo, folliculitis, cellulitis)

Viral (herpes zoster [shingles], herpes simplex, gingivitis, AIDS)

Fungal (ringworm [dermatophytosis], athlete's foot, vaginitis)

Related to decreased blood and nutrients to tissues secondary to:

Diabetes mellitus

Peripheral vascular
 alterations

Venous stasis

Arteriosclerosis

Hyperthermia

Obesity

Anemia

Cardiopulmonary disorders

Edema

Emaciation

Malnutrition

Nutritional alterations

Dehydration

Treatment-Related

Related to decreased blood and nutrients to tissues secondary to: NPO status, therapeutic extremes in body temperature, or surgery

Related to imposed immobility related to sedation

Related to mechanical trauma (e.g., therapeutic fixation devices, wired jaw, traction, casts, orthopedic devices/braces)

Related to effects of radiation on epithelial and basal cells

Related to effects of mechanical irritants or pressure secondary to:

Inflatable or foam "donuts"

Tourniquets

Foot boards

Restraints

Dressings, tape, solutions

External urinary catheters

Nasogastric tubes

Endotracheal tubes

Oral prostheses/braces

Contact lenses

Situational (Personal, Environmental)

Related to chemical trauma secondary to: excretions, secretions, or noxious agents/substances

Related to environmental irritants secondary to:

Radiation—sunburn

Temperature

Bites (insect, animal)

Inhalants

Humidity   Poisonous plants
Parasites

Related to the effects of pressure or immobility secondary to pain; fatigue; motivation; cognitive, sensory, or motor deficits
Related to inadequate personal habits (hygiene, dental, dietary, sleep)
Related to impaired mobility secondary to (specify)
Related to thin body frame

Maturational
Older Adult
Related to dry, thin skin and decreased dermal vascularity secondary to aging

Skin Integrity, Impaired

DEFINITION
Impaired Skin Integrity: The state in which an individual experiences or is at risk for altered epidermis and/or dermis.

DEFINING CHARACTERISTICS
Major (Must be Present)
Disruptions of epidermal and dermal tissue

Minor (May be Present)
Denuded skin
Erythema
Lesions (primary, secondary)
Pruritus

RELATED FACTORS
See *Impaired Tissue Integrity.*

NOC Tissue Integrity: Skin and Mucous Membrane

Goals

The person will demonstrate progressive healing of tissue.

Indicators

- Participate in risk assessment.
- Express willingness to participate in prevention of pressure ulcers.
- Describe etiology and prevention measures.
- Explain rationale for interventions.

NIC Pressure Management, Pressure Ulcer Care, Skin Surveillance, Positioning

Generic Interventions

Identify the Stage of Pressure Ulcer Development.

Stage I: Nonblanchable erythema of intact skin
Stage II: Ulceration of epidermis or dermis
Stage III: Ulceration involving subcutaneous fat
Stage IV: Extensive ulceration penetrating muscle, bone, or supporting structure

Assess Status of Ulcer.

Size—measure longest and widest wound surface
Depth:
　No break in skin
　Abrasion or shallow crater
　Deep crater
　Necrosis
Edges:
　Attached
　Not attached
　Fibrotic
Undermining:
　<2 cm
　2 to 4 cm
　More than 4 cm
　Tunneling

Necrotic tissue type (color, consistency, adherence) and
amount
Exudate type, amount
Surrounding skin color
Presence of peripheral tissue edema, induration
Granulation tissue
Epithelialization

**Wash Reddened Area Gently with a
Mild Soap, Rinse Thoroughly to
Remove Soap, and Pat Dry.**

**Gently Massage Healthy Skin Around
the Affected Area to Stimulate
Circulation; Do Not Massage
if Reddened.**

**Protect the Healthy Skin Surface with
One or a Combination of the Following:**

Apply a thin coat of liquid copolymer skin sealant.
Cover area with moisture-permeable film dressing.
Cover area with a hydrocolloid wafer barrier, and secure
with strips of 1-inch nonallergenic tape; leave in place
for 2 to 3 days.

**Increase Protein and Carbohydrate
Intake to Maintain a Positive
Nitrogen Balance; Weigh the Person
Daily, and Determine Serum Albumin
Level Weekly to Monitor Status.**

**Devise Plan for Pressure Ulcer
Management Using Principles
of Moist Wound-Healing.**

Débride necrotic tissue (collaborate with physician).
Flush ulcer base with sterile saline solution.
Protect granulating wound bed from trauma.
Cover pressure ulcer with a sterile dressing that main-
tains a moist environment over the ulcer base (e.g., film
dressing, hydrocolloid wafer dressing, moist gauze
dressing).
Avoid the use of drying agents (heat lamps, magnesium
hydroxide [Maalox], milk of magnesia).
Monitor for clinical signs of wound infection.

Consult with Nurse Specialist or Physician for Treatment of Stage IV Pressure Ulcers.

Refer to Community Nursing Agency if Additional Assistance at Home Is Needed.

Risk for Impaired Skin Integrity

DEFINITION
Refer to *Impaired Skin Integrity*.

RISK FACTORS
Refer to Related Factors in *Impaired Skin Integrity*.

Goals

The person will demonstrate skin integrity free of pressure ulcers (if able).

Indicators

- Participate in risk assessment.
- Express willingness to participate in prevention of pressure ulcers.
- Describe etiology and prevention measures.
- Explain rationale for interventions.

Generic Interventions

Maintain sufficient fluid intake for adequate hydration (approximately 2500 mL daily, unless contraindicated); check mucous membranes in mouth for moisture, and check urine specific gravity.

Establish a schedule for emptying bladder (begin with every 2 hours). If person is confused, determine incontinence pattern, and intervene before incontinence occurs. Explain problem to person, and secure cooperation for plan.

When incontinent, wash perineum with a liquid soap that will not alter skin pH, and apply a protective barrier to the perineal region (incontinence film barrier spray or wipes).

Encourage range-of-motion exercises and weight-bearing mobility, when possible.

Turn or instruct person to turn or shift weight every 30 minutes to 2 hours, depending on other causative factors present and the ability of the skin to recover from pressure.

Frequency of turning should be increased if any reddened areas that appear do not disappear within 1 hour after turning.

Keep bed as flat as possible to reduce shearing forces; limit Fowler's position to 30 minutes at a time.

Use enough personnel to lift person up in bed or chair rather than pull or slide skin surfaces.

Instruct person to lift self using chair arms every 10 minutes if possible, or assist person in rising up off the chair every 10 to 20 minutes, depending on risk factors present.

Observe for erythema and blanching, and palpate for warmth and tissue sponginess with each position change.

Do not rub reddened areas or over bony prominences.

Increase protein and carbohydrate intake to maintain a positive nitrogen balance; weigh the person daily, and determine serum albumin level weekly to monitor status.

Instruct person and family in specific techniques to use at home to prevent pressure ulcers.

🄖 Geriatric Interventions

Explain high-risk age-related factors:
  Decreased subcutaneous fat
  Drier skin, decreased elasticity
  Slowed rate of dermal healing
  Decreased skin strength (loss of collagen)
  Proteins, vitamins, and mineral deficiencies
  Immobility
  Urinary or bowel incontinence

Oral Mucous Membrane, Impaired

DEFINITION

Impaired Oral Mucous Membrane: The state in which an individual experiences or is at risk of experiencing disruptions in the oral cavity.

DEFINING CHARACTERISTICS
Major (Must be Present)

Disrupted oral mucous membranes

Minor (May be Present)

Coated tongue	Edema
Xerostomia (dry mouth)	Hemorrhagic gingivitis
Stomatitis	Purulent drainage
Leukoplakia	Taste changes

RELATED FACTORS
Pathophysiologic
Related to inflammation secondary to:

Diabetes mellitus	Periodontal disease
Oral cancer	Infection

Treatment-Related
Related to drying effects of:

NPO status for 24 hours
Radiation to head or neck
Prolonged use of steroids or other immunosuppressives
Use of antineoplastic drugs

Related to mechanical irritation secondary to: endotracheal or nasogastric intubation

Situational (Personal, Environmental)
Related to chemical irritants secondary to: acidic foods, drugs, noxious agents, alcohol, or tobacco
Related to mechanical trauma secondary to: broken or jagged teeth, ill-fitting dentures, braces
Related to malnutrition

Related to dehydration
Related to mouth breathing
Related to inadequate oral hygiene
Related to lack of knowledge of oral hygiene
Related to decreased salivation

NOC Oral Tissue Integrity, Oral Health

Goals

The person will demonstrate integrity of the oral cavity.

Indicators

- Be free of harmful plaque to prevent secondary infection.
- Be free of oral discomfort during food and fluid intake.
- Demonstrate optimal oral hygiene.

NIC Oral Health Restoration, Chemotherapy Management, Oral Health Maintenance

Generic Interventions

Discuss the importance of daily oral hygiene and periodic dental examinations.

Evaluate ability to perform oral hygiene.

Teach correct oral care.

Remove and clean dentures and bridges daily.

Floss teeth (every 24 hours).

Brush teeth (after meals and before sleep).

Inspect mouth for lesions, sores, or excessive bleeding.

Perform oral hygiene on person who is unconscious or at risk for aspiration, as often as needed.

Teach preventive oral hygiene to individuals at risk of developing stomatitis:

Perform the regimen after meals and before sleep (if there is excessive exudate, also perform regimen before breakfast).

Floss teeth only once in 24 hours.

Omit flossing if excessive bleeding occurs, and use extreme caution with persons with platelet counts of less than 50,000.

Avoid mouthwashes with high alcohol content, lemon/ glycerine swabs, or prolonged use of hydrogen peroxide.

Use an oxidizing agent to loosen thick, tenacious mucus (gargle and expectorate); for example, hydrogen peroxide and water quarter strength (avoid prolonged use), or sodium bicarbonate 1 teaspoon in 8 oz warm water (can flavor these with mouthwash or one drop of oil of wintergreen).

Rinse mouth with saline solution after gargling.

Apply lubricant to lips every 2 hours and as needed (e.g., lanolin, A&D ointment, petroleum jelly).

If person cannot tolerate brushing or swabbing, teach to irrigate mouth (every 2 hours and as needed):

With baking soda solution (4 teaspoons in 1 L warm water) using an enema bag (labeled for oral use only) with a soft irrigation catheter tip

By placing catheter tip in mouth and slowly increasing flow while standing over a basin or having a basin held under chin

Removing dentures before irrigation and not replacing in person with severe stomatitis

Inspect oral cavity three times daily with tongue blade and light; if stomatitis is severe, inspect mouth every 4 hours. Teach client to inspect mouth.

Ensure that oral hygiene regimen is done every 2 hours while awake and every 6 hours (4 if severe) during the night.

Instruct individual to:

Avoid commercial mouthwashes, citrus fruit juices, spicy foods, extremes in food temperature (hot, cold), crusty or rough foods, alcohol, mouthwashes with alcohol.

Eat bland, cool foods (sherbets).

Drink cool liquids every 2 hours and as needed.

Consult with physician or advanced practice nurse for an oral pain-relief solution.

Use lidocaine (Xylocaine Viscous) 2% oral swish and expectorant every 2 hours and before meals (if throat is sore, the solution can be swallowed; if swallowed, lidocaine produces local anesthesia and may affect the gag reflex).

Mix equal parts of lidocaine, 0.5 aqueous diphenhydramine (Benadryl) solution, and magnesium hydroxide; swish and swallow 1 oz of mixture every 2 to 4 hours as needed.

Mix equal parts of 0.5 aqueous diphenhydramine solution and kaolin (Kaopectate); swish and swallow every 2 to 4 hours as needed.

Teach person and family the factors that contribute to the development and progression of stomatitis.

Have individual describe or demonstrate home care regimen.

❖ Pediatric Interventions

If thrush (oral candidiasis) is present:
  Rinse mouth with plain water after each feeding.
  Boil nipples and bottles for at least 20 minutes.
  Boil pacifiers once a day.
  Apply topical medication as prescribed.

Explain the need to teach 2-year-olds how to brush their teeth after meals and before bedtime.

Encourage parent to have toddler accompany him or her to dentist office to meet personnel.

Discuss the importance of routine dental examinations every 6 months beginning at 3 to 4 years old.

🧑 Maternal Interventions

Stress the importance of good oral hygiene and dental examinations.

Remind to advise dentist of pregnancy.

Explain that gum hypertrophy and tenderness are normal during pregnancy.

© Geriatric Interventions

Explain high-risk age-related factors (Miller, 1999):
  Degenerative bone disease
  Diminished oral blood supply
  Dry mouth
  Vitamin deficiencies

Explain that some medications cause dry mouth:
  Laxatives

⊖ Geriatric Interventions (cont'd)

Antibiotics
Antidepressants
Analgesics
Iron sulfate
Cardiovascular
Anticholinergics
Determine the presence of barriers to dental care:
Financial
Mobility
Dexterity
Lack of knowledge

Relocation Stress (Syndrome)
Relocation Stress (Syndrome), Risk for

Relocation Stress (Syndrome)

DEFINITION

Relocation Stress (Syndrome): A state in which an individual
experiences physiologic and/or psychological disturbances as
a result of transfer from one environment to another.

⊗ **AUTHOR'S NOTE**

Relocation represents a disruption for all parties involved.
It can accompany a transfer from one unit to another or
from one facility to another. It can involve a permanent

> ○ **AUTHOR'S NOTE (continued)**
>
> move to a long-term care facility or to a new home. All age groups involved are disturbed by the relocation. When physiologic and psychological disturbances compromise functioning, the nursing diagnosis *Relocation Stress (Syndrome)* is appropriate.
>
> The optimal nursing approach to relocation stress is to initiate preventive measures, using *Risk for Relocation Stress* as the diagnosis.
>
> NANDA has accepted this diagnosis as a syndrome diagnosis. *Relocation Stress* as a syndrome diagnosis does not fit the criteria for a syndrome diagnosis, which is a cluster of actual or high-risk nursing diagnoses as defining characteristics. The defining characteristics associated with *Relocation Stress* are observable or reportable cues consistent with *Relocation Stress,* not *Relocation Stress Syndrome.* The author recommends deleting "syndrome" from the label.
>
> Other terms found in the literature that describe relocation stress include admission stress, post-relocation crisis, relocation crisis, relocation shock, relocation trauma, transfer stress, transfer trauma, translocation syndrome, and transplantation shock.

DEFINING CHARACTERISTICS
(Harkulich & Brugler, 1988)
Major (80% to 100%)

Responds to transfer or relocation with:

Loneliness	Apprehension
Depression	Anxiety
Increased confusion (older adult population)	Anger

Minor (50% to 79%)

Change in former eating habits
Change in former sleep patterns
Demonstration of dependency
Demonstration of insecurity
Demonstration of lack of trust
Gastrointestinal disturbances
Increased verbalization of needs

Need for excessive reassurance
Restlessness
Sad affect
Unfavorable comparison of post-transfer with pretransfer staff
Verbalization of being concerned/upset about transfer
Verbalization of insecurity in new living situation
Vigilance
Weight change
Withdrawal

RELATED FACTORS
Pathophysiologic
Related to compromised ability to adapt to changes secondary to:
Decreased physical health status
Decreased psychosocial health status
Increased/perceived stress before relocation
Depression
Decreased self-esteem

Situational (Personal, Environmental)
Related to moderate to high amount of environmental change secondary to:
Decreased control of individual care
Decrease and/or change in available caregivers
Decrease/increase in client-monitoring equipment
Increased noise/activities in post-transfer environment
Loss of privacy

Related to negative history with previous transfers secondary to:
Involuntary moves
Frequent moves within short time spans
Transfers occurring at evenings/nights

Related to concurrent, recent, and past interpersonal losses secondary to:
Negative experiences dealing with earlier separations (for adults as well as children)
Loss of social and familial ties
Abandonment
Perceived/actual rejection by caregivers
Anticipation of lengthy and/or permanent stay in new environment

Threat to financial security
Change in relationship with family members

Related to little or no preparation for the impending move
Lack of predictability in new environment
Little or no time between notification and move
Unrealistic expectations of individual/family members
  regarding facility and staff
Lack of decision-making and control on behalf of the person
  who is moving

Maturational
School-Age and Adolescents
Related to losses associated with moving secondary to fear of rejection, loss of peer group, or school-related problems
Related to decreased security in new adolescent peer group and school

NOC Anxiety Control, Coping, Loneliness, Psychosocial
         Adjustment: Life Changes, Quality of Life

Goals

The person will:

- Verbalize positive statements about acceptance of the
  new environment and reasons for leaving the previous
  environment
- Adjust to the new environment without physiologic
  and/or psychological disturbance

Indicators

- Participate in decision-making activities regarding the
  new environment.
- Establish bonds in the new environment.
- Become involved in activities in the new environment.
- Voice concerns regarding the move.
- Describe realistic expectations of the new environment.

NIC Anxiety Reduction, Coping Enhancement, Counseling, Family
         Involvement Promotion, Support System Enhancement,
         Anticipatory Guidance, Family Integrity Promotion

Generic Interventions

Reduce environmental differences between old and new settings; promote continuity of care in new environment:

Maintain person on same activity level and diet through pretransfer and post-transfer units.

Transfer person to similar, proximal area when possible.

Wean any monitoring equipment gradually before transfer.

Transfer all personal items (e.g., mobility aids, eyeglasses, hearing aids, dentures, prostheses, and belongings) with the person.

Transfer person during daytime hours.

Offer person decision-making opportunities throughout relocation experience.

Promote person's input about new environment when possible, such as use of decorations and arrangement of furniture.

Encourage family members to share their perceptions of relocation with one another.

Offer person help in maintaining contact with significant others by telephone calls, writing letters, and visits with previous roommates when applicable.

Provide follow-up visit with nurse from pretransfer unit to person on post-transfer unit.

Retain highly anxious person in pretransfer unit until anxiety decreases, when possible.

Identify individuals at high risk for selected physiologic responses:

Musculoskeletal/neurologic deficits

Advanced age

Infections

Changes in orientation

Cardiovascular deficits

Assess vital signs and level of orientation prior to relocation.

❖ Pediatric Interventions

Teach parents to assist their child with the move:

Remain positive about the move before, during, and after, with the acceptance that child may not be optimistic.

◈ Pediatric Interventions (cont'd)

Explore options with child on how to communicate with
   friends/families in previous environment.

Keep regular routines in the new environment.

Acknowledge the difficulty of peer losses with the adolescent.

Join the organizations to which child previously
   belonged (e.g., Girl Scouts, sports).

Plan a trip to school during a class and lunch period to
   reduce fear of unknown.

Ask teacher or counselor at new school to introduce
   child to a student who recently relocated to that
   school.

◉ Geriatric Interventions

Promote integration after transfer into a long-term care
   nursing facility.

Allow as many choices as possible.

Encourage person to bring familiar objects from home.

Encourage person to interact with other individuals in
   new facility.

Assist person to maintain previous interpersonal
   relationships.

Risk for Relocation Stress (Syndrome)

DEFINITION

Risk for Relocation Stress: A state in which an individual is at risk to experience physiologic and/or psychological disturbances as a result of transfer from one environment to another.

RISK FACTORS

Refer to *Relocation Stress,* Related Factors.

Goals

The person/family will continue to report adjustment to the new environment.

Indicators

- Verbalize positive aspects of relocation.
- Engage in decision-making regarding new environment.

Generic Interventions

Refer to *Relocation Stress.*

Respiratory Function, Risk for Impaired*
Dysfunctional Ventilatory Weaning Response
Dysfunctional Ventilatory Weaning Response,
  Risk for
Ineffective Airway Clearance
Ineffective Breathing Patterns
Impaired Gas Exchange
Inability to Sustain Spontaneous Ventilation

Respiratory Function, Risk for Impaired

DEFINITION

Risk for Impaired Respiratory Function: The state in which an individual is at risk of experiencing a threat to the passage of air through the respiratory tract and to the exchange of gases (O_2 and CO_2) between the lungs and vascular system.

⊚ AUTHOR'S NOTE

The author has added this diagnosis to describe a state in which the entire respiratory system may be affected, not just isolated areas, such as airway clearance or gas exchange. Smoking, allergy, and immobility are examples of factors that affect the entire system and thus make it incorrect to use *Impaired Gas Exchange related to immobility,* because immobility also affects airway clearance and breathing patterns. It is advised that *Risk for Impaired Respiratory Function* not be used to describe an actual problem, which is a collaborative problem, not a nursing diagnosis.

---

*This diagnosis is not currently on the NANDA list but has been included for clarity or usefulness.

> ⊗ **AUTHOR'S NOTE (continued)**
>
> The diagnoses *Ineffective Airway Clearance* and *Ineffective Breathing Patterns* can be used when the nurse can definitively alter the contributing factors that are influencing respiratory function—for example, ineffective cough, immobility, or stress. The nurse is cautioned not to use this diagnosis to describe acute respiratory disorders, which is the primary responsibility of physicians and nurses together (i.e., a collaborative problem). This can be labeled Potential Complication: Hypoxemia, or Potential Complication: Pulmonary Edema.

RISK FACTORS
Presence of risk factors that can change respiratory function (see Related Factors)

RELATED FACTORS
Pathophysiologic
Related to excessive or thick secretions secondary to: infection, cystic fibrosis, or influenza
Related to immobility, stasis of secretions, and ineffective cough secondary to:
Diseases of the nervous system (e.g., Guillain-Barré syndrome, multiple sclerosis, myasthenia gravis)
Central nervous system depression/head trauma
Cerebrovascular accident (stroke)
Quadriplegia

Treatment-Related
Related to immobility secondary to: sedating effects of medications (specify); anesthesia, general or spinal
Related to suppressed cough reflex secondary to (specify)
Related to decreased oxygen in the inspired air

Situational (Personal, Environmental)
Related to immobility secondary to: surgery or trauma, pain, fear, anxiety, fatigue, or perception/cognitive impairment
Related to extremely high or low humidity, exposure to cold, crying, allergens, smoke, laughing

Goals

The person will achieve maximum pulmonary function.

Indicators

- Perform hourly deep-breathing exercises (sigh) and cough sessions if needed.
- Relate importance of daily pulmonary exercises.

Generic Interventions

Assess for optimal pain relief with minimal period of fatigue or respiratory depression.

Encourage ambulation as soon as consistent with plan of care.

If client cannot walk, establish a regimen for being out of bed in a chair several times a day (e.g., 1 hour after meals and 1 hour before bedtime).

Increase activity gradually, explaining that respiratory function will improve and dyspnea will decrease with practice.

Assist client to reposition, turning frequently from side to side (hourly if possible).

Encourage deep-breathing and controlled-coughing exercises five times every hour.

Teach client to use blow bottle or incentive spirometer every hour while awake (with severe neuromuscular impairment, the person may have to be awakened during the night as well).

Auscultate lung field every 8 hours; increase frequency if altered breath sounds are present.

🔷 Pediatric Interventions

Observe for nasal flaring, retractions, or cyanosis.

Allow child to select the color of water in blow bottles.

Monitor intake, output, and urine specific gravity.

Provide age-appropriate explanation for deep-breathing exercises.

Dysfunctional Ventilatory Weaning Response

DEFINITION

Dysfunctional Ventilatory Weaning Response (DVWR): A state in which an individual cannot adjust to lowered levels of mechanical ventilator support, which interrupts and prolongs the weaning process.

⊚ AUTHOR'S NOTE

DVWR is a specific diagnosis within the category of *Risk for Impaired Respiratory Function. Ineffective Airway Clearance, Ineffective Breathing Patterns,* and *Impaired Gas Exchange* also can be encountered in the weaning situation, either as indicators of lack of weaning readiness or as factors related to the onset of *DVWR. DVWR* is a separate client state. Its distinctive etiologies and treatments arise from the process of separating the client from the mechanical ventilator.

DEFINING CHARACTERISTICS

DVWR is a progressive state, and experienced nurses have identified three levels of defining characteristics that can occur in response to weaning (Logan & Jenny, 1991):

Mild
Major (Must be Present, One or More)
Restlessness
Slight increase in respiratory rate from baseline

Minor (May be Present)
Expressed feelings of increased oxygen need, breathing discomfort, fatigue, warmth
Queries about possible machine dysfunction
Increased concentration on breathing

Moderate
Major (Must be Present, One or More)

Slight increase in blood pressure <20 mm Hg or less from
baseline

Slight increase in heart rate <20 beats/min or less from
baseline

Increase in respiratory rate <5 breaths/min or less from
baseline

Minor (May be Present)

Hypervigilance to activities
Inability to respond to coaching
Inability to cooperate
Apprehension
Diaphoresis
Eye-widening (wide-eyed look)
Decreased air entry heard on auscultation
Skin color changes: pale, slight cyanosis
Slight respiratory accessory muscle use

Severe
Major (Must be Present, One or More)

Agitation
Significant deterioration in arterial blood gases from baseline
Increase in blood pressure >20 mm Hg from baseline
Increase in heart rate >20 beats/min from baseline
Rapid, shallow breathing >25 breaths/min

Minor (May be Present)

Full respiratory accessory muscle use
Shallow, gasping breaths
Paradoxical abdominal breathing
Adventitious breath sounds
Cyanosis
Profuse diaphoresis
Discoordinated breathing with the ventilator
Decreased level of consciousness

RELATED FACTORS
Pathophysiologic

Related to muscle weakness and fatigue secondary to:
Unstable hemodynamic status
Decreased level of consciousness

Anemia
Infection
Metabolic abnormalities or acid-base imbalance
Fluid or electrolyte imbalance
Severe disease process
Chronic respiratory disease
Chronic neuromuscular disability
Multisystem disease
Chronic nutritional deficit
Debilitated condition

Related to ineffective airway clearance

Treatment-Related

Related to obstructed airway
Related to muscle weakness and fatigue secondary to:
Excess sedation, analgesia
Uncontrolled pain

Related to inadequate nutrition (deficit in calories, excess carbohydrates, inadequate fat and protein intake)
Related to prolonged ventilator dependence (>1 week)
Related to previous unsuccessful ventilator weaning attempt(s)
Related to too-rapid pacing of the weaning process

Situational (Personal, Environmental)

Related to insufficient knowledge of the weaning process
Related to excessive energy demands (self-care activities, diagnostic and treatment procedures, visitors)
Related to inadequate social support
Related to insecure environment (noisy, upsetting events, busy room)
Related to fatigue secondary to interrupted sleep patterns
Related to inadequate self-efficacy
Related to moderate to high anxiety related to breathing efforts
Related to fear of separation from ventilator
Related to feelings of powerlessness
Related to feelings of hopelessness

NOC Anxiety Control, Respiratory Status, Vital Signs Status, Knowledge: Weaning, Energy Conservation

Goals

The person will:

- Achieve progressive weaning goals
- Remain extubated *or*
- Demonstrate a positive attitude toward the next weaning trial

Indicators

- Collaborate willingly with the weaning plan.
- Communicate comfort status during the weaning process.
- Attempt to control the breathing pattern.
- Try to control emotional responses.

NIC Anxiety Reduction, Preparatory Sensory Information, Respiratory Monitoring, Ventilation Assistance, Presence, Endurance

Generic Interventions

If Applicable, Assess Causative Factors for Previous Unsuccessful Weaning Attempts.

Inadequate energy substrates: oxygen, nutrition, and rest
Inadequate comfort status
Excessive activity demands
Decreased self-esteem, confidence, feelings of control
Lack of knowledge of role in weaning
Lack of trust relationship with staff
Negative emotional state
Adverse weaning environment

Determine Readiness for Weaning (Geisman, 1989).

Oxygen concentration of 50% or less on the ventilator
Positive end-expiratory pressure less than 5 cm of water pressure

Respiratory rate less than 30 breaths/min
Minute ventilation of less than 10 L/min
Low dynamic and static pressures, with compliance of at
   least 35 cm of water pressure
Adequate respiratory muscle strength
Rested, controlled discomfort
Willingness to try weaning

If Readiness for Weaning is Determined to be Present, Engage Client in Establishing the Plan.

Explain the weaning process.
Jointly negotiate progressive weaning goals.
Explain that these goals will be reexamined daily with the
   client.

Refer to Unit Protocols for Specific Weaning Procedures.

Explain Client's Role in the Weaning Process.

Strengthen feelings of self-esteem, self-efficacy, and control.
Demonstrate confidence in client's ability to wean.
Maintain client's confidence by adopting a weaning pace
   (may require a doctor's order) that will ensure success
   and minimize setbacks.
Promote trust in the staff and environment.

Reduce Negative Effects of Anxiety and Fatigue.

Monitor status frequently to prevent undue fatigue and
   anxiety.
Provide regular periods of rest before fatigue is advanced.
If the client is starting to get agitated, try to help him or
   her calm down while remaining at the bedside.
If weaning trial is discontinued, address client's perceptions
   of weaning failure. Reassure him or her that the trial was
   good exercise and a useful form of training.

Create a Positive Weaning Environment, Which Increases the Client's Feelings of Security.

Coordinate Necessary Activities to Promote Adequate Time for Rest or Relaxation.

Coordinate Analgesia Schedule with the Weaning Schedule.

Start Weaning Trial When the Client Is Rested, Usually in the Morning after a Night's Sleep.

Discuss Elements of the Weaning Process with Other Clinicians to Maximize the Probability of Weaning Success:

Starting time

Pace of the weaning

Adherence to the care plan

Diversional activities (e.g., trips outside the unit)

Scheduling of activities and rest periods

❖ Pediatric Interventions

Withhold oral feedings 2 hours before weaning attempts and after extubation.

Dysfunctional Ventilatory Weaning Response, Risk for

DEFINITION

Risk for Dysfunctional Ventilatory Weaning Response: The state in which an individual is at risk for experiencing an inability to adjust to lowered levels of mechanical ventilator support during the weaning process, related to physical or psychological unreadiness to wean.

RISK FACTORS
Pathophysiologic
Related to airway obstruction
Related to muscle weakness and fatigue secondary to:

Impaired respiratory
  functioning
Anemia
Decreased level of
  consciousness
Infection
Metabolic abnormalities
Fluid or electrolyte
  imbalance

Unstable hemodynamic
  status
Dysrhythmia
Mental confusion
Fever
Acid-base abnormalities
Severe disease process
Multisystem disease

Treatment-Related
Related to ineffective airway clearance
Related to excess sedation, analgesia
Related to uncontrolled pain
Related to fatigue
Related to inadequate nutrition (deficit in calories, excess carbohydrates, inadequate fat and protein intake)
Related to prolonged ventilator dependence of more than 1 week
Related to previous unsuccessful ventilator weaning attempt(s)
Related to too-rapid pacing of the weaning process

Situational (Personal, Environmental)
Related to muscle weakness and fatigue secondary to:
Chronic nutritional deficit
Obesity
Ineffective sleep patterns

Related to deficient knowledge related to the weaning process
Related to inadequate self-efficacy related to weaning
Related to moderate to high anxiety related to breathing efforts
Related to fear of separation from ventilator
Related to feelings of powerlessness
Related to depressed mood
Related to feelings of hopelessness

Related to uncontrolled energy demands (self-care activities, diagnostic and treatment procedures, visitors)
Related to inadequate social support
Related to insecure environment (noisy, upsetting events, busy room)

NOC (Refer to Dysfunctional Ventilatory Weaning Response)

Goals

The person will demonstrate a willingness to start weaning.

Indicators

- Demonstrate a positive attitude about ability to succeed.
- Maintain emotional control.
- Collaborate with planning of the weaning.

NIC (Refer to Dysfunctional Ventilatory Weaning Response)

Generic Interventions

Assess for Causative and Contributory Factors of Inadequate Self-Efficacy About Weaning Readiness:

Verbalizes continued need for ventilator support

Uses excuses for delaying the start of weaning

Displays concern about ability to adjust to lowered level of ventilator support or about the probability of success of weaning

Is agitated when weaning is mentioned

Has elevated blood pressure, pulse, and respirations when weaning is discussed

Reduce Risk Factors.

Negotiate with the medical staff for a delayed start and a weaning plan with a slow pace that ensures success at each stage.

See *Dysfunctional Ventilatory Weaning Response.*

DEFINITION

Ineffective Airway Clearance: The state in which an individual experiences a threat to respiratory status related to inability to cough effectively.

DEFINING CHARACTERISTICS
Major (Must be Present, One or More)

Ineffective or absent cough
Inability to remove airway secretions

Minor (May be Present)

Abnormal breath sounds
Abnormal respiratory rate, rhythm, depth

RELATED FACTORS

See *Risk for Impaired Respiratory Function.*

NOC Aspiration Control, Respiratory Status

Goals

The person will not experience aspiration.

Indicators

- Demonstrate effective coughing.
- Demonstrate increased air exchange in lungs.

NIC Cough Enhancement, Airway Suctioning, Positioning, Energy Management

Generic Interventions

Instruct person on the proper method of controlled coughing.
  Breathe deeply and slowly while sitting up as high as possible.
  Use diaphragmatic breathing.

Hold breath for 3 to 5 seconds and then slowly exhale as much of this breath as possible through the mouth (lower rib cage and abdomen should sink down).

Take a second breath, hold, and cough forcefully from the chest (not from the back of the mouth or throat), using two short forceful coughs.

Assess present analgesic regimen. Is the client too lethargic? Is he or she still in pain?

Initiate coughing when client appears to have best pain relief with optimal level of alertness and physical performance.

Splint abdominal or chest incisions with hand, pillow, or both.

Maintain adequate hydration (increase fluid intake to 2 to 3 quarts a day if not contraindicated by decreased cardiac output or renal disease).

Maintain adequate humidity of inspired air.

Plan for rest periods (after coughing, before meals).

Vigorously coach and encourage coughing, using positive reinforcement.

Proceed with health teaching with constant reinforcement in principles of care.

Acknowledge and encourage good individual effort and progress.

❖ Pediatric Interventions

Position to prevent aspiration.
Suction secretions from airway as needed.
Provide humidified atmosphere.

DEFINITION

Ineffective Breathing Patterns: The state in which an individual experiences an actual or potential loss of adequate ventilation related to an altered breathing pattern.

⚰ AUTHOR'S NOTE

This diagnosis has limited clinical utility except to describe situations that nurses definitively treat, such as hyperventilation. For individuals with chronic pulmonary disease with *Ineffective Breathing Patterns,* refer to *Activity Intolerance.* Individuals with periodic apnea and hypoventilation have a collaborative problem that can be labeled Potential Complication: Hypoxemia to indicate that they are to be monitored for various respiratory dysfunctions. If the person is more vulnerable to a specific respiratory complication, the nurse can write the collaborative problem as Potential Complication: Pneumonia, or Potential Complication: Pulmonary embolism. Hyperventilation is a manifestation of anxiety or fear. The nurse can use *Anxiety* or *Fear related to (specify event) as manifested by hyperventilation* as a more descriptive diagnosis.

DEFINING CHARACTERISTICS
Major (Must be Present, One or More)

Changes in respiratory rate or pattern (from baseline)
Changes in pulse (rate, rhythm, quality)

Minor (May be Present)

Orthopnea
Tachypnea, hyperpnea, hyperventilation
Dysrhythmic respirations
Splinted/guarded respirations

RELATED FACTORS

See *Risk for Impaired Respiratory Function.*

NOC Respiratory Status, Vital Signs Status, Anxiety Control

Goals

The person will demonstrate an effective respiratory rate and experience improved gas exchange in the lungs.

Indicators

- Relate the causative factors, if known.
- Relate adaptive ways of coping with causative factors.

NIC Respiratory Monitoring, Progressive Muscle Relaxation, Teaching, Anxiety Reduction

Generic Interventions

For Hyperventilation:

Reassure person that measures are being taken to ensure safety.

Distract person from thinking about anxious state by having him or her maintain eye contact with you.
Say, "Now look at me, and breathe slowly with me like this."

Consider use of paper bag as means of rebreathing expired air.

Stay with person, and coach in taking slower, more effective breaths.

Explain that one can learn to overcome hyperventilation through conscious control of breathing, even when the cause is unknown.

Discuss possible causes, physical and emotional, and methods of coping effectively (see *Anxiety*).

❖ Pediatric Interventions

If child is prone to bronchospasm, medication may be indicated.

Impaired Gas Exchange

DEFINITION

Impaired Gas Exchange: The state in which an individual experiences an actual or potential decreased passage of gases (oxygen and carbon dioxide) between the alveoli of the lungs and the vascular system.

> ### ⊗ AUTHOR'S NOTE
>
> This diagnosis does not represent a situation for which nurses prescribe definitive treatment. Nurses do not treat *Impaired Gas Exchange,* but nurses can treat the functional health patterns that decreased oxygenation can affect, such as activity, sleep, nutrition, and sexual function. Thus, *Activity Intolerance related to insufficient oxygenation for activities of daily living* better describes the nursing focus. If an individual is at risk or has experienced respiratory dysfunction, the nurse can describe the situation as Potential Complication: Respiratory or be even more specific with Potential Complication: Embolism.

DEFINING CHARACTERISTICS
Major (Must be Present)

Dyspnea on exertion

Minor (May be Present)

Confusion/agitation
Tendency to assume a three-point position (sitting, one
  hand on each knee, bending forward)
Pursed-lip breathing with prolonged expiratory phase
Lethargy and fatigue

Increased pulmonary vascular resistance (increased pulmonary artery/right ventricular pressure)

Decreased gastric motility, prolonged gastric emptying

Decreased oxygen content, decreased oxygen saturation, increased P_{CO_2}, as measured by blood gas studies

Cyanosis

RELATED FACTORS

See *Risk for Impaired Respiratory Function.*

Inability to Sustain Spontaneous Ventilation

DEFINITION

Inability to Sustain Spontaneous Ventilation: A state in which an individual is unable to maintain adequate breathing to support life. This is measured by deterioration of arterial blood gases, increased work of breathing, and decreasing energy.

⊗ AUTHOR'S NOTE

This diagnosis represents respiratory insufficiency with corresponding metabolic changes that are incompatible with life. This situation requires rapid nursing and medical management, specifically resuscitation and mechanical ventilation. *Inability to Sustain Spontaneous Ventilation* is not appropriate as a nursing diagnosis; it is hypoxemia, a collaborative problem. Hypoxemia is insufficient plasma oxygen saturation from alveolar hypoventilation, pulmonary shunting, or ventilation-perfusion inequality. As a collaborative problem, physicians prescribe the definitive

---

ⓧ **AUTHOR'S NOTE (continued)**

treatments; however, both nursing and medical-prescribed interventions are required for management. The nursing accountability is to monitor status continuously and to manage changes in status with the appropriate interventions using protocols. (For interventions refer to Potential Complication: Hypoxemia, in Section III in Carpenito-Moyet, L. J. [2004]. *Nursing diagnosis: Application to clinical practice* [10th ed.]. Philadelphia: Lippincott Williams & Wilkins.)

DEFINING CHARACTERISTICS
Major (Must be Present)

Dyspnea   Increased metabolic rate

Minor (May be Present)

Increased restlessness   Increased heart rate
Apprehension   Decreased P_{O_2}
Increased use of accessory   Increased P_{CO_2}
  muscles   Decreased cooperation
Decreased tidal volume   Decreased Sa_{O_2}

Role Performance, Ineffective   ⓞ

DEFINITION

Ineffective Role Performance: The state in which an individual experiences or is at risk of experiencing a disruption in the way he or she perceives that his or her role performance matches norms or expectations.

ⓧ **AUTHOR'S NOTE**

This nursing diagnosis previously had been a subcategory under *Disturbed Self-Concept.* The use of this diagnosis in its present state may prove problematic. If a woman were unable to continue her household responsibilities because of illness and other family members assumed these responsibilities, the situations that might arise would better be described as *Risk for Disturbed Self-Concept related to recent loss of role responsibility secondary to illness* and *Risk for Impaired Home Maintenance Management related to lack of knowledge of family members.* Until clinical research defines this diagnosis more definitively, the nurse should use *Ineffective Role Performance* as a cause of *Disturbed Self-Concept* or *Risk for Impaired Home Maintenance.* If the role disturbance relates to parenting, the nurse should consider *Parental Role Conflict.*

DEFINING CHARACTERISTICS
Major (Must be Present)
Conflict related to role perception or performance

Minor (May be Present)
Change in self-perception of role
Denial of role
Change in others' perception of role
Change in physical capacity to resume role
Lack of knowledge of role
Change in usual patterns of responsibility

Sedentary Lifestyle

DEFINITION

Sedentary Lifestyle: The state in which an individual or group reports a habit of life that is characterized by a low physical activity level.

> ⓐ **AUTHOR'S NOTE**
>
> This is the first nursing diagnosis submitted by a nurse from another country and accepted by NANDA. Congratulations to J. Adolf Gulirao-Goris of Valencia Spain.

DEFINING CHARACTERISTICS
Major (must be present, one or more)

Chooses a daily routine lacking physical exercise
Demonstrates physical deconditioning
Verbalizes preference for activities low in physical activity

RELATED FACTORS
Pathophysiologic
Related to decreased endurance secondary to obesity

Situational (Personal, Environment)

Related to inadequate knowledge of health benefits of physical activity
Related to inadequate knowledge of exercise routines
Related to insufficient resources (money, facilities)
Related to perceived lack of time
Related to lack of motivation
Related to lack of interest
Related to lack of injury

NOC Knowledge: Health Behaviors, Physical Fitness

Goals

The person will verbalize intent to or engage in increased
physical activity.

Indicators

- Sets a goal for weekly exercise.
- Identifies a desired activity or exercise.

NIC Exercise Promotion, Exercise Therapy

Generic Interventions

Discuss Benefits of Exercise.

Reduces caloric absorption
Preserves lean muscle mass
Reduces depression, anxiety,
  stress
Improves body posture
Provides fun, recreation,
  diversion
Suppresses appetite
Increases oxygen uptake

Increases caloric
  expenditure
Maintains weight loss
Increases metabolic rate
Improves self-esteem
Increases restful sleep
Increases resistance to
  age-related degeneration

Assist Client to Identify Realistic Exercise Program.

Personality
Time of day
Safety
Physical size
Lifestyle
Season

Costs
Physical condition
Time factor
Occupation
Age

Discuss Aspects of Starting the Exercise Program.

Start slow and easy. Obtain clearance from physician.

Choose an activity that uses many body parts and is vigorous enough to cause "healthful fatigue."

Read, consult experts, and talk with friends/coworkers who
exercise.

Plan a daily walking program.
  Start at 5 to 10 blocks for 0.5 to 1 mile/day; increase
  1 block or 0.1 mile/week.

Gradually increase rate and length of walk; remember to progress slowly.

Stop immediately if any of the following occur:

Lightness or pain in chest	Dizziness
	Loss of muscle control
Severe breathlessness	Nausea
Lightheadedness	

If pulse is 120 beats/minute (bpm) at 5 min or 100 bpm at 10 min after stopping exercise, or if shortness of breath occurs 10 min after exercise, slow down either the rate or the distance of walking.

If client cannot walk 5 blocks or 0.5 mile without signs of overexertion, decrease length of walking for 1 week to point before signs appear and then start to add 1 block/0.1 mile each week.

Walk at same rate; time with stopwatch or second hand on watch; after reaching 10 blocks (1 mile), try to increase speed.

Remember, increase only the rate or the distance of walking at one time.

Establish a regular time for exercise, with the goal of three to five times/week for 15 to 45 min and a heart rate of 80% of stress test or gross calculation (170 bpm for 20 to 29 years of age; decrease 10 bpm for each additional decade [eg, 160 bpm for 30 to 39 years of age, 150 bpm for 40 to 49 years of age]).

Encourage significant others also to engage in walking program.

Add supplemental activity (eg, parking far from destination, gardening, using stairs, spending weekends at activities that require walking).

Work up to 1 h of exercise per day at least 4 days per week.

Avoid lapses of more than 2 days between exercise sessions.

Assist Client to Increase Interest and Motivation.

Develop contract listing realistic short- and long-term goals.

Keep intake/activity records.

Increase knowledge by reading and talking with health-conscious friends and coworkers.

Make new friends who are health conscious.

Get a friend to also follow program or be a source of support.

Be aware of rationalization (e.g., a lack of time may be a lack of prioritization).

Keep a list of positive outcomes.

Self-Care Deficit Syndrome
Feeding Self-Care Deficit
Bathing/Hygiene Self-Care Deficit
Dressing/Grooming Self-Care Deficit
Toileting Self-Care Deficit
Instrumental Self-Care Deficit*

Self-Care Deficit Syndrome

DEFINITION

Self-Care Deficit Syndrome: The state in which the individual experiences an impaired motor function or cognitive function, causing a decreased ability to perform each of the five self-care activities.

> ☒ **AUTHOR'S NOTE**
>
> Self-care encompasses the activities needed to meet daily needs, usually called *activities of daily living.* Activities of daily living are learned and become life-long habits. Enmeshed in the broad category of self-care activities are tasks that *are* to be done (hygiene, bathing, dressing, toileting, feeding), *how* these tasks are done, and *when, where,* and *with whom* they are to be done. *Self-Care Deficit Syndrome,* not currently on the NANDA list, has been added to describe a person with compromised ability in all five self-care activities. The nurse will assess functioning in each of the five areas and identify the level of participation of which the person is capable. The goal will be to maintain that functioning or to increase participation and independence. The syndrome distinction

---

*This diagnosis is not currently on the NANDA list but has been included for clarity or usefulness.

ⓦ **AUTHOR'S NOTE (continued)**

will cluster all five self-care deficits together to provide clustering of interventions when indicated (e.g., to ensure that the individual is wearing the corrective lenses required). It also will permit specialized interventions for one of the five activities (e.g., to lay out clothes in the order in which they will be put on by the person).

The danger of *Self-Care Deficit* diagnoses is that the nurse could prematurely label a person as unable to participate at any level. This would eliminate a rehabilitation focus. The nurse must classify the client's functional level to promote independence.

DEFINING CHARACTERISTICS*
Major (One Deficit Must Be Present in Each Activity)

Self-Feeding Deficits
Unable to cut food or open packages
Unable to bring food to mouth

Self-Bathing Deficits (Includes Washing Entire Body, Combing Hair, Brushing Teeth, Attending to Skin and Nail Care, and Applying Makeup)
Unable or unwilling to wash body or body parts
Unable to obtain a water source
Unable to regulate temperature or water flow
Inability to perceive need for hygienic measures

---

*Evaluate each of the activities of daily living using the following coding scale:

0 = Completely independent
1 = Requires use of assistive device
2 = Needs minimal help
3 = Needs assistance or some supervision
4 = Needs total supervision
5 = Needs total assistance or unable to assist

Self-Dressing Deficits (Including Donning Regular or Special Clothing, Not Nightclothes)
Impaired ability to put on or take off clothing
Unable to fasten clothing
Unable to groom self satisfactorily
Unable to obtain or replace articles of clothing

Self-Toileting Deficits
Unable or unwilling to get to toilet or commode
Unable or unwilling to carry out proper hygiene
Unable to transfer to and from toilet or commode
Unable to handle clothing to accommodate toileting
Unable to flush toilet or empty commode

Instrumental Self-Care Deficits
Difficulty using telephone
Difficulty accessing transportation
Difficulty laundering, ironing
Difficulty preparing meals
Difficulty shopping
Difficulty managing money
Difficulty with medication administration

RELATED FACTORS
Pathophysiologic
Related to lack of coordination secondary to (specify)
Related to spasticity or flaccidity secondary to (specify)
Related to muscular weakness secondary to (specify)
Related to partial or total paralysis secondary to (specify)
Related to atrophy secondary to (specify)
Related to muscle contractures secondary to (specify)
Related to visual disorders secondary to (specify)
Related to nonfunctioning or missing limb(s)
Related to regression to an earlier level of development
Related to excessive ritualistic behavior
Related to somatoform deficits (specify)

Treatment-Related
Related to external devices (specify), e.g., cast, splints, braces, IV equipment
Related to postoperative fatigue and pain

Situational (Personal, Environmental)

Related to cognitive deficits
Related to pain
Related to decreased motivation
Related to fatigue
Related to confusion
Related to disabling anxiety

Maturational

Older Adult
Related to decreased visual and motor ability, muscle weakness

Assessment

Subjective/Objective Data

Observed or reported inability or difficulty in performing some activity in each of the five areas of self-care.

NOC (See Bathing/Hygiene, Feeding, Dressing/Grooming, Toileting, and/or Instrumental Self-Care Deficit)

Goals

The person will participate in feeding, dressing, toileting, bathing activities.

Indicators

- Identify preferences in self-care activities (e.g., time, products, location).
- Demonstrate optimal hygiene after assistance with care.

NIC (See Feeding, Bathing/Hygiene, Dressing/Grooming, Toileting, and/or Instrumental Self-Care Deficit)

Generic Interventions

Assess Causative or Contributing Factors.

Visual deficits
Impaired cognition
Decreased motivation

Impaired mobility
Lack of knowledge
Inadequate social support
Regression
Excessive ritualistic behavior

Promote Optimal Participation.

Promote Self-Esteem and Self-Determination.

During self-care activities, provide choices and request preferences.

Evaluate Ability to Participate in Each Self-Care Activity.

Encourage Client to Express Feelings About Self-Care Deficits.

For Self-Care Deficits Associated with Mental Disorders:

Encourage independence and involvement. Praise involvement.

Provide assistance with self-care activities. Remain nonjudgmental.

Avoid increasing person's dependency by doing for the person when he or she has demonstrated the ability to do independently.

Explore person's feelings about his or her disability and the need for help. Gently explore the disability and its purpose.

Refer to Interventions under Each Diagnosis, *Feeding, Bathing/Hygiene, Dressing/Grooming, Toileting,* and *Instrumental Self-Care Deficit,* as Indicated.

DEFINITION

Feeding Self-Care Deficit: A state in which the individual experiences an impaired ability to perform or complete feeding activities for himself or herself.

DEFINING CHARACTERISTICS

Unable to cut food or open packages
Unable to bring food to mouth

RELATED FACTORS

See *Self-Care Deficit Syndrome.*

NOC Nutritional Status, Self-Care: Eating, Swallowing Status

Goals

The person will demonstrate increased ability to feed self or report that he or she needs assistance.

Indicators

- Demonstrate ability to make use of adaptive devices, if indicated.
- Demonstrate increased interest and desire to eat.
- Describe rationale and procedure for treatment.
- Describe causative factors for feeding deficit.

NIC Feeding, Self-Care Assistance: Feeding, Swallowing Therapy, Teaching: Aspiration Precautions

Generic Interventions

Ascertain from Person or Family Members What Foods the Person Likes or Dislikes.

Have Client Take Meals in the Same Setting, with Pleasant Surroundings that are Not Too Distracting.

**Maintain Correct Food Temperatures
(Hot Foods Hot, Cold Foods Cold).**

**Provide Pain Relief, Because Pain
Can Affect Appetite and Ability to
Feed Self.**

**Provide Good Oral Hygiene Before
and After Meals.**

**Encourage Person to Wear Dentures
and Eyeglasses.**

**Place Person in the Most Normal
Eating Position Suited to His or Her
Physical Disability (Best is Sitting in
a Chair at a Table).**

Provide Social Contact During Eating.

For Perceptual Deficits:

Choose different-colored dishes to help distinguish items
(e.g., red tray, white plates).

Ascertain person's usual eating patterns and provide food
items according to preference (or arrange food items in
clocklike pattern); record on care plan the arrangement
used (e.g., meat, 6 o'clock; potatoes, 9 o'clock; vegetables,
12 o'clock).

Encourage eating of "finger foods" (e.g., bread, bacon, fruit,
hot dogs) to promote independence.

**To Enhance Maximum Independence,
Provide Necessary Adaptive Devices:**

Plate guard to avoid pushing food off plate

Suction device under plate or bowl for stabilization

Padded handles on utensils for a more secure grip

Wrist or hand splints with clamp to hold eating utensils

Special drinking cup

Rocker knife for cutting

**Assist with Setup if Necessary,
Opening Containers, Napkins,
Condiment Packages; Cutting Meat;
Buttering Bread.**

For People With Cognitive Deficits:
Provide isolated, quiet atmosphere until person can attend
to eating and is not easily distracted from the task.
Orient person to location and purpose of feeding
equipment.
Place person in the most normal eating position he or she
is physically able to assume.
Encourage person to attend to the task, but be alert for
fatigue, frustration, or agitation.

For People Who Are Fearful of Being Poisoned:
Allow person to open canned foods.
Eat one cookie first.
Have family-style meals.

Assess to Ensure that Both Person and Family Understand the Reason for and Purpose of All Interventions.

Bathing/Hygiene Self-Care Deficit

DEFINITION
Bathing / Hygiene Self-Care Deficit: A state in which the individual experiences an impaired ability to perform or complete
bathing/hygiene activities for himself or herself.

DEFINING CHARACTERISTICS
Self-bathing deficits (including washing entire body, combing hair, brushing teeth, attending to skin and nail care,
and applying makeup)

Unable or unwilling to wash body or body parts
Unable to obtain a water source
Unable to regulate temperature or water flow
Inability to perceive need for hygienic measures

RELATED FACTORS
See *Self-Care Deficit Syndrome.*

NOC Self-Care: Activities of Daily Living, Self-Care: Bathing, Self-Care: Hygiene

Goals

The person will perform bathing activity at expected optimal level or report satisfaction with accomplishments despite limitations.

Indicators

- Relate feeling of comfort and satisfaction with body cleanliness.
- Demonstrate ability to use adaptive devices.
- Describe causative factors of bathing deficit.

NIC Self-Care Assistance: Bathing/Hygiene, Teaching: Individual

Generic Interventions

Encourage Person to Wear Prescribed Corrective Lenses or Hearing Aid.

Keep Bathroom Temperature Warm; Ascertain Client's Preferred Water Temperature.

Provide for Privacy During Bathing Routine.

Provide All Bathing Equipment Within Easy Reach.

Provide for Safety in the Bathroom (Nonslip Mats, Grab-Bars).

When person is physically able, encourage use of either tub or shower stall, depending on which facility is at home (the person should practice in the hospital in preparation for going home).

Provide for Adaptive Equipment as Needed.

Chair or stool in bathtub or shower
Long-handled sponge to reach back or lower extremities
Grab-bars on bathroom walls where needed to assist in
  mobility
Bath board for transferring to tub chair or stool
Safety treads or nonslip mat on floor of bathroom, tub, and
  shower
Washing mitts with pocket for soap
Adapted toothbrushes
Shaver holders
Hand-held shower spray

For People With Visual Deficits:

Place bathing equipment in location most suitable to
  individual.
Keep call bell within reach if person is to bathe alone.
Give the visually impaired individual the same degree of
  privacy and dignity as any other person.
Verbally announce yourself before entering or leaving the
  bathing area.
Observe the person's ability to locate all bathing utensils.
Observe the person's ability to perform mouth care, hair
  combing, and shaving tasks.
Provide place for clean clothing within easy reach.

For People With Affected or Missing Limbs:

Bathe early in morning or before bed at night to avoid
  unnecessary dressing and undressing.
Encourage person to use a mirror during bathing to
  inspect the skin of paralyzed areas.
Encourage person with amputation to inspect remaining
  foot or stump for good skin integrity.
Provide only the amount of supervision or assistance necessary for relearning the use of extremity or adaptation
  to the handicap.

For People with Cognitive Deficits:

Provide a consistent time for the bathing routine as part of
  a structured program to help decrease confusion.
Keep instructions simple and avoid distractions; orient to
  purpose of bathing equipment.

If person is unable to bathe the entire body, have the individual bathe one part until it is done correctly; give positive reinforcement for success.

Supervise activity until person can safely perform the task unassisted.

Encourage attention to the task, but be alert for fatigue that may increase confusion.

Evaluate Bathing Facilities at Home, and Assist in Determining if There Is Any Need for Adaptations; Refer to Occupational Therapy or Social Service for Help in Obtaining Needed Home Equipment.

Dressing/Grooming Self-Care Deficit

DEFINITION

Dressing/Grooming Self-Care Deficit: A state in which the individual experiences an impaired ability to perform or complete dressing and grooming activities for himself or herself.

DEFINING CHARACTERISTICS

Self-dressing deficits (including donning regular or special clothing, not nightclothes)

Impaired ability to put on or take off clothing

Unable to fasten clothing

Unable to groom self satisfactorily

Unable to obtain or replace articles of clothing

RELATED FACTORS

See *Self-Care Deficit Syndrome.*

NOC Self-Care: Activities of Daily Living, Self-Care: Dressing, Self-Care: Grooming

Goals

The person will demonstrate increased ability to dress self or the need for having someone else assist him or her in performing the task.

Indicators

- Demonstrate ability to learn how to use adaptive devices to facilitate optimal independence in the task of dressing.
- Demonstrate increased interest in wearing street clothes.
- Describe causative factors for dressing deficit.
- Relate rationale and procedures for treatments.

NIC Self-Care Assistance: Dressing/Grooming, Teaching: Individual Dressing

Generic Interventions

Encourage Person to Wear Prescribed Corrective Lenses or Hearing Aid.

Promote Independence in Dressing Through Continual and Unaided Practice.

Choose Clothing that is Loose-Fitting, With Wide Sleeves and Pant Legs and Front Fasteners.

Allow Sufficient Time for Dressing and Undressing, Because the Task May Be Tiring, Painful, or Difficult.

Plan for Person to Learn and Demonstrate One Part of an Activity Before Progressing Further.

Lay Clothes Out in the Order in Which They Will Be Needed to Dress.

Provide Dressing Aids as Necessary (Some Commonly Used Aids Include Dressing Stick, Swedish Reacher, Zipper Pull, Buttonhook, Long-Handled Shoehorn, and Shoe Fasteners Adapted With Elastic Laces, Velcro Closures, or Flip-Back Tongues; All Garments with Fasteners May Be Adapted with Velcro Closures).

Encourage Person to Wear Ordinary or Special Clothing Rather Than Nightclothes.

Provide for Privacy During Dressing Routine.

For People with Visual Deficits:

Allow person to ascertain the most convenient location for clothing, and adapt the environment to accomplish the task (e.g., remove unnecessary barriers).

Verbally announce yourself before entering or leaving the dressing area.

For People with Cognitive Deficits:

Establish a consistent dressing routine to provide a structured program to decrease confusion.

Keep instructions simple, and repeat them frequently; avoid distractions.

Introduce one article of clothing at a time.

Encourage attention to the task; be alert for fatigue, which may increase confusion.

Assess Understanding and Knowledge of Individual and Family for Above Instructions and Rationale.

Toileting Self-Care Deficit

DEFINITION

Toileting Self-Care Deficit: A state in which the individual experiences an impaired ability to perform or complete toileting activities.

DEFINING CHARACTERISTICS

Unable or unwilling to get to toilet or commode
Unable or unwilling to carry out proper hygiene
Unable to transfer to and from toilet or commode
Unable to handle clothing to accommodate toileting
Unable to flush toilet or empty commode

RELATED FACTORS

See *Self-Care Deficit Syndrome.*

> **NOC** Self-Care: Activities of Daily Living, Self-Care: Hygiene, Self-Care: Toileting

Goals

The person will demonstrate increased ability to toilet self or report the need to have someone assist him or her to perform the task.

Indicators

- Demonstrate ability to make use of adaptive devices to facilitate toileting.
- Describe causative factors for toileting deficit.
- Relate rationale and procedures for treatment.

> **NIC** Self-Care Assistance: Toileting, Self-Care Assistance: Hygiene, Teaching: Individual Mutual Goal Setting

Generic Interventions

Encourage Person to Wear Prescribed Corrective Lenses or Hearing Aid.

Obtain Bladder and Bowel History from Client or Significant Other (See *Constipation* or *Impaired Urinary Elimination*).

Ascertain Communication System Person Uses to Express the Need to Toilet.

Maintain Bladder and Bowel Record to Determine Toileting Patterns.

Avoid Development of "Bowel Fixation" by Less Frequent Discussion and Inquiries about Bowel Movements.

Be Alert to Possibility of Falls when Toileting Person (Be Prepared to Ease Him or Her to Floor Without Injuring Either of You).

Achieve Independence in Toileting by Continual and Unaided Practice.

Allow Sufficient Time for Toileting to Avoid Fatigue (Lack of Sufficient Time to Use the Toilet May Cause Incontinence or Constipation).

Avoid Use of Indwelling Catheters and Condom Catheters to Expedite Bladder Continence (if Possible).

For People with Visual Deficits:
Keep call bell easily accessible so person can quickly obtain help to get to toilet; answer call bell promptly to decrease anxiety.
If bedpan or urinal is necessary for toileting, be sure it is within person's reach.

Verbally announce yourself before entering or leaving
toileting area.

Observe person's ability to obtain equipment or get to the
toilet unassisted.

Provide for a safe and clear pathway to toilet area.

For People with Affected or Missing Limbs:

Provide only the amount of supervision and assistance necessary for relearning or adapting to the prosthesis.

Encourage person to look at affected area or limb and use
it during toileting tasks.

Encourage useful transfer techniques taught by occupational or physical therapy (the nurse should familiarize
himself or herself with planned mode of transfer).

Provide the necessary adaptive devices to enhance independence and safety (commode chairs, spill-proof urinals,
fracture bedpans, raised toilet seats, support side rails
for toilets).

Provide for a safe and clear pathway to toilet area.

For People with Cognitive Deficits:

Offer toileting reminders every 2 hours, after meals, and
before bedtime.

When person is able to indicate the need to use toilet,
begin toileting at 2-hour intervals, after meals, and
before bedtime.

Answer call bell immediately to avoid frustration and
incontinence.

Encourage wearing ordinary clothes (many confused individuals are continent while wearing regular clothing).

Avoid the use of bedpans and urinals; if physically possible, provide a normal atmosphere of elimination in bathroom (the toilet used should remain constant to promote
familiarity).

Give verbal cues as to what is expected of the individual,
and give positive reinforcement for success.

See *Impaired Urinary Elimination* for additional information on incontinence.

**Ascertain Home Toileting Needs, and
Refer to Occupational Therapy or
Social Services for Help in Obtaining
Necessary Equipment.**

Instrumental Self-Care Deficit*

DEFINITION
Instrumental Self-Care Deficit: A state in which the individual experiences an impaired ability to perform certain activities or access certain services essential for managing a household.

⚭ AUTHOR'S NOTE

Instrumental Self-Care Deficit describes problems in performing certain activities or accessing certain services needed to live in the community (e.g., telephone use, shopping, money management). This diagnosis is important to consider in discharge planning and during assessment by the community nurse.

DEFINING CHARACTERISTICS
Major (Must Be Present, One or More)
Observed or reported difficulty in:
Using a telephone
Accessing transportation
Laundering, ironing
Preparing meals
Shopping (food, clothes)
Managing money
Medication administration

RELATED FACTORS
See *Self-Care Deficit Syndrome.*

---

*This diagnosis is not currently on the NANDA list but has been included for clarity or usefulness.

NOC Self Care: Instrumental Activities of Daily Living

Goals

The person, family will report satisfaction with household management.

Indicators

- Demonstrate use of adaptive devices (e.g., telephone, cooking aids).
- Describe a method to ensure adherence to medication schedule.
- Report ability to call on and answer telephone.
- Report regular laundering by self or others.
- Report daily intake of two nutritious meals.
- Identify transportation options to stores, physician, house of worship, social activities.
- Demonstrate management of simple money transactions.
- Identify individuals who will assist with money matters.

NIC Teaching: Individual, Family Involvement Promotion

Generic Interventions

Assess for Causative and Contributing Factors.

Visual, hearing deficits
Impaired cognition
Impaired mobility
Lack of knowledge
Inadequate social support

Assist Client to Identify Self-Help Devices.

Promote Self-Care and Safety with Clients Who Have Cognitive Deficits.

Evaluate activities that are achievable.
Evaluate ability to procure, select, and prepare nutritious food daily.
Teach hints for adherence to medicine schedule (e.g., 7-day pill holder, separate pill for each time to be taken).

Evaluate ability to understand money, budget money, and pay bills.

Determine Sources of Transportation (e.g., Church Groups, Neighbors).

Determine Sources of Social Support (Transportation, Laundry, Money Matters).

Discuss the Importance of Identifying Need for Assistance (e.g., Department of Social Services, Agency on Aging).

Disturbed Self-Concept*
Disturbed Body Image
Disturbed Personal Identity
Disturbed Self-Esteem
Chronic Low Self-Esteem
Situational Low Self-Esteem
Risk for Situational Low Self-Esteem

Disturbed Self-Concept

DEFINITION

Disturbed Self-Concept: The state in which an individual experiences, or is at risk of experiencing, a negative state of change about the way he or she feels, thinks, or views himself or herself. It may include a change in body image, self-esteem, or personal identity (Boyd, 2005).

---

*This diagnosis is not currently on the NANDA list but has been included for clarity or usefulness.

⚛ AUTHOR'S NOTE

Disturbed Self-Concept represents a broad category under which more specific categories fall. Initially the nurse may not have sufficient clinical data to validate a more specific diagnosis as *Chronic Low Self-Esteem* or *Disturbed Body Image;* thus, he or she can use *Disturbed Self-Concept* until more specific diagnoses can be supported with data.

DEFINING CHARACTERISTICS

Because a self-concept disturbance may include a change in any one or a combination of its three component parts (body image, self-esteem, personal identity) and the nature of the change causing the alteration can be so varied, there is no "typical" response for this diagnosis. Reactions may include the following:

Refusal to touch or look at a body part
Refusal to look into a mirror
Unwillingness to discuss a limitation, deformity,
   or disfigurement
Inappropriate attempts to direct own treatment
Denial of the existence of a deformity or disfigurement
Increasing dependence on others
Signs of grieving: weeping, despair, anger
Self-destructive behavior (alcohol, drug abuse)
Displaying hostility toward the healthy
Showing change in ability to estimate relationship of body
   to environment

RELATED FACTORS

A self-concept disturbance can occur as a response to a variety of health problems, situations, and conflicts. Some common sources include the following.

Pathophysiologic
Related to change in appearance, lifestyle, role, and response of others secondary to:

Loss of body part(s)   Chronic disease
Loss of body function(s)   Pain
Severe trauma

Situational (Personal, Environmental)
Related to feelings of abandonment or failure secondary to:
Divorce, separation from, or death of significant other
Loss of job or ability to work

Related to immobility or loss of function
Related to unsatisfactory relationships (parental, spousal)
Related to change in usual patterns of responsibilities

Maturational
Older Adult
Related to multiple losses (job, roles, etc.)

 Quality of Life, Coping, Depression, Violence Control, Self-Esteem

Goals

The person will demonstrate healthy adaptation and coping skills.

Indicators

- Appraise situations in a realistic manner without distortions.
- Verbalize and demonstrate increased positive feelings.

NIC Hope Instillation, Mood Management, Values Clarification, Counseling, Referrals, Support Group, Coping Enhancement

Generic Interventions

Encourage Person to Express Feelings, Especially about the Way Person Feels, Thinks, or Views Self.

Encourage Person to Ask Questions about Health Problem, Treatment, Progress, Prognosis.

Provide Reliable Information and Reinforce Information Already Given.

Elicit Areas that He or She Would Like to Change. Encourage to Consider Options.

Clarify Any Misconceptions the Person Has about Self, Care, or Caregivers.

Avoid Criticism.

Provide Privacy and a Safe Environment.

If Indicated, Refer to *Disturbed Self-Esteem* or *Disturbed Body Image* for Interventions.

Teach Person What Community Resources Are Available, if Needed (e.g., Mental Health Centers, Self-help Groups Such as Reach for Recovery, Make Today Count).

◈ Pediatric Interventions

Allow the Child to Bring His or Her Own Experiences Into the Situation (e.g., Some Children Say that an Injection Feels Like a Insect Sting, and Some Say They Don't Feel Anything). "After We Do This, You Can Tell Me How It Felt."

Avoid Using "Good" or "Bad" to Describe Behavior. Be Specific and Descriptive (e.g., "You Really Helped Me by Holding Still. Thank You for Helping.").

❖ Pediatric Interventions (cont'd)

Connect a Previous Experience with the Present One (e.g., "The X-ray Camera Will Look Different from the Last Time. You Will Have to Hold Real Still Again. The Table Will Move Too.").

Convey Optimism with Positive Self-talk (e.g., "I Am So Busy Today. I Wonder if I Will Get All My Work Done? I Bet I Can." "When You Come Back from Surgery, You Will Need to Stay in Bed. What Would You Like to Do When You Come Back?").

Help the Child Plan Playtime with Choices. Encourage Crafts that Produce a Product.

Encourage Interaction with Peers and Supportive Adults.

Encourage Decoration of Room with Crafts and Personal Items.

Disturbed Body Image

DEFINITION
Disturbed Body Image: The state in which an individual experiences, or is at risk to experience a disruption in the way he/she perceives his/her body.

DEFINING CHARACTERISTICS
Major (Must Be Present)
Verbal or nonverbal negative response to actual or perceived change in structure or function (e.g., shame, embarrassment, guilt, revulsion)

Minor (May Be Present)
Not looking at body part
Not touching body part
Hiding or overexposing body part
Change in social involvement
Negative feelings about body, feelings of helplessness, hopelessness, powerlessness, vulnerability
Preoccupation with change or loss
Refusal to verify actual change
Depersonalization of part or loss
Self-destructive behaviors (e.g., mutilation, suicide attempts, overeating, undereating)

RELATED FACTORS
Pathophysiologic
Related to changes in appearance secondary to:
Chronic disease
Loss of body part
Loss of body function
Severe trauma

Related to unrealistic perceptions of appearance secondary to:
Psychoses
Anorexia nervosa or bulimia

Treatment-Related

Related to changes in appearance secondary to:

Hospitalization

Surgery

Chemotherapy or radiation

Situational

Related to physical trauma secondary to:

Sexual abuse or rape (perpetrator known or unknown)

Related to effects of (specify) on appearance (e.g., obesity, pregnancy, immobility)

Maturational

Related to developmental changes

NOC   Body Image Child Development (specify age), Grief Resolution, Psychosocial Adjustment, Life Change, Self-Esteem

Goals

The person will implement new coping patterns and verbalize and demonstrate acceptance of appearance (grooming, dress, posture, eating patterns, presentation of self).

Indicators

- Demonstrate a willingness and ability to resume self-care/role responsibilities.
- Initiate new or reestablish contacts with existing support systems.

NIC   Self-Esteem Enhancement, Counseling, Presence, Active Listening, Body Image Enhancement, Grief Work Facilitation, Support Group Referral

Generic Interventions

Encourage Person to Express Feelings, Especially about the Way He or She Feels, Thinks, or Views Self.

**Encourage Person to Ask Questions
about Health Problem, Treatment,
Progress, Prognosis.**

**Provide Reliable Information,
and Reinforce Information
Already Given.**

**Clarify Any Misconceptions the
Person Has about Self, Care,
or Caregivers.**

**Prepare Significant Others for
Physical and Emotional Changes.
Support Family Members as
They Adapt.**

**Encourage Visits from Peers and
Significant Others. Advise Them
to Share with the Person How
Important He or She Is to Them.**

**Encourage Contact (Letters,
Telephone) with Peers and Family.**

**Provide Opportunity to Share
with People Going Through
Similar Experiences.**

For Loss of Body Part or Function:

Assess the meaning of the loss for the individual and significant others, as related to visibility of loss, function of
  loss, and emotional investment.

Expect the individual to respond to the loss with denial,
  shock, anger, and depression.

Be aware of the effect of the responses of others to the
  loss; encourage sharing of feelings among significant
  others.

Allow individual to ventilate feelings and grieve.

Use role-playing to assist with sharing.

Explore realistic alternatives and provide
  encouragement.

Explore strengths and resources with person.

**Assist with the Resolution of a
Surgically Created Alteration
of Body Image.**

Replace the lost body part with prosthesis as soon as
possible.

Encourage viewing of site.

Encourage touching of site.

**For Changes Associated with
Chemotherapy (Cooley et al., 1986):**

Discuss the possibility of hair loss, absence of menses, temporary or permanent sterility, decreased estrogen levels,
vaginal dryness, mucositis.

Encourage person to share concerns, fears, and perception
of the impact of these changes on his or her life.

Explain where hair loss may occur (head, eyelashes, eye-
brows, and axillary, pubic, and leg hair).

Explain that hair will grow back after treatment but may
change in color and texture.

Have person select a wig and wear it before hair loss. Consult a beautician for tips on how to vary the look of the
wig (e.g., combs, clips).

Encourage the wearing of scarves, turbans when wig is
not on.

Teach to minimize the amount of hair loss.

Avoid excessive shampooing; use a conditioner twice
weekly.

Pat hair dry gently.

Avoid electric curlers, dryers, and curling irons.

Avoid pulling hair with bands, clips, or bobby pins.

Avoid hair spray and hair dye.

Use a wide-tooth comb; avoid vigorous brushing.

Refer to American Cancer Society for information regarding new or used wigs. Inform that the wig is a tax-
deductible item.

**Discuss the Difficulty that Others
(Spouse, Friends, Coworkers) May
Have with Visible Changes.**

**Allow Significant Others Opportunities
to Share Feelings and Fears.**

**Assist Significant Others to Identify
Positive Aspects of the Client and
Ways This Can Be Shared.**

Teach Person What Community Resources Are Available if Needed (e.g., Mental Health Centers, Self-Help Groups Such as Reach for Recovery, Make Today Count).

🔅 Pediatric Interventions

Discuss with Parents How Body Image Develops and What Interactions Contribute to Their Child's Self-Perceptions.

Teach the names and functions of body parts.
Acknowledge changes (e.g., height).
Allow some choices of what to wear.

Ask Child to Draw a Picture of His or Her Body Just after a Bath (Naked). Ask to Describe Picture.

Focus Child on Body Changes (e.g., "What Can You Do Now That You Couldn't Do When You Were Little?").

Adolescent Interventions

Discuss with Parents the Adolescent's Need to "Fit In."

Do not dismiss adolescent's concerns too quickly.
Be flexible and compromise when possible (e.g., clothes are temporary, tattoos are not).
Negotiate a time to think about it (e.g., 4 to 6 weeks).
Provide reasons for denying a request. Elicit adolescent's reasons. Compromise if possible (e.g., curfew parents want, 11:00; adolescent, 12:00; compromise 11:30).

Provide Opportunities to Discuss Concerns When Parents Are Not Present.

Ask to Describe Best Features and Those He or She Dislikes.

Prepare for Impending Development Changes.

🔱 Maternal Interventions

Teach Couples about Anticipated Physiologic Changes and Possible Changes In Sexual Response.

Allow Woman Opportunities to Discuss Her Feelings Regarding Body Changes.

Disturbed Personal Identity

DEFINITION

Disturbed Personal Identity: The state in which an individual experiences, or is at risk of experiencing, an inability to distinguish between self and nonself.

> ℀ **AUTHOR'S NOTE**
>
> This diagnosis is a subcategory under *Disturbed Self-Concept.* Until clinical research defines and differentiates this diagnosis from others, refer to *Disturbed Self-Concept* or *Delayed Growth and Development* for assessment criteria and interventions.

DEFINING CHARACTERISTICS

See Defining Characteristics for *Disturbed Self-Concept* or *Delayed Growth and Development.*

DEFINITION

Disturbed Self-Esteem: The state in which an individual experiences, or is at risk of experiencing, negative self-evaluation about self or capabilities.

> **⊛ AUTHOR'S NOTE**
>
> Self-esteem is one of the four components of self-concept. *Disturbed Self-Esteem* is the general diagnostic category. *Chronic Low Self-Esteem* and *Situational Low Self-Esteem* represent specific types of *Disturbed Self-Esteem,* thus involving more specific interventions. Initially, the nurse may not have sufficient clinical data to validate a more specific diagnosis, such as *Chronic Low Self-Esteem* or *Situational Low Self-Esteem.* Refer to the major defining characteristics under these diagnoses for validation.

DEFINING CHARACTERISTICS

Overt or Covert:
Self-negating verbalization*
Expressions of shame or guilt*
Evaluation of self as unable to deal with events*
Rationalizing away/rejecting positive feedback and
   exaggerating negative feedback about self*
Inability to set goals
Indecisiveness
Lack of/poor problem-solving
Signs of depression (sleeping, eating)
Seeking approval or reassurance excessively
Poor body presentation (posture, eye contact, movements)
Self-abusive behavior (mutilation, suicide attempts, nail
   biting, substance abuse, becoming a victim)

*Norris, J., & Kunes-Connell, M. (1987). Self-esteem disturbance: A clinical validation study. In A. McLane (Ed.), *Classification of nursing diagnoses: Proceedings of the seventh NANDA national conference.* St. Louis: C. V. Mosby.

Hesitation to try new things/situations*
Denial of problems obvious to others
Projection of blame/responsibility for problems*
Rationalization of personal failures*
Hypersensitivity to slight criticism*
Grandiosity*

RELATED FACTORS

Disturbed Self-Esteem can be either an episodic event or a chronic problem. Failure to resolve a problem or multiple sequential stresses can result in *Chronic Low Self-Esteem.* Factors that occur with time and are associated with *Chronic Low Self-Esteem* are indicated by CLSE.

Pathophysiologic
Related to change in appearance secondary to:
Loss of body part(s)
Loss of body function(s)
Disfigurement (trauma, surgery, birth defects)

Situational (Personal, Environmental)
Related to unmet dependency needs
Related to lack of positive feedback
Related to feelings of abandonment secondary to:
Death of significant other
Child abduction/murder
Separation from significant other

Related to feelings of failure secondary to:
Unemployment
Financial problems
Loss of job or ability to work
Relationship problems
Marital discord
Separation
Step-parents
In-laws
Increase/decrease in weight
Premenstrual syndrome

Related to failure in school
Related to history of ineffective relationship with own parents (CLSE)
Related to history of abusive relationships (CLSE)

Related to unrealistic expectations of child by parent (CLSE)
Related to unrealistic expectations of self (CLSE)
Related to unrealistic expectations of parent by child (CLSE)
Related to parental rejection (CLSE)
Related to inconsistent punishment (CLSE)
Related to feelings of helplessness or failure secondary to: institutionalization (e.g., mental health facility, jail, orphanage, halfway house)
Related to history of numerous failures (CLSE)

Maturational
Infant/Toddler/Preschool
Related to lack of stimulation or closeness (CLSE)
Related to separation from parents/significant others (CLSE)
Related to continual negative evaluation by parents
Related to inadequate parental support (CLSE)
Related to inability to trust significant other (CLSE)

School Age
Related to failure to achieve grade-level objectives
Related to loss of peer group
Related to repeated negative feedback (CLSE)

Adolescent
Related to loss of independence and autonomy secondary to (specify)
Related to disruption of peer relationships
Related to scholastic problems
Related to loss of significant others

Middle Age
Related to changes associated with aging

Older Adult
Related to losses (people, function, financial, retirement)

Goals

The person will express a positive outlook for the future and resume previous level of functioning.

Indicators

- Identify source of threat to self-esteem and work through that issue.
- Identify positive aspects of self.
- Analyze own behavior and its consequences.
- Identify one positive aspect of change.

Generic Interventions

Establish a Trusting Nurse–Client Relationship.

Encourage person to express feelings, especially about way he or she thinks or views self.

Encourage person to ask questions about health problem, treatment, progress, prognosis.

Provide reliable information and reinforce information already given.

Clarify any misconceptions the person has about self, care, or caregivers.

Avoid criticism.

Provide privacy and a safe environment.

Promote Social Interaction.

Assist person to accept help from others.

Avoid overprotection while still limiting the demands made on the individual.

Encourage movement.

Support family as they adapt.

Explore Strengths and Resources with Person.

Discuss Expectations.

Discuss if realistic.

Explore realistic alternatives.

Refer to Community Resources as Indicated (e.g., Counseling, Assertiveness Courses).

DEFINITION

Chronic Low Self-Esteem: The state in which an individual experiences a long-standing negative self-evaluation about self or capabilities.

DEFINING CHARACTERISTICS
(Norris & Kunes-Connell, 1987)
Major (80% to 100%)

Long-Standing or Chronic:
Self-negating verbalization
Expressions of shame/guilt
Evaluation of self as unable to deal with events
Rationalizing away/rejecting positive feedback and
  exaggerating negative feedback about self
Hesitation to try new things/situations

Minor (50% to 79%)

Frequent lack of success in work or other life events
Overly conforming, dependent on opinions of others
Poor body presentation (eye contact, posture, movements)
Nonassertive/passive
Indecisive
Excessively seeking reassurance

RELATED FACTORS

See *Disturbed Self-Esteem.*

NOC Depression Level, Self-Esteem, Quality of Life

Goals

The individual will identify positive aspects of self and report freedom from symptoms of depression.

Indicators

- Modify excessive and unrealistic self-expectations.
- Verbalize acceptance of limitations.
- Verbalize nonjudgmental perceptions of self.

- Cease self-abusive behavior.
- Begin to take verbal and behavioral risks.

NIC Hope Instillation, Anxiety Reduction, Self-Enhancement, Coping Enhancement, Socialization Enhancement, Referral

Generic Interventions

Assist the Person to Reduce Anxiety Level.

Enhance the Person's Sense of Self.
Be attentive.
Respect individual's personal space.
Validate your interpretation of what person is saying or experiencing ("Is this what you mean?").

Provide Encouragement as a Task or Skill Is Attempted. Allow Person to Perform as Independently as Possible.

Assist Person in Expressing Thoughts and Feelings.

Encourage Visits/Contact with Peers and Significant Others (Letters, Telephone).

Be a Role Model in One-to-one Interactions.

Involve in Activities, Especially When Strengths Can Be Used.

Do Not Allow Person to Isolate Self (Refer to *Social Isolation* for Further Interventions).

Set Limits on Problematic Behavior, Such as Aggression, Poor Hygiene, Ruminations, and Suicidal Preoccupation. Refer to *Risk for Suicide* or *Risk for Violence* if These Are Assessed as Problems.

Encourage Activities That Exercise Large Muscles (e.g., Walking, Biking, Swimming). Avoid Competitive Activities.

Provide for Development of Social and Vocational Skills.

Refer for Vocational Counseling if Indicated.

❖ Pediatric Interventions

Provide Opportunities for Child to Be Successful and Needed.

Personalize the Child's Environment with Pictures, Possessions, and Crafts Made.

Provide Structured and Unstructured Playtime.

Ensure Continuance of Academic Experiences in the Hospital or Home. Provide Uninterrupted Time for School Work.

● Geriatric Interventions (Miller, 2004)

Acknowledge Person by Name.

Use Tone of Voice That You Would Use for Own Peer Group.

Avoid Words Associated with Babies (e.g., Diapers).

Ask about Family Pictures, Personal Items, and Past Experiences.

Avoid Attributing Disabilities to "Old Age."

Knock on Door of Bedrooms and Bathrooms.

Allow Person Enough Time to Accomplish Tasks at Own Pace.

Situational Low Self-Esteem

DEFINITION

Situational Low Self-Esteem: The state in which an individual who previously had positive self-esteem experiences negative feelings about self in response to an event (loss, change).

 AUTHOR'S NOTE

Although *Situational Low Self-Esteem* is an episodic event, repeated occurrences or the continuation of these negative self-appraisals over time can lead to *Chronic Low Self-Esteem* (Willard, 1991; personal communication).

DEFINING CHARACTERISTICS
(Norris & Kunes-Connell, 1987)
Major (80% to 100%)

Episodic occurrence of negative self-appraisal in response to life events in a person with a previously positive self-evaluation

Verbalization of negative feelings about self (helplessness, uselessness)

Minor (50% to 79%)

Self-negating verbalizations
Expressions of shame/guilt
Evaluation of self as unable to handle situations/events
Difficulty making decisions
Self-neglect
Social isolation

RELATED FACTORS

See *Disturbed Self-Esteem.*

NOC	Decision Making, Grief Resolution, Psychosocial Adjustment, Life Change, Self-Esteem

Goals

The person will express a positive outlook for the future and resume previous level of functioning.

Indicators

- Identify source of threat to self-esteem and work through that issue.
- Identify positive aspects of self.
- Analyze own behavior and its consequences.
- Identify one positive aspect of change.

NIC	Active Listening, Presence, Counseling, Cognitive Restructuring, Family Support, Support Group, Coping Enhancement

Generic Interventions

Assist the Individual In Identifying and Expressing Feelings.

Practice Self-Talk (Murray, 2000).

Write a brief description of the change and the consequence that it has created (e.g., "My spouse has had an affair. I am betrayed.").

Write three things that may be useful about this situation.

Communicate that the Person Can Handle the Change.

Challenge the Person to Imagine Positive Futures and Outcomes.

Examine and Reinforce Positive Abilities and Traits (e.g., Hobbies, Skills, School, Relationships,

Appearance, Loyalty, Industriousness).

Encourage an Activity that Exercises Large Muscles (e.g., Walking, Swimming, Biking). Avoid Competitive Situations.

Help Individual Accept Positive and Negative Feelings.

Encourage Examination of Current Behavior and Its Consequences (e.g., Dependency, Procrastination, Isolation).

Help to Identify Negative Automatic Thoughts and Overgeneralizing.

Assist in Identifying Own Responsibility and Control in a Situation (e.g., When Continually Blaming Others for Problems).

Assess and Mobilize Current Support System.

Refer to Community Resources as Indicated (e.g., Reach for Recovery).

Risk for Situational Low Self-Esteem

DEFINITION

Risk for Situational Low Self-Esteem: The state in which an individual who previously had a positive self-esteem is at risk to experience negative feelings about self in response to an event (loss, change).

RISK FACTORS

Refer to *Situational Low Self-Esteem.*

Goals

The person will continue to express a positive outlook for the future to identify positive aspects of self.

Indicators

- Identify threats to self-esteem.
- Identify one positive aspect of change.

NIC (See Situational Low-Self-Esteem)

General Interventions

Refer to *Situational Low Self-Esteem.*

Risk for Self-Harm*
Risk for Self-Abuse*
Self-Mutilation
Risk for Self-Mutilation
Risk for Suicide*

Risk for Self-Harm*

DEFINITION

Risk for Self-Harm: A state in which an individual is at risk for inflicting direct harm on himself or herself. This may include one or more of the following: self-abuse, self-mutilation, suicide.

> ### ⊛ AUTHOR'S NOTE
>
> *Risk for Self-Harm* represents a broad diagnosis that can encompass self-abuse, self-mutilation, or risk for suicide. Although initially they may appear the same, the distinction lies in the intent. "Self-mutilation and self-abuse are pathological attempts to relieve stress (temporary reprieve), whereas suicide is an attempt to die (to relieve stress permanently)" (Casscadden, 1992; personal communication). *Risk for Self-Harm* can also be a useful early diagnosis when insufficient data are present to differentiate one from the other.

DEFINING CHARACTERISTICS
Major (Must Be Present, One or More)

Expresses desire or intent to harm self
Expresses desire to die or commit suicide
Has history of attempts to harm self

---

*This diagnosis is not currently on the NANDA list but has been included for clarity or usefulness.

Minor
Reports or Observed:

Depression

Poor self-concept

Hallucinations/delusion

Substance abuse

Poor impulse control

Agitation

Hopelessness

Helplessness

Lack of support system

Emotional pain

Hostility

RELATED FACTORS
Risk for Self-Harm can occur as a response to a variety of health problems, situations, and conflicts. Some sources are listed below.

Pathophysiologic
Related to feelings of helplessness, loneliness, or hopelessness secondary to:

Disabilities

Chemical dependency

Terminal illness

Substance abuse

Chronic illness

Mental impairment (organic or traumatic)

Chronic pain

Psychiatric disorder

   Schizophrenia

   Bipolar disorder

   Post-traumatic stress disorder

   Personality disorder

   Adolescent adjustment disorder

   Somatoform disorders

New diagnosis of positive HIV status

TREATMENT-RELATED
Related to unsatisfactory outcome of treatment (medical, surgical, psychological)

Related to prolonged dependence on, e.g., dialysis, insulin injections, chemotherapy/radiation, ventilator

Situational (Personal, Environmental)
Related to:

Depression

Ineffective individual coping skills

Child abuse (present, past)

Parental/marital conflict

Substance abuse in family

Related to real or perceived loss secondary to:

Finances/job

Threat of abandonment

Death of significant others

Status/prestige

Separation/divorce

Someone leaving home

Related to wish for revenge on real or perceived injury (body or self-esteem)

Related to multiple losses associated with AIDS

Maturational

Adolescent

Related to feelings of abandonment

Related to unrealistic expectations of child by parents

Related to peer pressure or rejection

Related to depression

Related to relocation

Related to significant loss

Older Adult

Related to multiple losses secondary to retirement, social isolation, significant loss, or illness

NOC Aggression Control, Impulse Control

Goals

The person will choose alternatives that are not harmful.

Indicators

- Acknowledge self-harm thoughts.
- Admit to use of self-harm behavior if it occurs.
- Be able to identify personal triggers.
- Learn to properly identify and tolerate uncomfortable feelings.

NIC Presence, Anger Control, Environmental Management: Violence Prevention, Behavior Modification, Security Enhancement, Therapy Group, Coping Enhancement, Impulse Control Training, Crisis Intervention

Generic Interventions

Demonstrate an Acceptance of the Individual as a Worthwhile Person Through the Use of Nonjudgmental Statements and Behavior.

Actively listen or provide support by just being there if the person is silent.

Label the behavior, not the person.

Assist in Recognizing the Presence of Hope and the Element of Alternatives.

Orient Individual as Required. Point Out Sensory or Environmental Misperceptions Without Belittling Fears or Indicating Disapproval of Verbal Expressions.

Help Reframe Old Thinking/ Feeling Patterns

Assist in identifying thought–feeling–behavior concept.

Help assess payoffs and drawbacks to self-harm.

Encourage identification of personal triggers.

Facilitate the development of new behaviors.

Validate Good Coping Skills Already in Existence.

Encourage the Use of Positive Affirmations, Meditation and Relaxation Techniques, and Other Esteem-Building Exercises.

Encourage Journaling, Keeping a Diary of Triggers, Thoughts, and Feelings, and Alternatives That Do or Do Not Work.

Assist in Developing Body Awareness as a Method of Ascertaining Triggers and Determining Levels of Impending Self-Harm.

Introduce "Contracting" to Individual.

Assist in Role Playing to Solve Problems in Situations/Relationships.

Reduce Excessive Stimuli.

Intervene at Earliest Stages to Assist Person to Regain Control, Prevent Escalation, and Allow Treatment in the Least Restrictive Manner.

Promote the Use of Alternatives.

Stress that there are always alternatives.
Stress that self-harm is a choice, not something uncontrollable.
Allow opportunities for verbal expression of thoughts and feelings.
Provide acceptable physical outlets.

Initiate Support Systems to Community When Indicated.

Teach Family:

Constructive expression of feelings
How to recognize levels of impending self-harm
How to assist with appropriate interventions
How to deal with self-harm behavior/results

Supply Phone Number of 24-Hour Emergency Hotlines.

Recommend Counseling, as Appropriate.

Leisure/vocational counseling
Halfway houses
Other community resources

Risk for Self-Abuse

DEFINITION

Risk for Self-Abuse: A state in which an individual is at risk to perform a deliberate act upon self, without the intent to kill, which may or may not cause harm to the body.

DEFINING CHARACTERISTICS
Major (Must Be Present, One or More)

Expresses a desire or intent to harm self

Evidence of self-abuse: e.g.,
    Head banging
    Slapping
    Picking
    Scratching
    Nonlethal use of drugs/poison
    Anorexic/bulimic behaviors
    Swallowing foreign objects (glass, needles, safety pins,
        straight pins, various hardware [e.g., nails, screws])

RELATED FACTORS

See *Risk for Self-Harm.*

Goals

See *Risk for Self-Harm.*

Generic Interventions

See *Risk for Self-Harm.*

❖ Pediatric Interventions

**Redirect Child Back to the Activity
or Task.**

**Praise His or Her Attention to the
Activity.**

**If Applicable, Look Away from the
Child; Make No Eye Contact.**

**If Quiet Room Is Used, Limit as Much
as Possible.**

DEFINITION

Self-Mutilation: The state in which an individual has performed a deliberate act on the self with the intent to injure, not kill, that produces immediate tissue damage.

DEFINING CHARACTERISTICS

Express desire or intent to harm self
Past history of attempts to harm self, including:

Cutting	Scratching
Slashing	Picking
Stabbing	Gouging

RELATED FACTORS

See *Risk for Self-Harm.*

Goals

See *Risk for Self-Harm.*

Generic Interventions

See *Risk for Self-Harm.*

Risk for Self-Mutilation

DEFINITION

Risk for Self-Mutilation: A state in which an individual is at risk to perform a deliberate act upon the self with the intent to injure, not kill, which produces immediate tissue damage to the body.

DEFINING CHARACTERISTICS
Major (Must Be Present, One or More)

Expresses desire or intent to harm self
History of attempts to harm self, e.g.,
   Cutting
   Slashing
   Stabbing
   Scratching
   Picking
   Gouging

RELATED FACTORS

See *Risk for Self-Harm.*

Goals

See *Risk for Self-Harm.*

Generic Interventions

See *Risk for Self-Harm.*

Risk for Suicide

Definition

Risk for Suicide: The state in which an individual is at risk for killing himself or herself.

⚛ AUTHOR'S NOTE

Risk for Suicide is not currently on the NANDA list but has been added for clarity. *Risk for Violence: Self-directed* is included under *Risk for Violence.* The term *violence* is described as a swift and intense force or a rough or injurious physical force. Suicide can be violent, but it can also be nonviolent (overdose of barbiturates). Using the term *violence* unfortunately can cause the risk for suicide to be undetected because of the belief that an individual is not capable of violence.

   Risk for Suicide clearly denotes an individual at high risk for suicide and the need for protection. The treatment of the diagnosis comprises validation, contracting, and protection. The treatment of the underlying depression and hopelessness should be addressed with other nursing diagnoses (e.g., *Ineffective Coping, Hopelessness*).

RISK FACTORS
Major (Must Be Present, One or More)
Suicidal ideation
Previous suicidal attempts

Minor (May Be Present)
See *Risk for Self-Harm.*

RELATED FACTORS
See *Risk for Self-Harm.*

NOC Impulse Control, Suicide, Self-Restraint

Goals

The person will not commit suicide.

Indicators

- State the desire to live.
- Verbalize feelings of anger, loneliness, hopelessness.
- Identify persons to contact if suicidal thoughts occur.
- Identify alternative coping mechanisms.

> **NIC** Active Listening, Coping Enhancement, Suicide Prevention,
> Impulse Control Training, Behavior Control Training,
> Behavior Management: Self-Harm, Hope Instillation,
> Contracting, Surveillance: Safety

Generic Interventions

Assess Level of Risk (Table I-3) (High, Moderate, Low).

Assess Level of Long-Term Risk: Lifestyle, Lethality of Plan, Usual Coping Mechanisms. Support Available.

Provide Closely Supervised Environment for High-Risk Person.

Restrict glass, nail files, scissors, nail polish remover, mirrors, needles, razors, soda cans, plastic bags, lighters, electrical equipment, belts, hangers, knives, tweezers, alcohol, guns.

Meals should be provided in a closely supervised area.

When administering oral medications, check to ensure that all medications are swallowed.

Provide checks on the person per institution policy.

Restrict the individual to the unit unless specifically ordered by physician. When off unit, provide a staff member to accompany the person.

Instruct visitors on restricted items.

The acutely suicidal person may be required to wear a hospital gown to prevent unauthorized leaving.

Room searches should be done periodically per institution policy.

TABLE I.3 Assessing the Degree of Suicidal Risk

Behavior or Symptom	Intensity of Risk		
	LOW	**MODERATE**	**HIGH**
Anxiety	Mild	Moderate	High or panic state
Depression	Mild	Moderate	Severe
Isolation/withdrawal	Some feelings of isolation; no withdrawal	Some feelings of hopelessness, withdrawal	Hopeless, withdrawn, and self-deprecating; isolation
Daily functioning	Effective	Moody	Depressed
	⚛ Good grades in school	⚛ Variable grades	⚛ Poor grades
	Close friends	Some friends	Few or no close friends
	No prior suicide attempt	Prior suicidal thoughts	Prior suicide attempts
	Stable job		Erratic or poor work history
Lifestyle	Stable	Moderately stable	Unstable
Alcohol/drug use	Infrequently to excess	Frequently to excess	Continual abuse
Previous suicide attempts	None or of low lethality (few pills)	One or more (pills, superficial wrist slash)	One or more (entire bottle of pills, gun, hanging)

(table continues on p. 436)

⚛ Applies only to children and adolescents.

435

TABLE I.3 Assessing the Degree of Suicidal Risk (continued)

Behavior or Symptom	Intensity of Risk		
Associated events	None or an argument	⚔ Disciplinary action	Relationship breakup
		⚔ Failing grades	Death of a loved one
		Work problems	Loss of job
		Family illness	Pregnancy
Purpose of act	None or not clear	Relief of shame or guilt	Wants to die
		To punish others	Escape to join deceased
		To get attention	Debilitating disease
Family's reaction and structure	Supportive	Mixed reaction	Angry and unsupportive
	Intact family	Divorced/separated	Disorganized
	Good coping and mental health	Usually copes and understands	Rigid/abusive
	No history of suicide		History of suicide in family
Suicide plan (method, location, time)	No plan	Frequent thoughts, occasional ideas about a plan	Specific plan

⚔ Applies only to children and adolescents.

(Adapted from Hatton, C. L., & McBride, S. [1984]. *Suicide: Assessment and intervention.* Norwalk, CT: Appleton-Century-Crofts and Jackson, D. B., & Saunders, R. B. [1993]. *Child health nursing.* Philadelphia: J. B. Lippincott.)

Use seclusion and restraint if necessary (refer to *Risk for Violence* for discussion).
Notify police if the person leaves and is at risk for suicide.

Notify All Staff that This Person Is at Risk for Suicide.

Make a No-Suicide Contract with the Individual (Include Family if Person Is at Home).
Written contract
Mutual agreement

Encourage Appropriate Expression of Anger and Hostility.

Set Limits on Ruminations about Suicide or Previous Attempts.

Assist in Recognizing Predisposing Factors: "What Was Happening Before You Started Having These Thoughts?"

Facilitate Examination of Life Stresses and Past Coping Mechanisms.

Explore Alternative Behaviors.

Anticipate Future Stresses and Assist in Planning Alternatives.

Involve Person in Planning the Treatment Goals and Evaluating Progress.

Instruct Significant Others in How to Recognize an Increase in Risk: Change in Behavior, Verbal, Nonverbal Communication, Withdrawal, Signs of Depression.

Supply Phone Numbers of 24-hour Emergency Hotlines.

Refer to Community Agency for Ongoing Therapy.

❖ Pediatric Interventions

Take All Suicide Threats Seriously.

Engage Parents, Friends, School Personnel, and the Individual in Behavior Contracts to "Keep Safe."

Explore Feelings and Reason for Suicidal Feelings.

Consult with a Psychiatric Expert Regarding the Most Appropriate Environment for Treatment.

Participate in Programs in Schools to Teach about the Symptoms of Depression and Signs of Suicidal Behavior.

Ⓒ Geriatric Interventions (Miller, 2004)

Be Direct (e.g., "Are You Thinking of Hurting Yourself?").

Acknowledge the Intent with Concern; Remain Nonjudgmental.

Help to Identify Other Options.

Accept the Person's Feelings of Helplessness and Hopelessness.

Discuss the Problem with Family.

Disturbed Sensory Perception

DEFINITION

Disturbed Sensory Perception: The state in which an individual/group experiences, or is at risk of experiencing, a change in the amount, pattern, or interpretation of incoming stimuli.

ⓧ AUTHOR'S NOTE

The diagnosis *Disturbed Sensory Perception* describes a person with altered perception and cognition influenced by physiologic factors (e.g., pain, sleep deprivation, immobility, and excessive or decreased meaningful stimuli from the environment). *Impaired Thought Processes* also can manifest with altered perception and cognition. *Disturbed Sensory Perception* results when barriers or factors interfere with a person's ability to interpret stimuli accurately. When personality or mental disorders interfere with one's ability to interpret stimuli accurately, *Impaired Thought Processes* is more accurate than *Disturbed Sensory Perception.*

The diagnosis *Disturbed Sensory Perception* has six subcategories: visual, auditory, kinesthetic, gustatory, tactile, and olfactory. When a person has a visual or hearing deficit, how does the nurse intervene with the diagnosis *Disturbed Sensory Perception: Visual related to effects of glaucoma*? What would the goals be? The nurse should assess for the individual's response to the visual loss and specifically label the response, not the deficit.

The diagnosis *Disturbed Sensory Perception* is more clinically useful without the addition of the specific sense. Examples of responses to sensory deficits may be:

Visual
    Risk for Injury   *Self-Care Deficit*
Auditory
    Impaired Communication   *Social Isolation*
Kinesthetic
    Risk for Injury

⊙ AUTHOR'S NOTE (continued)

Olfactory
Imbalanced Nutrition
Tactile
Risk for Injury
Gustatory
Imbalanced Nutrition

DEFINING CHARACTERISTICS
Major (Must Be Present, One or More)
Inaccurate interpretation of environmental stimuli *and/or*
Negative change in amount or pattern of incoming stimuli

Minor (May Be Present)
Disorientation about time or place

Auditory or visual hallucinations

Altered problem-solving ability

Altered behavior or communication pattern

Restlessness

Disorientation about people

Irritability

Poor concentration

RELATED FACTORS
Many factors in an individual's life can contribute to *Disturbed Sensory Perception*. Some common factors are listed below.

Pathophysiologic
Related to misinterpretations secondary to:
Sensory organ alterations
Visual, gustatory, auditory, olfactory, and tactile deficits

Neurologic alterations
Cerebrovascular accident   Neuropathies
Encephalitis/meningitis

Metabolic alterations
Fluid and electrolyte   Acidosis
  imbalance   Alkalosis
Elevated blood urea
  nitrogen

Impaired oxygen transport

Cerebral	Respiratory
Cardiac	Anemia

Related to mobility restrictions secondary to paraplegia or quadriplegia

Treatment-Related

Related to misinterpretations secondary to:
Medications (sedatives, tranquilizers)
Surgery (glaucoma, cataract, detached retina)

Related to physical isolation (reverse isolation, communicable disease, prison)
Related to immobility
Related to mobility restrictions (bed rest, traction, casts, Stryker frame, CircOlectric bed)

Situational (Personal, Environmental)

Related to misinterpretations secondary to pain or stress
Related to socially restricted environment
Related to excessive noise
Related to complex environment (noise, lights, constant changes, excess activity, frequent demands)
Related to monotonous environment
Related to loss of socialization

NOC Cognitive Orientation, Distorted Thought Control

Goals

The person will demonstrate decreased symptoms of sensory overload as evident by (specify).

Indicators

- Identify and eliminate the potential risk factors, if possible.
- Describe the rationale for the treatment modality.

NIC Cognitive Stimulation, Reality Orientation

Generic Interventions

Reduce Excess Noise or Light.

Share with Person the Source of the Noise.

Discuss the Use of a Radio with Earplugs to Provide Soft, Relaxing Music.

Share with Personnel the Need to Reduce Noise and Provide Individuals with Uninterrupted Sleep for at Least 2 to 4 Hours.

Attempt to Reduce Fears and Concerns by Explaining Equipment, Its Purpose, and Noises.

Encourage Person to Share Perceptions of Noises.

Orient to All Three Spheres (Person, Place, Time).

Offer Simple Explanations of Each Task.

Allow Person to Participate in Task, Such as Washing Own Face.

Promote Movement In and Out of Bed.

Avoid Isolation of the Person; Change Environment Daily (e.g., Move Into Hall).

Provide at Least Four Undisturbed Sleep and Rest Periods for 100 Minutes Every 24 Hours.

Use a Variety of Methods to Stimulate Senses (e.g., Perfume, Pet Therapy, Ambulate to Window).

Ask Family to Bring in Familiar Possessions.

Limit Use of Sedation.

If at Risk for Injury, Refer to *Risk for Injury*.

Sexuality Patterns, Ineffective

DEFINITION

Ineffective Sexuality Patterns: The state in which an individual experiences, or is at risk of experiencing, a change in sexual health. Sexual health is the integration of somatic, emotional, intellectual, and social aspects of sexual being in ways that are enriching and that enhance personality, communication, and love.

> **Ⓔ AUTHOR'S NOTE**
>
> The diagnoses *Ineffective Sexuality Patterns* and *Sexual Dysfunction* are difficult to differentiate. *Ineffective Sexuality Patterns* is a broad diagnosis of which sexual dysfunction can be one part. Sexual health is the integration of somatic, emotional, intellectual, and social aspects of sexual being in ways that are enriching and that enhance personality, communication, and love (World Health Organization).
>
> *Sexual Dysfunction* may be more appropriately used by a nurse with advanced preparation in sex therapy. Until *Sexual Dysfunction* is differentiated from *Ineffective Sexuality Patterns,* it is unnecessary for most nurses to use this diagnosis.

DEFINING CHARACTERISTICS
Major (Must Be Present)

Actual or anticipated negative changes in sexual functioning or sexual identity

Minor (May Be Present)

Expression of concern about sexual functioning or sexual
  identity
Inappropriate sexual verbal or nonverbal behavior
Changes in primary and/or secondary sexual characteristics

RELATED FACTORS

Altered sexuality patterns can occur as a response to a variety of health problems, situations, and conflicts. Some common sources are listed below.

Pathophysiologic
Related to biochemical effects on energy and libido secondary to:
Endocrine

Diabetes mellitus   Hyperthyroidism
Decreased hormone   Addison's disease
  production   Myxedema
Acromegaly

Genitourinary
Chronic renal failure

Neuromuscular and skeletal
Arthritis
Multiple sclerosis
Amyotrophic lateral sclerosis
Disturbances of the nerve supply to the brain, spinal cord,
  sensory nerves, and autonomic nerves

Cardiorespiratory
Myocardial infarction   Congestive heart failure
Peripheral vascular   Chronic respiratory
  disorders   disorders

Related to fears associated with (specify) (sexually transmitted diseases)
HIV/AIDS   Human papilloma virus
Herpes   Chlamydia
Syphilis   Gonorrhea

Related to the effects of alcohol on performance
Related to decreased vaginal lubrication secondary to (specify)
Related to fear of premature ejaculation
Related to painful intercourse

Treatment-Related

Related to the effects of medications or radiation treatment

Related to altered self-concept from change in appearance (trauma, radical surgery)

Situational (Personal, Environmental)

Related to partner problem (specify), for example, unwilling, uninformed, abusive, not available, separated, divorced

Related to no privacy

Related to stressors secondary to job problems, financial worries, conflicting values, or religious conflict

Related to misinformation or lack of knowledge

Related to fatigue

Related to fear of rejection secondary to obesity

Related to pain

Related to fear of sexual failure

Related to fear of pregnancy

Related to depression

Related to anxiety

Related to guilt

Related to history of unsatisfactory sexual experiences

Maturational

Adolescent

Related to ineffective role models

Related to negative sexual teaching

Related to absence of sexual teaching

Adult

Related to adjustment to parenthood

Related to effects of pregnancy on energy levels and body image

Related to values conflict

NOC Body Image, Self-Esteem, Role Performance, Sexual Identity: Acceptance

Goals

The person will resume previous sexual activity or engage in alternative satisfying sexual activity.

NIC Behavioral Management: Sexual, Counseling, Sexual Counseling,
Emotional Support, Active Listening, Teaching: Sexuality

Indicators

- Identify impact of stressors, loss, or change on sexual functioning.
- Modify behavior to reduce stressors.
- Identify limitations on sexual activity caused by health problem.
- Identify appropriate modifications in sexual practices in response to these limitations.
- Report satisfying sexual activity.

Generic Interventions

Acquire a Sexual History.

Usual sexual pattern
Satisfaction (individual, partner)
Sexual knowledge
Problems (sexual, health)
Expectations
Mood, energy level

Encourage Client to Ask Questions about Sexuality or Sexual Functioning that May Be Disturbing Him or Her.

Explore His or Her Relationship with Partner.

If Stressors or a Stressful Lifestyle Have Decreased Functioning:

Assist person in modifying lifestyle to reduce stress.
Encourage identification of present stressors in life; group as those the person can control and those the person cannot, e.g.,
Can control:
    Personal lateness
    Involvement in community activities
Cannot control:
    Report due
    Daughter's illness

Initiate a Regular Exercise Program for Stress Reduction. See *Health Seeking Behaviors* for Interventions.

Identify Alternative Methods for Dispersing Sexual Energy when Partner Is Unavailable or Unwilling.

Use masturbation, if acceptable to individual.

Teach the physical and psychological benefits of regular physical activity (at least three times a week for 30 minutes).

If partner is deceased, explore opportunities to meet and socialize with others (night school, singles club, community work).

If a Change or Loss of Body Part Has Decreased Functioning:

Assess the stage of adaptation of the individual and partner to the loss (denial, depression, anger, resolution; see *Grieving*).

Explain the normality of the foregoing responses to loss.

Explain the need to share concerns with partner:
    Imagined response of partner
    Fear of rejection
    Fear of future losses
    Fear of physically hurting partner

Encourage the Partner to Discuss the Strengths of Their Relationship and to Assess the Influence of the Loss on Their Strengths.

Encourage Person to Resume Sexual Activity as Close to Previous Pattern as Possible.

Identify Barriers to Satisfying Sexual Functioning (e.g., Hypoxia, Pain, Impaired Mobility, Pregnancy, Side Effects of Medications).

Teach Techniques to:

Reduce oxygen consumption.

Use oxygen during sexual activity if indicated.

Engage in sexual activity after intermittent positive-pressure breathing treatment or postural drainage.

Plan sexual activities for time of day person is most rested.

Use positions for intercourse that are comfortable and permit unrestricted breathing.

Reduce Cardiac Workload.

Clients with Cardiac Problems Should Avoid Sexual Activity:

In extremes of temperature
Directly after eating or drinking
When intoxicated
When tired
With unfamiliar partner
Rest before engaging in sexual activity (mornings are best)

Clients with Cardiac Problems Should Terminate Sexual Activity if Chest Discomfort or Dyspnea Occurs.

Reduce or Eliminate Pain.

If vaginal lubrication is decreased, use a water-soluble
  lubricant.
Take medication for pain before beginning sexual activity.
Use whatever relaxes individual before beginning sexual
  activity (hot packs, hot shower).

Initiate Health Teaching and Referrals As Indicated; Discuss with Individuals or Couples the Availability of Self-Help Groups (e.g., Reach for Recovery, United Ostomy Association).

❖ Pediatric Interventions

Clarify the Confidentiality of the Discussion.

Strive to Be Open, Warm, Objective, Unembarrassed, and Reassuring.

Explore Feelings and Sexual Experiences. Encourage Questions. Clarify Myths.

Discuss How Bacteria Are Transferred (Vaginally, Anally, Orally).

For Young Women, Explain the Relationship of Sexually Transmitted Diseases and Pelvic Inflammatory Disease, Infertility, and Ectopic Pregnancies.

◆ Pediatric Interventions (cont'd)

Show a Diagram of Reproductive Structures.

Emphasize that Most Sexually Transmitted Diseases Have No Symptoms Initially.

Discuss Abstinence from Sexual Perspective (e.g., Right to Say No, Commitment, Unwanted Pregnancies, Sexually Transmitted Diseases).

Discuss Contraceptive Methods Available (e.g., Pill, Depo-Provera, Intrauterine Device, Condoms, Foam, Diaphragm, Spermicides):
How it works
Effectiveness
Cost
Prevention of sexually transmitted diseases

Explain and Provide Written Instructions for Method Chosen.

◆ Maternal Interventions

Discuss Body Changes During Pregnancy.

Encourage Couple to Share Their Feelings.

Reassure that Unless Problems Exist (Preterm Labor, Previous Early Loss, Bleeding or Rupture of Membranes) Intercourse Is Allowed Until Labor Begins.

Suggest Alternative Sexual Positions for Later Pregnancy to Prevent Abdominal Pressure (e.g., Side-Lying, Woman Kneeling, Woman on Top).

🏃 Maternal Interventions (cont'd)

Give Reassurance about Postpartum Changes. Reassure that This Is a Temporary State and Will Resolve in 2 to 3 Months.

Reassure that Sexual Attitudes Change Throughout Pregnancy from Feeling Very Desirous of Sex to Wanting Only to Be Cuddled.

Discuss Techniques to Enhance the Couple's Relationship (Polomeno, 1999).

Explore Fears and Anxieties (Separately).

Discuss Barriers to Disclosing Fears and Anxieties.

Role-Play Disclosure.

Encourage Client to Share the "Little Things" that Represent Caring.

Instruct on "Heart Talks." One Partner Talks for 5 Minutes with No Interruption or Argument. The Other Partner then Has a Chance to Talk. At the End the Couple Hugs and Says, "I Love You" (Polomeno, 1999).

Instruct on "Sexual Conversation" (Gray, 1995). Useful Questions Are:

What do you like about having sex with me?
Would you like more sex?
Would you like more or less foreplay?
Is there a way that you would like me to touch you?

Discuss Methods to Keep Romance Alive (Gray, 1995):

Set aside regular time with each other.
Hold hands.
Send messages that partner is appreciated.

▲ Maternal Interventions (cont'd)

Acknowledge Fatigue, Especially During First Trimester, Last Month, and Postpartum.

Encourage Person to Make Time for Her Relationship in Sexual and Other Contexts.

Teach Couples to Abstain from Any Sex Play or Intercourse and Seek the Advice of their Health Care Provider If Any of the Following Situations Are Present (Pillitteri, 2003):

Vaginal bleeding	Premature dilation
Multiple pregnancy	Engaged fetal head
Placenta previa	or lightening
History of premature	Rupture of membranes
delivery	History of miscarriage

ⓒ Geriatric Interventions

Explain that Normal Aging Affects Reproductive Abilities but Has Little Effect on Sexual Functioning.

Explore Interest, Activity, Attitude, and Knowledge Regarding Sexual Functioning.

If Pertinent, Discuss the Effects of Chronic Diseases on Functioning.

Explain the Effects of Certain Medications on Sexual Functioning (e.g., Cardiovascular, Antidepressants, Antihistamine, Gastrointestinal, Sedatives, Alcohol).

If Sexual Dysfunction Is Related to Medications, Explore Alternatives (e.g., Medication Change, Dose Reduction).

⊜ Geriatric Interventions (cont'd)

With Women, Discuss the Quality of Vaginal Lubrication and Available Water-Soluble Lubricants.

Encourage Questions. If Needed, Refer to Urologist or Other Specialist.

Sexual Dysfunction

DEFINITION
Sexual Dysfunction: The state in which an individual experiences, or is at risk of experiencing, a change in sexual function that is viewed as unrewarding or inadequate.

> ℗ **AUTHOR'S NOTE**
> Refer to *Ineffective Sexuality Patterns.*

DEFINING CHARACTERISTICS
Major (Must Be Present, One or More)
Verbalization of problem with sexual function
Reports limitations on sexual performance imposed by disease or therapy

Minor (May Be Present)
Fears future limitations on sexual performance
Is misinformed about sexuality
Lacks knowledge about sexuality and sexual function
Has value conflicts involving sexual expression (cultural, religious)
Experiences altered relationship with significant other
Is dissatisfied with sex role (perceived or actual)

Disturbed Sleep Pattern

DEFINITION

Disturbed Sleep Pattern: The state in which an individual experiences or is at risk of experiencing a change in the quantity or quality of his or her rest pattern that causes discomfort or interferes with desired lifestyle.

DEFINING CHARACTERISTICS
ADULTS
Major (Must Be Present)

Difficulty falling or remaining asleep

Minor (May Be Present)

Fatigue on awakening   Agitation
  or during the day   Dozing during the day
Mood alterations

CHILDREN

Sleep disturbances in children are frequently related to fear, enuresis, or inconsistent responses of parents to the child's requests for changes in sleep rules, such as requests to stay up late.

Reluctance to retire
Frequent awakening during the night
Desire to sleep with parents

RELATED FACTORS

Many factors in life can contribute to *Disturbed Sleep Pattern.* Some common factors are listed below.

Pathophysiologic
Related to frequent awakenings secondary to:

Angina   Retention

Peripheral arteriosclerosis
Respiratory disorders
Circulatory disorders
Diarrhea
Constipation
Incontinence

Dysuria
Frequency
Hyperthyroidism
Gastric ulcers
Hepatic disorders

Treatment-Related
Related to difficulty assuming usual position secondary to:

Casts
Pain

Traction
Intravenous therapy

Related to excessive daytime sleeping secondary to medications, e.g.:

Tranquilizers
Sedatives
Hypnotics
Antidepressants
Barbiturates
Corticosteroids

Soporifics
Monoamine oxidase
    inhibitors
Antihypertensives
Amphetamines

Situational (Personal, Environmental)
Related to excessive hyperactivity secondary to:

Bipolar disorder
Attention-deficit disorder

Panic anxiety

Related to excessive daytime sleeping
Related to inadequate daytime activities
Related to depression
Related to pain
Related to anxiety response
Related to discomforts secondary to pregnancy
Related to lifestyle disruptions (e.g., occupational, emotional, social, sexual, financial)
Related to environmental changes (e.g., hospitalization [noise, disturbing roommate, fear] or travel)
Related to circadian rhythm changes
Related to fears

Maturational
Child
Related to fear of the dark

Adult Women
Related to hormonal changes (e.g., perimenopausal)

NOC Rest, Sleep, Well-being

Goals

The person will report an optimal balance of rest and activity.

Indicators

- Describe factors that prevent or inhibit sleep.
- Identify techniques to induce sleep.

NIC Energy Management, Sleep Enhancement, Environmental Management

Generic Interventions

Reduce Noise.

Organize Procedures to Provide the Fewest Number of Disturbances During Sleep Period (e.g., When Individual Awakens for Medication, Also Administer Treatments and Obtain Vital Signs).

If Voiding During the Night Is Disruptive, Have Person Limit Nighttime Fluids and Void before Retiring.

Establish with Person a Schedule for a Daytime Program of Activity (Walking, Physical Therapy).

Limit Amount and Length of Daytime Sleeping If Excessive (i.e., >1 Hour).

Assess with Person, Family, or Parents the Usual Bedtime Routine— Time, Hygiene Practices, Rituals (Reading, Toy)—and Adhere to It as Closely as Possible.

Limit Intake of Caffeinated Drinks after Midafternoon.

Explain to Person and Significant Others the Causes of Sleep/Rest Disturbance and Possible Ways to Avoid It (Boyd, 2004).

Avoid alcohol.

Keep regular bedtimes and rising times.

Set a relaxing routine to prepare for sleep (e.g., herbal tea, warm bath).

Keep bedroom slightly cool.

Wear ear plugs if noise is a problem.

Do not exercise within 3 hours of bedtime.

Pediatric Interventions

Explain Night to the Child (Stars and Moon).

Discuss How Some Persons (Nurses, Factory Workers) Work at Night.

Compare the Contrast that When Night Comes for Him or Her, Day Is Coming for Persons in Another Country.

If a Nightmare Occurs, Encourage the Child to Talk about it if Possible. Reassure Child that it Is a Dream, Even if It Seems so Real. Share with Child that You Have Dreams Too.

Provide Child with a Night Light or a Flashlight to Use to Give Child Control over the Dark.

Reassure Child that You Will Be Nearby All Night.

Explain the Possible Problems of Sleeping with Child.

Maternal Interventions

Explain Some Reasons for Sleeping Difficulties During Pregnancy (e.g., Leg Cramps, Backache).

Teach How to Position Pillows in Side-Lying Position (One between Legs, One under Abdomen, One under Top Arm, One under Head).

Teach to Avoid Caffeine and Large Meals Within 2 to 3 Hours of Bedtime.

Advise to Exercise Daily and Take a Warm Bath at Bedtime.

Geriatric Interventions

Explain the Effects of Alcohol on Sleep (e.g., Nightmares, Frequent Awakenings).

Explain that Sleeping Pills (Prescribed or over the Counter) Are Not Effective after 1 Month and that They Interfere with the Quality of Sleep and Daytime Functioning.

Instruct to Avoid Over-the-Counter Sleeping Pills Because of their Antihistamine Effects.

If Sleeping Pills Are Needed for a Few Days, Advise to Consult Primary Care Provider for a Type with a Short Half-Life.

DEFINITION

Sleep Deprivation: The state in which an individual experiences prolonged periods of time without sustained, natural, periodic states of relative unconsciousness.

ⓒ AUTHOR'S NOTE

This diagnostic label represents a situation in which insufficient sleep is achieved. It is the most common type of sleep pattern disturbance and will probably be used for most clinical situations.

DEFINING CHARACTERISTICS

Refer to *Disturbed Sleep Pattern.*

RELATED FACTORS

Refer to *Disturbed Sleep Pattern.*

Goals

Refer to *Disturbed Sleep Pattern.*

Generic Interventions

Refer to *Disturbed Sleep Pattern.*

DEFINITION

Impaired Social Interaction: The state in which an individual experiences, or is at risk of experiencing, negative, insufficient, or unsatisfactory responses from interactions.

DEFINING CHARACTERISTICS
Major (Must Be Present, One or More)

Reports inability to establish and/or maintain stable supportive relationships
Is dissatisfied with social network

Minor (May Be Present)

Social isolation
Superficial relationships
Blaming others for interpersonal problems
Feelings of rejection
Others reporting problematic patterns of interaction

Feelings of being misunderstood
Avoidance of others
Interpersonal difficulties at work

RELATED FACTORS

Impaired Social Interaction can result from a variety of situations and health problems that are related to the inability to establish and maintain rewarding relationships. Some common sources are as follows:

Pathophysiologic

Related to embarrassment or limited physical mobility or energy secondary to loss of body function, terminal illness, or loss of body part
Related to communication barriers secondary to hearing deficits, mental retardation, visual deficits, speech impediments, or chronic mental illness

Treatment-Related

Related to surgical disfigurement
Related to therapeutic isolation

Situational (Personal, Environmental)
Related to alienation from others secondary to:

Constant complaining

Rumination

Overt hostility

Manipulative behaviors

Mistrust or suspicions

Illogical ideas

Egocentric behavior

Emotional immaturity

Aggressive responses

High anxiety

Impulsive behavior

Delusions

Hallucinations

Disorganized thinking

Dependent behavior

Strong unpopular beliefs

Depressive behavior

Related to language/cultural barriers
Related to lack of social skills
Related to change in usual social patterns secondary to divorce, relocation, or death

Maturational
Child/Adolescent
Related to impulse control
Related to altered appearance
Related to speech impediments

Adult
Related to loss of ability to practice vocation

Older Adult
Related to change in usual social patterns secondary to:

Death of spouse

Retirement

Functional deficits

NOC Family Environment: Internal, Social Interaction Skills, Social Involvement

Goals

The person/family will report increased satisfaction with socialization.

Indicators

• Identify problematic behavior that deters socialization.

- Substitute constructive behaviors for disruptive social behaviors (specify).
- Describe strategies to promote effective socialization.

NIC Anticipatory Guidance, Behavior Modification, Family Integrity: Promotion, Counseling, Behavior Management, Family Support, Self-Responsibility, Facilitation

Generic Interventions

Provide an Individual, Supportive Relationship.

Help to Identify How Stress Precipitates Problems.

Support Healthy Defenses.

Help to Identify Alternative Courses of Action.

Assist in Analyzing Approaches that Work Best.

Role Play Situations that Are Problematic. Discuss Feelings.

If in Group Therapy:

Focus on here and now.

Establish group norms that discourage inappropriate behavior.

Encourage testing of new social behavior.

Use snacks or coffee to decrease anxiety during sessions.

Role model certain accepted social behaviors (e.g., responding to a friendly greeting versus ignoring it).

Foster development of relationships among members through self-disclosure and genuineness.

Use questions and observations to encourage persons with limited interaction skills.

Encourage members to validate their perception with others.

Identify strengths among members and ignore selected weaknesses.

For Family Members of Persons with Chronic Mental Illness:

Assist in understanding and providing support.

Provide factual information concerning illness, treatment, and progress.

Validate feelings of frustration when dealing with daily problems.

Provide guidance on overstimulating or understimulating environments.

Allow families to discuss their feelings of guilt and how their behavior affects the person.

Develop an alliance with family.

Arrange for periodic respite care.

For Individuals with Chronic Mental Illness, Teach (McFarland & Wasli, 2000):

Responsibilities of his or her role as a client (making requests clearly known, participating in therapies)

To outline activities of the day and focus on accomplishing them

How to approach others to communicate

To identify which interactions encourage others to give him or her consideration and respect

To identify how he or she can participate in formulating family roles and responsibility to comply

To recognize signs of anxiety and methods to relieve them

To identify his or her positive behavior and experience satisfaction with self in selecting constructive choices

As Indicated, Refer to Community Agencies (e.g., Social Service, Occupational Counseling, Family Therapy, Crisis Intervention).

❖ Pediatric Interventions

If Impulse Control Is a Problem:

Set firm, responsible limits.

Do not lecture.

State limits simply and back them up.

Maintain routines.

Limit play to one playmate to learn appropriate play skills (e.g., relative, adult, quiet child).

❖ Pediatric Interventions (cont'd)

Gradually increase number of playmates.
Provide immediate and constant feedback.

Teach Parents To:

Avoid harsh criticism.
Do not disagree in front of child.
Establish eye contact before giving instructions and ask
  child to repeat what was said.

**Teach Older Child to Self-Monitor
Target Behaviors and to Develop
Self-Reliance.**

**If Antisocial Behavior Is Present,
Help To:**

Describe behaviors that interfere with socialization.
Role play alternative responses.
Limit social circle to a manageable size.
Elicit peer feedback for positive and negative behavior.

Social Isolation

DEFINITION

Social Isolation: The state in which an individual or group
experiences or perceives a need or desire for increased involvement with others but is unable to make that contact.

> ⊗ **AUTHOR'S NOTE**
>
> In 1994, NANDA added a new diagnosis, *Risk for Loneli-
> ness*. Although this diagnosis is only in stage 1 of a four-
> stage developmental process, it more accurately adheres

> ○ **AUTHOR'S NOTE (continued)**
>
> to the NANDA definition of "response to." Social isolation is not a response but a cause or contributing factor to loneliness. In addition, one can experience loneliness even with many persons around. I recommend deleting *Social Isolation* from clinical use and using *Loneliness* or *Risk for Loneliness.*

DEFINING CHARACTERISTICS

Because social isolation is a subjective state, all inferences made about a person's feelings of aloneness must be validated because the causes vary and people show their aloneness in different ways.

Major (Must Be Present, One or More)

Expresses feelings of aloneness, rejection
Desire for more contact with people
Reports insecurity in social situations*
Describes a lack of meaningful relationships*

Minor (May Be Present)

Time passing slowly ("Mondays are so long for me.")
Inability to concentrate and make decisions
Feelings of uselessness
Feelings of rejection
Underactivity (physical or verbal)
Appearing depressed, anxious, or angry
Failure to interact with others nearby
Sad, dull affect*
Uncommunicative*
Withdrawn*
Poor eye contact*
Preoccupied with own thoughts and memories

RELATED FACTORS

A state of social isolation can result from a variety of situations and health problems that are related to a loss of

---

*Elsen, J., & Blegen, M. (1991). Social isolation. In M. Maas, K. Buckwalter, & M. Hardy (Eds.), *Nursing diagnoses and interventions for the elderly.* Redwood City, CA: Addison-Wesley Nursing.

established relationships or to a failure to generate these relationships. Some common sources follow.

Pathophysiologic
Related to fear of rejection secondary to:
Obesity

Cancer (disfiguring surgery of head or neck, superstitions of others)

Physical handicaps (paraplegia, amputation, arthritis, hemiplegia)

Emotional handicaps (extreme anxiety, depression, paranoia, phobias)

Incontinence (embarrassment, odor)

Communicable diseases (AIDS, hepatitis)

Psychiatric illness (schizophrenia, bipolar affective disorder, personality disorders)

Treatment-Related
Therapeutic isolation

Situational (Personal, Environmental)
Related to death of a significant other
Related to divorce
Related to disfiguring appearance
Related to fear of rejection secondary to:

Obesity	Unemployment
Hospitalization or terminal illness (dying process)	Extreme poverty

Related to moving to another culture (e.g., unfamiliar language)
Related to history of unsatisfying relationships secondary to:

Drug abuse	Alcohol abuse
Immature behavior	Unacceptable social
Delusional thinking	behavior

Related to loss of usual means of transportation

Maturational
Child
Related to protective isolation or a communicable disease

Older Adult
Related to loss of usual social contacts

DEFINITION

Chronic Sorrow: The state in which a person experiences, or is at risk of experiencing, permanent sadness, variable in intensity, in response to loss of a loved one or a loved one forever changed by an event or condition, and the ongoing losses of normality (Teel, 1991).

> ## ⓒⓐ AUTHOR'S NOTE
>
> *Chronic Sorrow* was identified in 1962 by Olchansky. *Chronic Sorrow* is different from *Grieving. Grieving* is time-limited and ends in adaptation to the loss. *Chronic Sorrow* will vary in intensity, but persists as long as the person with the disability or chronic sorrow condition lives (Eakes, 1995). Chronic sorrow can also occur in an individual with a chronic disease that regularly impairs the person's ability to live a "normal life" (e.g., paraplegic, AIDS, sickle cell disease).

DEFINING CHARACTERISTICS

Life-long episodic sadness due to the loss of a loved one or the loss of normality in a loved one who is disabled
Variable in intensity

RELATED FACTORS
Situational (Personal, Environmental)
Related to the chronic loss of normality secondary to child's condition

Autism	Mental retardation
Down syndrome	Psychiatric condition
Severe scoliosis	Spina bifida
HIV	Sickle cell disease
Type I diabetes mellitus	

Related to lifetime losses associated with infertility
Related to ongoing losses associated with a degenerative condition

Multiple sclerosis	Alzheimer's disease

Related to untimely loss of a loved one (e.g., child)
Related to losses associated with caring for a child
with a fatal illness

NOC	Depression Control, Coping, Mood Management, Acceptance: Health Status

Goals

The person will be assisted to anticipate developmental events that can trigger heightened sadness.

Indicators

- Express sadness.
- Discuss the loss periodically.

NIC	Anticipatory Guidance, Coping Enhancement, Referral, Active Listening, Presence, Resiliency Promotion

Generic Interventions

**Explain the Difference between
Chronic Sorrow and Chronic Grieving:**
Normal response
Focused on loss of normality
Not time-limited
Persists throughout life

**Encourage to Share His or Her
Feelings Since the Change
(e.g., Birth of Child, Accident).**

**Gently Encourage to Share Lost
Dreams or Hopes.**

**Assist to Identify Developmental
Milestones that Will Exacerbate the
Loss of Normality (e.g., School Play,
Sports, Prom, Dating).**

**Encourage to Participate in Support
Groups with Others Experiencing
Chronic Sorrow.**

Link the Family with Appropriate Services (e.g., Home Health, Respite Counselor).

Clarify that His or Her Feelings Will Fluctuate (Intensify, Diminish) Through the Years, but the Sorrow Will Not Disappear.

Stress the Importance of Maintaining Support Systems and Friendships.

Share the Difficulties of:
Living worried
Treating child like other children
Staying in the struggle

Refer also to Caregiver rule strain.

Spiritual Distress
Spiritual Distress, Risk for
Spiritual Well-Being, Readiness for Enhanced
Religiosity, Impaired
Religiosity, Risk for Impaired

Spiritual Distress

DEFINITION

Spiritual Distress: The state in which an individual or group experiences, or is at risk of experiencing, a disturbance in the belief or value system that provides strength, hope, and meaning to life.

DEFINING CHARACTERISTICS
Major (Must Be Present)
Experiences a disturbance in belief system

Minor (May Be Present)
Questions meaning of life, death, and suffering
Questions credibility of belief system
Demonstrates discouragement or despair
Chooses not to practice usual religious rituals
Has ambivalent feelings (doubts) about beliefs
Expresses that he or she has no reason for living
Feels a sense of spiritual emptiness
Shows emotional detachment from self and others
Expresses concern—anger, resentment, fear—about the
  meaning of life, suffering, death
Requests spiritual assistance for a disturbance in belief
  system

RELATED FACTORS
Pathophysiologic
**Related to challenges to belief system or separation
from spiritual ties secondary to:**

Loss of body part or function	Pain
Terminal illness	Trauma
Debilitating disease	Miscarriage, stillbirth

Treatment-Related
**Related to conflict between (specify prescribed regi-
men) and beliefs**

Abortion	Surgery
Blood transfusion	Dietary restrictions
Isolation	Amputation
Medications	Medical procedures

Situational (Personal, Environmental)
Related to death or illness of significant other
**Related to embarrassment at practicing spiritual
rituals**
Related to barriers to practicing spiritual rituals
Intensive care restrictions
Confinement to bed or room
Lack of privacy
Lack of availability of special foods/diet

**Related to beliefs opposed by family, peers, health care
providers**
Related to divorce, separation from loved ones

NOC Hope, Spiritual Well-Being

Goals

The person will express satisfaction with spiritual condition.

Indicators

- Continue spiritual practices not detrimental to health.
- Express decreasing feelings of guilt and anxiety.

NIC Spiritual Growth Facilitation, Hope Instillation, Active
Listening, Presence, Emotional Support, Spiritual Support

Generic Interventions

**Communicate Acceptance of Various
Spiritual Beliefs and Practices.**

Convey Nonjudgmental Attitude.

**Acknowledge Importance
of Spiritual Needs.**

**Express Willingness of Health Care
Team to Help in Meeting
Spiritual Needs.**

**Provide Privacy and Quiet As Needed
for Daily Prayer, Visit of Spiritual
Leader, and Spiritual Reading
and Contemplation.**

**Contact Spiritual Leader to Clarify
Practices and Perform Religious
Rites or Services if Desired.**

**Maintain Diet with Religious
Restrictions When Not
Detrimental to Health.**

Encourage Spiritual Rituals
Not Detrimental to Health.

Provide Opportunity for Individual
to Pray with Others or Be Read to
by Members of Own Religious Group
or a Member of the Health Care
Team Who Feels Comfortable
with These Activities.

Give "Permission" to Discuss
Spiritual Matters with Nurse by
Bringing Up Subject of Spiritual
Welfare if Necessary.

Use Questions about Past Beliefs and
Spiritual Experiences to Assist Person
in Putting this Life Event Into
Wider Perspective.

Offer to Pray/Meditate/Read with
Client If You Are Comfortable with
This, or Arrange for Another
Member of Health Care Team
if More Appropriate.

Be Available and Willing to Listen
When Client Expresses Self-Doubt,
Guilt, or Other Negative Feelings.

Offer to Contact Other Spiritual
Support Person (e.g., Pastoral Care,
Hospital Chaplain) if Person Cannot
Share Feelings with Usual
Spiritual Leader.

❖ Pediatric Interventions

Provide Child with Opportunity to
Engage in Usual Spiritual Practices
(e.g., Bedtime Prayers, Visit to
Chapel).

Discuss if Being Sick Has Changed His
or Her Beliefs (e.g., Prayer Requests).

❖ Pediatric Interventions (cont'd)

Clarify that Accidents or Illnesses Are Not Punishments for "Bad" Acts.

Support an Adolescent Who May Be Struggling for Understanding of Spiritual Teachings.

For Parental Conflict about Treatment of Child:

If parents refuse treatment of child, encourage consideration of alternative methods of therapy (e.g., use of Christian Science nurses and practitioners; special surgeons and techniques for surgery without blood transfusions); support individual making informed decision even if decision conflicts with own values.

If treatment is still refused, physician or hospital administrator may obtain court order appointing temporary guardian to consent to treatment.

Call spiritual leader to support parents (and possibly child).

Encourage expression of negative feelings.

Spiritual Distress, Risk for

DEFINITION

Risk for Spiritual Distress: The state in which the individual or group is at risk of experiencing a disturbance in the belief or value system that provides strength, hope, and meaning to life.

RISK FACTORS

Refer to *Spiritual Distress* for related factors.

NOC Hope, Spiritual Well-Being

Goals

The person will express continued spiritual harmony.

Indicators

- Continue to practice usual spiritual rituals.
- Describe increased comfort after assistance.

NIC Refer to Spiritual Distress

Generic Interventions

Refer to *Spiritual Distress* for interventions.

Spiritual Well-Being, Readiness for Enhanced

DEFINITION

Readiness for Enhanced Spiritual Well-Being: An individual who experiences affirmation of life in a relationship with a higher power (as defined by the person), self, community, and environment that nurtures and celebrates wholeness (The National Interfaith Coalition on Aging, 1980, as cited in Carson, 1989).

> ⚙ **AUTHOR'S NOTE**
> Refer to *Spiritual Distress.*

DEFINING CHARACTERISTICS (CARSON, 1989)

Inner Strengths That Nurture

Sense of awareness	Sacred source
Trust relationships	Inner peace
Unifying force	

Intangible motivation and commitment directing toward
  ultimate values of love, meaning, hope, beauty, and truth
Trust relations with or in the transcendent that provide
  bases for meaning and hope in life's experiences and love
  in one's relationships
Has meaning and purpose to one's existence

RISK FACTORS
Refer to Related Factors.

RELATED FACTORS
Because this is a diagnosis of positive functioning, the use of
related factors is not warranted.

`NOC` Hope, Spiritual Well-Being

Goals
The person will express enhanced spiritual harmony and
wholeness.

Indicators
• Maintain previous relationship with higher being.
• Continue spiritual practices not detrimental to health.

`NIC` Spiritual Growth Facilitation, Spiritual Support

Generic Interventions
**Support the Person's Spiritual
Practices. Refer to Interventions to
Reduce Barriers for Spiritual
Practices under *Spiritual Distress*.**

DEFINITION

Impaired religiosity: The state in which a person or group has impaired ability to exercise reliance on beliefs of a particular denomination or faith community and to participate in related rituals.

DEFINING CHARACTERISTICS

Individual experiences distress because of difficulty in adhering to prescribed religious rituals.

Examples
- Religious ceremonies
- Dietary regulations
- Certain clothing
- Prayer
- Request to worship
- Holiday observances
- Expresses emotional distress because of separation from fifth community
- Expresses emotional distress regarding religious beliefs and/or religious social network
- Expresses a need to reconnect with previous belief patterns and customs
- Questions religious belief patterns and customs

RELATED FACTORS

Pathophysiologic
Related to sickness/illness
Related to suffering
Related to pain

Situational
Related to personal crisis related to activity
Related to fear of death
Relate to embarrassment at practicing spiritual rituals
Related to barriers to practicing spiritual rituals
Intensive care restrictions
Confinement to bed or room

Lack of privacy
Lack of availability of special foods/diets

NOC Spiritual Well-being

Goal

The person will express satisfaction with spiritual condition.

Indicators

- Continue spiritual practices not detrimental to health.
- Express decreasing feelings of guilt and anxiety.

NIC Spiritual Support, Presence

General Interventions

Explore Whether the Client Desires to Engage in an Allowable Religious or Spiritual Practice or Ritual; If So, Provide Opportunities To Do So.

Express Your Understanding and Acceptance of the Importance of the Client's Religious or Spiritual Beliefs and Practices.

Assess for Causative and Contributing Factors.

Hospital or nursing home environment

Limitations related to disease process or treatment regimen (eg, cannot kneel to pray owing to traction; prescribed diet differs from usual religious diet)

Fear of imposing on or antagonizing medical and nursing staff with requests for spiritual rituals

Embarrassment over spiritual beliefs or customs (especially common in adolescents)

Separation from articles, texts, or environment of spiritual significance

Lack of transportation to spiritual place or service

Spiritual leader unavailable because of emergency or lack of time

**Eliminate or Reduce Causative and
Contributing Factors, if Possible.**

Limitations Imposed by the Hospital or Nursing Home Environment

Provide privacy and quiet as needed for daily prayer, visit of
spiritual leader, and spiritual reading and contemplation.
  Pull curtains or close door.
  Turn off television and radio.
  Ask desk to hold calls, if possible.
  Note spiritual interventions on Kardex and include in
  care plan.
Contact spiritual leader to clarify practices and perform
religious rites or services, if desired.
  Communicate with spiritual leader concerning person's
  condition.
  Address Roman Catholic, Orthodox, and Episcopal
  priests as "Father," other Christian ministers as
  "Pastor," and Jewish rabbis as "Rabbi."
  Prevent interruption during visit, if possible.
  Offer to provide table or stand covered with clean white
  cloth.
  Chart visit and client's response.

Inform about religious services and materials available within the institution

Limitations Related to Disease Process or Treatment Regimen

Encourage spiritual rituals not detrimental to health (see
Table II-26).
  Assist clients with physical limitations in prayer and
  spiritual observances (eg, help to hold rosary; help to
  kneeling position, if appropriate).
  Assist in habits of personal cleanliness.
  Avoid shaving if beard is of spiritual significance.
  Allow client to wear religious clothing or jewelry when-
  ever possible.
  Make special arrangements for burial of resected limbs
  or body organs.
  Allow family or spiritual leader to perform ritual care of
  body.
  Make arrangements as needed for other important spiri-
  tual rituals (eg, circumcisions).
Maintain diet with spiritual restrictions when not detri-
mental to health (see Table II-26).
  Consult with dietitian.

Allow fasting for short periods, if possible.*

Change therapeutic diet as necessary.*

Have family or friends bring in special food, if possible.

Have members of spiritual group supply meals to the person at home.

Be as flexible as possible in serving methods, times of meals, and so forth.

Fear of Imposing or Embarrassment

Communicate acceptance of various spiritual beliefs and practices.

Convey nonjudgmental, respectful attitude.

Acknowledge importance of spiritual needs.

Express willingness of health care team to help in meeting spiritual needs.

Provide privacy and ensure confidentiality.

Separation from Articles, Texts, or Environment of Spiritual Significance

Question person about missing religious or spiritual articles or reading material (see Table II-26).

Obtain missing items from clergy in hospital, spiritual leader, family, or members of spiritual group.

Treat these articles and books with respect.

Allow person to keep spiritual articles and books within reach as much as possible, or where they can be easily seen.

Protect from loss or damage (eg, medal pinned to gown can be lost in laundry).

Recognize that articles without overt religious meaning may have spiritual significance for person (eg, wedding band).

Use spiritual texts in large print, in Braille, or on tape when appropriate.

Provide opportunity for person to pray with others or be read to by members of own religious group or member of the health care team who feels comfortable with these activities.

Jews and Seventh-Day Adventists would find Psalms 23, 24, 42, 63, 71, 103, 121, and 127 appropriate.

Christians would also appreciate I Corinthians 13, Matthew 5:3–11, Romans 12, and the Lord's Prayer.

---

* May require a primary care professional's order.

Lack of Transportation

Take person to chapel or quiet environment on hospital
  grounds.

Arrange transportation to church or synagogue for person
  in home.

Provide access to spiritual programming on radio and television when appropriate.

Spiritual Leader Unavailable Because of Emergency or Lack of Time

Baptize critically ill newborn of Greek Orthodox, Episcopal, or Roman Catholic parents (see Table II-26).

Perform other mandatory spiritual rituals, if possible.

Rationales

- For a client who places a high value on prayer or other
  spiritual practices, these practices can provide meaning
  and purpose and can be a source of comfort and strength
  (Carson, 1989).
- Conveying a nonjudgmental attitude may help reduce
  the client's uneasiness about expressing his beliefs
  and practices.

Religiosity, Risk for Impaired

DEFINITION

Risk for Impaired Religiosity: the state in which an individual is at risk for impaired ability to exercise reliance on
beliefs of a particular denomination or faith community and
to participate in related rituals.

RISK FACTOR

Refer to Impaired Religiosity

NOC Spiritual Well-being

Goals

The person will express continued satisfaction with religious activities.

Indication

- Continue to practice religious rituals.
- Describe increased comfort after assessment.

Interventions

Refer to Impaired Religiosity for interventions.

Sudden Infant Death Syndrome, Risk for

DEFINITION

Risk for Sudden Infant Death Syndrome: The state in which an infant younger than 1 year old is at risk to experience sudden death, unexpected by history and unexplained by postmortem examination.

RISK FACTORS

Presence of risk factors (refer to Related Factors)

RELATED FACTORS (MCMILLAN ET AL., 1999)

Pathophysiologic

Related to increased vulnerability secondary to:

Cyanosis	Tachypnea
Poor feeding	*Prematurity
Tachycardia	Fever
*Small for gestational age	Respiratory distress

*Widely accepted; general agreement among investigators.

Hypothermia
Irritability
History of diarrhea, vomiting,
  or listlessness 2 weeks
  before death

*Low birth weight
Low apgar score (<7)

Related to increased vulnerability secondary to prenatal maternal:

*Anemia
Sexually transmitted
  infections

Urinary tract infection
Poor weight gain

Situational (Personal, Environmental)

Related to increased vulnerability secondary to maternal:

*Cigarette smoking
*Inadequate prenatal care
Multiparity
Drug use during pregnancy
*Low educational levels

*Young maternal age (<20)
*Lack of breastfeeding
*Single mother
*Young maternal age with
first pregnancy

Related to increased vulnerability secondary to:

*Crowded living conditions
Cold environment

*Sleeping on stomach
  (prone)
Poor family financial status

Related to increased vulnerability secondary to:

*Male gender
*Black/Native Americans
Previous SIDS death in family

Multiple births

NOC Knowledge: Maternal–Child Health, Risk Control:
Tobacco Use, Risk Control Knowledge: Infant Safety

Goals

The caregiver will reduce or eliminate risk factors that are modifiable.

Indicators

- Position infant on back.
- Eliminate smoking in the home, near the infant, and during pregnancy.

---

*Widely accepted, general agreement among investigators.

- Participate in prenatal and newborn medical care.
- Improve maternal health (e.g., treat anemia, promote optimal nutrition).
- Enroll in drug and alcohol programs, if indicated.
- Avoid giving over-the-counter medications to infant.

Generic Interventions

Explain SIDS to Caregivers and Identify Risk Factors Present.

Reduce or Eliminate Risk Factors that Can Be Modified.

Determine If Home Cardiorespiratory Monitoring Is Indicated. Consult With Pediatrician or Neonatal/ Pediatric Nurse Practitioner (McMillan et al., 1999).

Teach parents to focus on the infant when alarm sounds, not the machine.

Teach to assess:

Infant's color pink?
Infant's breathing

Teach Environmental Practices to Reduce SIDS.

Position infant on back.
Avoid overheating infant during sleep.
Avoid soft bedding (e.g., mattresses).
Avoid pillows.
Avoid sleeping with infant (Anderson, 2000).

Initiate Health Teaching and Referrals as Indicated.

Provide instructions on use of home monitor, if appropriate.
Refer client to drug and alcohol treatment programs as indicated.
Discuss strategies to stop smoking (refer to the index under *Smoking*).
Provide emergency numbers as indicated.
Refer to social agencies as indicated.

DEFINITION

Delayed Surgical Recovery: The state in which an individual experiences, or is at risk of experiencing, an extension of the number of postoperative days required to initiate and perform self-care activities.

⊚ AUTHOR'S NOTE

This newly accepted diagnosis represents an individual who has not achieved recovery from a surgical procedure during the expected time period. As one reviews the defining characteristics from NANDA, there is some confusion regarding the difference between defining characteristics (signs and symptoms) and related factors. Those preceded by an asterisk (*) are not defining characteristics, but are factors that can cause or contribute to *Delayed Surgical Recovery.* Currently the diagnosis has not been developed sufficiently for clinical use. This author recommends utilizing other nursing diagnoses, such as *Self-Care Deficit, Acute Pain,* or *Imbalanced Nutrition.*

DEFINING CHARACTERISTICS
(NANDA, 2001)

Postpones resumption of activities (home, work)
Perception that more time is needed to recover
Requires help to complete self-care
*Evidence of interrupted healing of surgical area
*Loss of appetite with or without nausea
*Difficulty in moving about
*Reports pain or discomfort

---

*Refer to Author's Note for explanation of asterisk.

Thought Processes, Disturbed

DEFINITION

Disturbed Thought Processes: The state in which an individual experiences a disruption in such mental activities as conscious thought, reality orientation, problem solving, judgment, and comprehension related to coping, personality, and/or mental disorder.

⚭ AUTHOR'S NOTE

The diagnosis *Disturbed Thought Processes* describes an individual with altered perception and cognition that interferes with daily living. Causes are biochemical or psychological disturbances (e.g., depression, personality disorders). The focus of nursing is to reduce disturbed thinking and promote reality orientation.

The nurse should be cautioned when using this diagnosis as a "wastebasket" diagnosis for all clients with disturbed thinking or confusion. Frequently, confusion in older adults is erroneously attributed to aging. Confusion in the older adult can be caused by a single factor or multiple factors (e.g., dementia, medication side effects, depression, or metabolic disorder). Depression causes impaired thinking in older adults more frequently than dementia (Miller, 2004). Refer to *Confusion* for additional information.

DEFINING CHARACTERISTICS
Major (Must Be Present)

Inaccurate interpretation of stimuli, internal or external

Minor (May Be Present)

Cognitive deficits, including abstraction, problem solving, memory deficits

Suspiciousness

Delusions

Hallucinations

Phobias

Obsessions

Confusion/disorientation

Ritualistic behavior

Impulsivity

Inappropriate social behavior

Distractibility

Lack of consensual validation

RELATED FACTORS
Pathophysiologic
Related to physiologic changes secondary to:
Drug or alcohol withdrawal

Related to biochemical alterations

Situational (Personal, Environmental)
Related to emotional trauma
Related to abuse (physical, sexual, mental)
Related to torture
Related to childhood trauma
Related to repressed fears
Related to panic level of anxiety
Related to continued low levels of stimulation
Related to decreased attention span and ability to process information secondary to:

Depression

Fear

Anxiety

Grieving

Maturational
Older Adult
Isolation, late-life depression

NOC Cognitive Ability, Cognitive Orientation, Concentration, Distorted Thought Control, Information Processing, Memory, Decision Making

---

Goals

The person will maintain reality orientation and communicate clearly with others.

Indicators

- Recognize changes in thinking/behavior.
- Identify situations that occur before hallucinations/
  delusions.
- Use coping strategies to deal effectively with
  hallucinations/delusions (specify).
- Participate in unit activities (specify).
- Express delusional material less frequently.

NIC Cognitive Stimulation, Dementia Management, Reality
Orientation, Family Support, Decision-Making Support,
Hallucination Management, Anxiety Reduction, Memory
Training, Environmental Management: Safety

Generic Interventions

**Approach in a Calm,
Nurturing Manner.**

**Recognize When Person Is Testing the
Trustworthiness of Others.**

**Avoid Making Promises that Cannot
Be Fulfilled.**

**Initial Staff Contact Should Be
Minimal and Brief With Suspicious
Person; Increase Time As
Suspicion Decreases.**

**Verify Your Interpretation of What
Person Is Experiencing ("I Understand
You Are Fearful of Others.").**

**Use Communication that Helps
Person Maintain Own Individuality
(e.g., "I" Instead of "We").**

For Hallucinations:

Observe for verbal and nonverbal hallucinations—inappropriate laughter, delayed verbal response, eye movements,
moving lips without sound, increased motor movements,
grinning.

Direct the focus from delusional expression to discussion of
reality-centered situations.

Encourage differentiation of stimuli arising from inner sources from those from outside (e.g., in response to "I hear voices," say, "Those are the voices of persons on television" or "I hear no one speaking now; they are your own thoughts.").

Avoid the impression that you confirm or approve reality distortions; tactfully express doubt.

Set limits for discussing repetitive delusional material ("You've already told me about that; let's talk about something realistic.").

Identify the underlying needs being met by the delusions/hallucinations.

Help connect false beliefs with increased levels of anxiety.

Assist in Communicating More Effectively.

Ask for the meaning of what is said; do not assume that you understand.

Validate your interpretation of what is being said ("Is this what you mean?").

Clarify all global pronouns—we, they ("Who is *they*?").

Refocus when person changes the subject in the middle of an explanation or thought.

Tell the person when you are not following his or her train of thought.

Do not mimic or restate words or phrases that you do not understand.

Teach the person to validate consensually with others.

Ask yes, no, or multiple choice questions.

Keep sentences short and clear.

Assist Person to Set Limits on Own Behavior.

Discuss alternative methods of coping (e.g., taking a walk instead of crying).

Confront person with the attitude that regression is not acceptable behavior.

Help delay gratification (e.g., "I want you to wait 5 minutes before you repeat your request for help in making your bed.").

Encourage person to achieve realistic expectations.

Pace expectations to avoid frustration.

Encourage and Support Person in the Decision-Making Process.

Compliment the person who assumes more responsibility.
Provide opportunity for person to contribute to own treatment plan.
Help establish future goals that are realistic; examine problems in achieving a goal, and suggest various alternatives.

Assist Person to Differentiate between Needs and Demands.

Explain the difference between needs and demands (e.g., food and clothing are needs; expectations that others dress and feed person, if he or she can do it, are demands).
Assist person to examine the effects of behavior on others; encourage a change in behavior if it evokes negative responses.

Help Person Recognize Behaviors that Stimulate Rejection.

Identify activities that reduce interpersonal anxiety (e.g., exercise, controlled-breathing exercises).
Set limits firmly and kindly on destructive behavior.
Allow expression of negative emotions, verbally or in constructive activity.
Help person accept responsibility for responses he or she elicits from others.
Encourage discussion of problems in relating after visits with family members.
Help person test new skills in relating to others in role-playing situations.

Anticipate Difficulties in Adjusting to Community Living; Discuss Concerns about Returning to Community, and Elicit Family Reaction to Individual's Discharge.

Provide Health Teaching that Will Prepare Person to Deal with Life Stresses (Methods of Relaxation, Problem-Solving Skills, How to Negotiate With Others, How to Express Feelings Constructively).

Inform Person of Social Agencies that Offer Help in Adjusting to Community Living.

Provide Sensory Input that Is Sufficient and Meaningful.

Keep person oriented to time and place.

Refer to time of day and place each morning.

Provide person with a clock and calendar large enough to see.

Provide person with opportunity to see daylight and dark through a window, or take person outdoors.

Single out holidays with cards or pins (e.g., wear a red heart for Valentine's Day).

Encourage family to bring in familiar objects from home (photographs, afghan).

Discuss current events, seasonal events (snow, water activities); share your interests (travel, crafts).

Assess if person can perform an activity with own hands (e.g., latch rugs, wood crafts).

Provide reading materials, audio tapes, puzzles (manual, computer, crossword).

Encourage person to keep own records if possible (e.g., intake and output).

Provide tasks to perform (addressing envelopes, occupational therapy).

Refer to *Risk for Injury* for Strategies for Assessing and Manipulating the Environment for Hazards.

❖ Pediatric Interventions

For Children With Thought Disturbance, Assess for Signs of Dissociative Disorder:

Abusive history (physical, sexual)

Amnesic periods

Switching between alter personalities

Affect disturbances

Abrupt behavioral changes

Refer for Multidisciplinary Evaluation.

DEFINITION

Impaired Memory: The state in which an individual experiences a temporary or permanent inability to remember or recall bits of information or behavioral skills.

> ⚱ **AUTHOR'S NOTE**
>
> This diagnosis is useful when the person can be helped to function better because of improved memory. If the person's memory cannot be improved because of cerebral degeneration, this diagnosis is not appropriate. Instead the nurse should evaluate the effects of impaired memory on functioning as *Self-Care Deficits* or *Risk for Injury*. The focus of interventions would be on improving self-care or protection, not on improving memory.

DEFINING CHARACTERISTICS
Major (Must Be Present, One or More)

Observed or reported experiences of forgetting
Inability to determine if a behavior was performed
Inability to learn or retain new skills or information
Inability to perform a previously learned skill
Inability to recall factual information
Inability to recall recent or past events

RELATED FACTORS
Pathophysiologic
Related to central nervous system changes secondary to:

Degenerative brain disease	Lesion
Head injury	Cerebrovascular accident

Related to reduced quantity and quality of information processed secondary to:

Visual deficits	Poor physical fitness
Learning habits	Educational level
Hearing deficits	Fatigue
Intellectual skills	

Related to nutritional deficiencies (e.g., vitamins C, B$_{12}$, folate, niacin, thiamine)

Treatment-Related

Related to effects of medication (specify) on memory storage

Situational (Personal, Environmental)

Related to self-fulfilling expectations
Related to excessive self-focusing and worrying secondary to grieving, depression, or anxiety
Related to alcohol consumption
Related to lack of motivation
Related to lack of stimulation
Related to difficulty concentrating secondary to:

Stress	Sleep disturbances
Lack of intellectual stimulation	Distractions
	Pain

NOC Cognitive Orientation, Memory

Goals

The person will report increased satisfaction with memory.

Indicators

- Identify three techniques to improve memory.
- Relate factors that deter memory.

NIC Reality Orientation, Memory Training, Environmental Management

Generic Interventions

Discuss the Person's Beliefs about Memory Deficits:

Correct misinformation.
Explain that negative expectations can result in memory deficits.
If a person is older, provide accurate information about age-related changes.

Explain that if One Wants to Improve Memory, the Intent to Remember and the Knowledge about Techniques for Remembering Are Needed (Miller, 2004).

If the Person Has Difficulty Concentrating, Explain the Favorable Effects of Relaxation and Imagery.

Teach the Person Two or Three Methods for Improving Memory Skills (Maier-Lorentz, 2000; Miller, 2004):

Write things down (e.g., use lists, calendars, and notebooks).

Use auditory cues (e.g., timers, alarm clocks) in conjunction with written cues.

Have specific places for specific items, and keep the items in their proper place (e.g., keep keys on a hook near the door).

Put reminders in appropriate places (e.g., place shoes to be repaired near the door).

Use active observation—pay attention to details of what's going on around you, and be alert to the environment.

Make associations between names and mental images (e.g., Carol and Christmas carol).

Rehearse items you want to remember by repeating them aloud or writing the information on paper.

Divide information into small "chunks" that can be remembered easily (e.g., to remember an address or a zip code, divide it into groups ["seven hundred sixty, fifty five"]).

Search the alphabet while focusing on what you are trying to remember (e.g., to remember that someone's name is Martin, start with names that begin with "A" and continue naming names through the alphabet until your memory is jogged for the correct one).

Explain that When One Is Trying to Learn or Remember Something:

Minimize distractions.

Do not rush.

Maintain some form of organization of routine tasks.

Carry a note pad or calendar or use written cues.

**When Teaching (Miller, 2004; Stanley
& Beare, 2000):**

Eliminate distractions.
Present information as concretely as possible.
Use practical examples.
Allow learner to pace the learning.
Use visual, auditory aids.
Provide advance organizers: outlines, written cues.
Encourage use of aids.
Make sure glasses are clean and lights are soft-white.
Correct wrong answers immediately.
Encourage verbal responses.

⊙ Geriatric Interventions

**Encourage Client to Share Concerns
about Memory Problems.**

**Explain that Short-Term Memory May
Decline With Aging.**

**Explain that Memory Aids Can
Improve Memory. Refer to
Generic Interventions.**

Tissue Perfusion, Ineffective

DEFINITION

Ineffective Tissue Perfusion: The state in which an individual experiences, or is at risk of experiencing, a decrease at the capillary level in oxygenation.

> ℗ **AUTHOR'S NOTE**
>
> This nursing diagnosis is restricted to represent only diminished peripheral tissue perfusion situations in which nurses prescribe definitive treatment to reduce, eliminate, or prevent the problem.
>
> In the other situations of diminished cardiopulmonary, cerebral, renal, or gastrointestinal tissue perfusion, the nurse should focus on the functional abilities of the individual that are or may be compromised because of the decreased tissue perfusion. The nurse should also monitor to detect physiologic complications of decreased tissue perfusion and label these situations as collaborative problems. The following illustrates examples of a compromised functional health problem (nursing diagnosis) and a potential complication (collaborative problem) for an individual with compromised cerebral tissue perfusion:
>
> *Risk for Injury related to vertigo secondary to recent head injury* (nursing diagnosis)
>
> *PC: Increased Intracranial Pressure* (collaborative problem)
>
> Refer to Chapter 2 of Carpenito, L. J. (2006). *Nursing Diagnosis: Application to Clinical Practice* (11th ed.), Philadelphia, Lippincott Williams & Wilkins, for additional information on collaborative problems. For additional examples of nursing diagnoses and collaborative problems grouped under medical conditions, refer to Section Two of this handbook.

Ineffective Peripheral Tissue Perfusion

DEFINITION
Ineffective Peripheral Tissue Perfusion: The state in which an individual experiences, or is at risk of experiencing, a decrease in nutrition and respiration at the peripheral cellular level because of a decrease in capillary blood supply.

DEFINING CHARACTERISTICS
Major (Must Be Present, One or More)
Presence of One of the Following Types:
Claudication (arterial)   Aching pain (arterial)
Rest pain (arterial)

Diminished or Absent Arterial Pulses
Skin Color Changes
Pallor (arterial)   Reactive hyperemia
Cyanosis (venous)   (arterial)

Skin Temperature Changes
Cooler (arterial)   Warmer (venous)

Decreased Blood Pressure (Arterial)
Capillary Refill Greater than 3 Seconds (Arterial)

Minor (May Be Present)
Edema (venous)
Change in sensory function (arterial)
Change in motor function (arterial)
Trophic tissue changes (arterial)
   Hard, thick nails
   Loss of hair
   Nonhealing wound

RELATED FACTORS
Pathophysiologic
Related to compromised blood flow secondary to:
Vascular disorders
   Arteriosclerosis   Raynaud's disease/syndrome
   Hypertension   Aneurysm
   Varicosities   Arterial thrombosis

495

Buerger's disease	Deep vein thrombosis
Sickle cell crisis	Collagen vascular disease
Cirrhosis	Rheumatoid arthritis
Alcoholism	Leriche's syndrome

Diabetes mellitus
Hypotension
Blood dyscrasias (platelet disorders)
Renal failure
Cancer/tumor

Treatment-Related

Related to immobilization
Related to invasive lines
Related to pressure sites/constriction (Ace bandages, stockings)
Related to blood vessel trauma or compression

Situational (Personal, Environmental)

Related to pressure of enlarging uterus on peripheral circulation
Related to pressure of enlarged abdomen on pelvic and peripheral circulation
Related to dependent venous pooling
Related to hypothermia
Related to vasoconstricting effects of tobacco
Related to decreased circulating volume secondary to dehydration
Related to pressure of muscle mass secondary to weightlifting

NOC Sensory Function: Cutaneous, Tissue Integrity, Tissue Perfusion: Peripheral

Goals

The individual will report a decrease in pain.

Indicators

- Define peripheral vascular problem in own words.
- Identify factors that improve peripheral circulation.
- Identify necessary lifestyle changes.
- Identify medical regimen, diet, medications, activities that promote vasodilatation.

- Identify factors that inhibit peripheral circulation.
- State when to contact physician or health care professional.

NIC Peripheral Sensation Management, Circulatory Care: Venous Insufficiency, Circulatory Care: Arterial Insufficiency, Positioning, Exercise Promotion

Generic Interventions

Teach Person to:

Keep extremity in a dependent position.

Keep extremity warm. (Do not use heating pad or hot water bottle, because the individual with a peripheral vascular disease may have a disturbance in sensation and will not be able to determine if the temperature is hot enough to damage tissue; the use of external heat may also increase the metabolic demands of the tissue beyond its capacity.)

Reduce Risk for Trauma:

Change positions at least every hour.

Avoid leg crossing.

Reduce external pressure points (inspect shoes daily for rough lining).

Avoid sheepskin heel protectors (they increase heel pressure and pressure across dorsum of foot).

Encourage range-of-motion exercises.

Plan a Daily Walking Program.

Instruct individual in reasons for program.

Teach individual to avoid fatigue.

Instruct to avoid increase in exercise until assessed by physician for cardiac problems.

Reassure individual that walking does not harm the blood vessels or the muscles; "walking into the pain," resting, and resuming walking assists in developing collateral circulation.

Teach Factors that Improve Venous Blood Flow.

Elevate extremity above the level of the heart (may be contraindicated if severe cardiac or respiratory disease is present).

Avoid standing or sitting with legs dependent for long
periods.

Consider the use of Ace bandages or below-knee elastic
stockings to prevent venous stasis.

Reduce or remove external venous compression that
impedes venous flow.

Avoid pillows behind the knees or Gatch bed that is elevated at the knees.

Avoid leg crossing.

Change positions; move extremities or wiggle fingers
and toes every hour.

Avoid garters and tight elastic stockings above the knees.

Measure Baseline Circumference of Calves and Thighs if Individual Is at Risk for Deep Venous Thrombosis or if It Is Suspected.

Teach Person to:

Avoid long car or plane rides (get up and walk around at
least every hour).

Keep dry skin lubricated (cracked skin eliminates the
physical barrier to infection).

Wear warm clothing during cold weather.

Wear cotton or wool socks.

Avoid dehydration in warm weather.

Give special attention to feet and toes:

Wash feet and dry well daily.

Do not soak feet.

Avoid harsh soaps or chemicals (including iodine) on feet.

Keep nails trimmed and filed smooth.

Inspect feet and legs daily for injuries and pressure points.

Wear clean socks.

Wear shoes that offer support and fit comfortably.

Inspect the inside of shoes daily for rough lining.

Teach Risk-Factor Modification.

Diet:

Avoid foods high in cholesterol.

Modify sodium intake to control hypertension.

Refer to dietitian.

Relaxation techniques to reduce effects of stress

Smoking cessation

Exercise program

Maternal Interventions

Explain that Uterine Pressure Can Cause Pooling of Venous Blood in Lower Extremities.

Teach to Report Immediately Signs and Symptoms of Thrombosis:

Pain in leg, groin
Unilateral leg swelling
Pale skin

Refer to Generic Interventions for Specific Techniques to Reduce Edema.

Unilateral Neglect

DEFINITION

Unilateral Neglect: The state in which a person cannot attend to or ignores the hemiplegic side of the body and/or, on the affected side, objects, persons, or sounds in the environment.

DEFINING CHARACTERISTICS
Major (Must Be Present, One or More)

Neglect of involved body parts and/or extrapersonal space (hemispatial neglect) *and/or*
Denial of the existence of the affected limb or side of the body (anosognosia)

Minor (May Be Present)

Difficulty with spatial–perceptual tasks
Hemiplegia (usually of the left side)

RELATED FACTORS
Pathophysiologic
Related to impaired perceptual abilities secondary to:

Cerebrovascular accident	Cerebral tumors
Brain injury/trauma	Cerebral aneurysms

NOC Body Image, Body Positioning: Self-Initiated, Self-Care: Activities of Daily Living

Goals

The person will demonstrate an ability to scan the visual field to compensate for loss of function/sensation in affected limbs.

Indicators

- Identify safety hazards in the environment.
- Describe the deficit and rationale for treatment.

NIC Unilateral Neglect Management, Self-Care Assistance

Generic Interventions

Initially Adapt the Environment to the Deficit.

Position call light, bedside stand, television, telephone, and personal items on the unaffected side.

Position bed so unaffected side is toward the door.

Approach and speak to person from unaffected side.

If you must approach from affected side, announce your presence as soon as you enter the room to avoid startling the person.

Gradually Change the Environment As You Teach Person to Compensate and Learn to Recognize the Forgotten Field; Move Furniture and Personal Items out of Visual Field.

For a Person in a Wheelchair, Obtain a Lapboard (Preferably Plexiglas), and Position Affected Arm on Lapboard With Fingertips at Midline; Encourage Person to Look for Arm on Board.

For an Ambulatory Person, Obtain an Arm Sling to Prevent the Arm from Dangling and Causing Shoulder Subluxation.

Constantly Cue Person to the Environment.

Encourage Person to Wear Prescribed Corrective Lenses or Hearing Aids.

For Bathing, Dressing, and Toileting:

Instruct person to attend to affected extremity/side first when performing activities of daily living.

Instruct person always to look for affected extremity when performing activities of daily living, to know where it is at all times.

Encourage person to integrate affected extremity during bathing; encourage person to feel extremity by rubbing and massage.

For Eating:

Instruct person to eat in small amounts; place food on unaffected side of mouth.

Instruct person to use tongue to sweep out pockets of food from affected side after every bite.

Check oral cavity for pocketed food/medication after meals/medications.

Provide oral care three times per day and as needed.

Initially place food in visual field; gradually move food out of field and teach person to scan entire visual field.

Retrain Person to Scan Entire Environment.

Have Person Stroke Involved Side With Uninvolved Hand; the Person Should Watch Arm or Leg As He or She Strokes It.

Evaluate that Both Person and Family Understand the Purpose and Rationale of All Interventions.

Impaired Urinary Elimination
Maturational Enuresis*
Functional Incontinence
Reflex Incontinence
Stress Incontinence
Total Incontinence
Urge Incontinence
Urge Incontinence, Risk for
Urinary Retention

⊙ **AUTHOR'S NOTE**

All of these diagnoses pertain to urine elimination, not urine formulation. Anuria, oliguria, and renal failure should be labeled collaborative problems, such as Potential Complication: Anuria. *Impaired Urinary Elimination* represents a broad diagnosis, probably too broad for clinical use. It is recommended that a more specific diagnosis such as *Stress Incontinence* be used instead. When the etiologic or contributing factors have not been identified for incontinence, the diagnosis can temporarily be written *Incontinence related to unknown etiology*.

---

*This diagnosis is not currently on the NANDA list but has been included for clarity or usefulness.

Impaired Urinary Elimination

DEFINITION
Impaired Urinary Elimination: The state in which an individual experiences, or is at risk of experiencing, urinary elimination dysfunction.

DEFINING CHARACTERISTICS
Major (Must Be Present, One or More)
Reports or experiences a urinary elimination problem, such as:

Urgency	Dribbling
Frequency	Bladder distention
Hesitancy	Incontinence
Nocturia	Large residual urine
Enuresis	volumes

RELATED FACTORS
Pathophysiologic
Related to incompetent bladder outlet secondary to congenital urinary tract anomalies

Related to decreased bladder capacity or irritation to bladder secondary to infection, trauma, urethritis, glucosuria, or carcinoma

Related to diminished bladder cues or impaired ability to recognize bladder cues secondary to:

Cord injury/tumor/infection	Diabetic neuropathy
Brain injury/tumor/infection	Alcoholic neuropathy
Cerebrovascular accident	Tabes dorsalis
Demyelinating diseases	Parkinsonism
Multiple sclerosis	

Treatment-Related
Related to effects of surgery on bladder sphincter secondary to postprostatectomy or extensive pelvic dissection

Related to diagnostic instrumentation

Related to decreased bladder muscle tone secondary to:

General or spinal anesthesia

Drug therapy (iatrogenic)

Antihistamines	Immunosuppressant therapy
Epinephrine	Diuretics
Anticholinergics	Tranquilizers
Sedatives	Muscle relaxants

Post-indwelling catheters

Situational (Personal, Environmental)
Related to weak pelvic floor muscles secondary to:

Obesity	Aging
Recent substantial weight loss	Childbirth

Related to inability to communicate needs
Related to bladder outlet obstruction secondary to fecal impaction or chronic constipation
Related to decreased bladder muscle tone secondary to dehydration
Related to decreased attention to bladder cues secondary to:

Depression	Confusion
Intentional suppression	Delirium

Related to environmental barriers to bathroom:

Distant toilets	Poor lighting
Unfamiliar surroundings	Bed too high, or side rails

Related to inability to access bathroom on time secondary to:

Impaired mobility	Caffeine/alcohol use

Maturational
Child
Related to small bladder capacity
Related to lack of motivation

Goals

The person will be continent (specify during day, night, 24 hours).

Indicators

- Be able to identify the cause of incontinence.
- Provide rationale for treatments.

Generic Interventions

Determine if There Is Acute Cause of Problem.

Infection (e.g., urinary tract, sexually transmitted disease, gonorrhea)
Renal disease
Renal calculi
Medication effects
Anesthesia effects

Refer to a Urologist if Acute Cause Is Determined.

If Incontinence Is the Problem, Determine Type. Assess:

History of continence
Onset and duration (day, night, just certain times)
Factors that increase incidence (Newman et al., 1991):
    Coughing
    Laughing
    Standing
    Turning in bed
    Delay in getting to bathroom
    When excited
    Leaving bathroom
    Running
Perception of need to void: present, absent, diminished
Ability to delay urination after urge
Relief after voiding
    Complete
    Continued desire to void after bladder is emptied

Using Data from Assessment, Refer to Specific Type of Incontinence.

Maturational Enuresis*

DEFINITION

Maturational Enuresis: The state in which a child experiences involuntary voiding during sleep, which is not pathophysiologic in origin.

> ⓧ **AUTHOR'S NOTE**
>
> This diagnosis would represent enuresis that is not caused by pathophysiologic or structural deficits, such as strictures.

DEFINING CHARACTERISTICS
Major (Must Be Present)

Reports or demonstrates episodes of involuntary voiding during sleep

RELATED FACTORS
Situational (Personal, Environmental)

Related to stressors (school, siblings)
Related to inattention to bladder cues
Related to unfamiliar surroundings

Maturational

Child
Related to small bladder capacity
Related to lack of motivation
Related to attention-seeking behavior

> **NOC** Urinary Continence, Knowledge: Enuresis, Family Functioning

Goals

The child will remain dry during the sleep cycle.

---

*This diagnosis is not currently on the NANDA list but has been included for clarity or usefulness.

Indicator

The child and family will be able to list factors that decrease enuresis.

> **NIC** Urinary Incontinence Care: Enuresis, Urinary Habit Training, Anticipatory Guidance, Family Support

❖ Pediatric Interventions

Explain the Nature of Enuresis and Its High Rate of Spontaneous Remission to Parents and Child.

Explain to Parents that Disapproval (Shaming, Punishing) Is Useless in Stopping Enuresis but Can Make Child Shy, Ashamed, and Afraid.

Offer Reassurance to Child that Other Children Wet the Bed at Night and Child Is Not Bad or Sinful.

Teach:
After child drinks fluids, encourage him or her to postpone voiding to help stretch the bladder.
Have child void before retiring.
Restrict fluids at bedtime.
If child is awakened later (about 11 P.M.) to void, attempt to awaken child fully for positive reinforcement.
Teach child awareness of sensations that occur when it is time to void.
Teach child ability to control urination (have child start and stop the stream; have child "hold" the urine during the day, even if only for a short time).

Have Child Keep a Record of Progress; Emphasize Dry Days or Nights (e.g., Stars on a Calendar).

Explain How Nocturnal Enuresis Alarm Works.

❖ Pediatric Interventions (cont'd)

Teach Child and Family Techniques to Control the Adverse Effects of Enuresis (e.g., Use of Plastic Mattress Covers, Use of Child's Own Sleeping Bag [Machine Washable] When Staying Overnight Away from Home).

Seek Opportunities to Teach the Public about Enuresis and Incontinence (e.g., School and Parent Organizations, Self-Help Groups).

Functional Incontinence

DEFINITION
Functional Incontinence: The state in which an individual experiences incontinence because of a difficulty or inability to reach the toilet in time.

DEFINING CHARACTERISTICS
Major (Must Be Present)
Incontinence before or during an attempt to reach the toilet

RELATED FACTORS
Pathophysiologic
Related to diminished bladder cues and impaired ability to recognize bladder cues secondary to:

Brain injury/tumor/infection	Alcoholic neuropathy
Cerebrovascular accident	Parkinsonism
Demyelinating diseases	Progressive dementia
Multiple sclerosis	

Treatment-Related
Related to decreased bladder tone secondary to:

Antihistamines	Immunosuppressant therapy

Epinephrine	Diuretics
Anticholinergics	Tranquilizers
Sedatives	Muscle relaxants

Situational (Personal, Environmental)
Related to impaired mobility
Related to decreased attention to bladder cues

Depression	Intentional suppression
Confusion	(self-induced deconditioning)

Related to environmental barriers to bathroom:

Distant toilets	Poor lighting
Unfamiliar surroundings	Bed too high, side rails

Maturational
Older Adult
Related to motor and sensory losses

NOC Tissue Integrity, Urinary Continence, Urinary Elimination

Goals

The person will report no or fewer episodes of incontinence.

Indicators

- Remove or minimize environmental barriers from home.
- Use proper adaptive equipment to assist with voiding, transfers, and dressing.
- Describe causative factors for incontinence.

NIC Perineal Care, Urinary Incontinence Care, Prompted Voiding, Urinary Habit Training, Urinary Elimination Management, Teaching: Procedure/Treatment

Generic Interventions

Determine if There Is Another Cause Contributing to Incontinence (e.g., Stress, Urge or Reflex Incontinence, Urinary Retention, Infection).

Assess for Sensory/Cognitive Deficits.

Assess for Motor/Mobility Deficits.

Reduce Environmental Barriers:

Obstacles, lighting, and distance
Adequacy of toilet height and need for grab-bars

**Provide a Commode between
Bathroom and Bed, if Needed.**

**For an Individual With Cognitive
Deficits, Offer Toileting Reminders
Every 2 Hours, after Meals, and
before Bedtime.**

**For Persons With Limited
Hand Function:**

Assess person's ability to remove and replace clothing.
  Clothing that is loose is easier to manipulate.
Provide dressing aids as necessary: Velcro closures in
  seams for wheelchair patients, zipper pulls; all garments
  with fasteners may be adapted with Velcro closures.

**Initiate Referral to Visiting Nurse
(Occupational Therapy Department)
for Assessment of Bathroom Facilities
at Home.**

◉ Geriatric Interventions

**Emphasize that Incontinence Is Not
an Inevitable Age-Related Event.**

**Explain Not to Restrict Fluid Intake
for Fear of Incontinence.**

**Explain Not to Rely on Thirst As a
Signal to Drink Fluids.**

**Teach the Need to Have Easy Access
to Bathroom at Night. If Needed,
Consider Commode Chair or Urinal.**

DEFINITION
Reflex Incontinence: The state in which an individual experiences predictable, involuntary loss of urine with no sensation of urge, voiding, or bladder fullness.

DEFINING CHARACTERISTICS
Major (Must Be Present, One or More)
Uninhibited bladder contractions
Involuntary reflexes that produce spontaneous voiding
Partial or complete loss of sensation of bladder fullness or
  urge to void

RELATED FACTORS
Pathophysiologic
Related to impaired conduction of impulses above the reflex arc level secondary to:
Cord injury   Tumor
Infection

NOC See Functional Incontinence

Goals

The person will report a state of dryness that is personally satisfactory.

Indicators

- Have a residual urine volume of less than 50 mL.
- Use triggering mechanisms to initiate reflex voiding.

NIC (See also Functional Retention Care)

Generic Interventions

Explain to Person Rationale for Treatment.

Teach Cutaneous Triggering Mechanisms:

Repeated deep, sharp suprapubic tapping (most effective)
Instruct individual to:
    Position self in a half-sitting position.
    Tapping is aimed directly at bladder wall.
    Rate is seven or eight times for 5 seconds (40 single blows).
    Use only one hand.
    Shift site of stimulation over bladder to find most successful site.
    Continue stimulation until a good stream starts.
    Wait approximately 1 minute, then repeat stimulation until bladder is empty.
    One or two series of stimulations without response signifies that nothing more will be expelled.

If the above Is Ineffective, Perform Each of the Following for 2 to 3 Minutes Each. Wait 1 Minute between Facilitation Attempts:

Stroking glans penis
Punching abdomen above inguinal ligaments (lightly)
Stroking inner thigh

Encourage Person to Void or Trigger at Least Every 3 Hours.

Persons with Abdominal Muscle Control Should Use Valsalva's Maneuver During Triggered Voiding.

Indicate on Intake and Output Sheet Which Mechanism Was Used to Induce Voiding.

Teach Person that if Fluid Intake Is Increased, He or She Also Needs to Increase the Frequency of Triggering to Prevent Overdistention.

If Needed, Schedule Intermittent Catheterization Program.

Instruct Person in Signs and Symptoms of Dysreflexia:

Elevated blood pressure, decreasing pulse
Flushing and sweating above the level of the lesion
Cool and clammy below the level of the lesion
Pounding headache
Nasal stuffiness
Anxiety, feeling of impending doom
Goose pimples
Blurred vision

Instruct Person in Measures to Reduce or Eliminate Symptoms:

Elevate head.
Check blood pressure.
Rule out bladder distention; empty bladder by catheter (do not trigger); use lidocaine lubricant for catheter.

If Condition Persists after Emptying Bladder, Check for Bowel Distention. If Stool Is Present in the Rectum, Use a Dibucaine (Nupercainal) Suppository to Desensitize the Area before Removing Stool.

If Condition Persists or Person Has Not Been Able to Identify Cause, Notify Physician Immediately, or Seek Help in an Emergency Room.

Instruct Person to Carry an Identification Card that States Signs, Symptoms, and Management in the Event that He or She Cannot Direct Others.

Stress Incontinence

DEFINITION
Stress Incontinence: The state in which an individual experiences an immediate involuntary loss of urine during an increase in intra-abdominal pressure.

DEFINING CHARACTERISTICS
Major (Must Be Present)
The individual reports loss of urine (usually less than 50 mL) occurring with increased abdominal pressure from standing, sneezing, coughing, running, or lifting heavy objects.

RELATED FACTORS
Pathophysiologic
Related to incompetent bladder outlet secondary to congenital urinary tract anomalies
Related to degenerative changes in pelvic muscles and structural supports secondary to estrogen deficiency

Situational (Personal, Environmental)
Related to high intra-abdominal pressure and weak pelvic muscles secondary to:

Obesity	Pregnancy
Sex	Poor personal hygiene

Related to weak pelvic muscles and sphincter incompetence secondary to:

Recent substantial weight loss	Childbirth

Maturational
Older Adult
Related to loss of muscle tone

NOC (See Functional Incontinence)

Goals

The person will report a reduction or elimination of stress incontinence.

Indicator

Be able to explain the cause of incontinence and rationale for treatment.

> **NIC** (See also Functional Incontinence), Pelvic Muscle Exercise, Weight Management

Generic Interventions

Assess Pattern of Voiding/ Incontinence and Fluid Intake.

Explain the Effect of Incompetent Floor Muscles on Continence.

Teach Person to Identify Pelvic Floor Muscles and Strengthen Them With Exercise (Kegel Exercises).

For posterior pelvic floor muscles: "Imagine you are trying to stop the passage of stool and tighten your anal muscles without tightening your legs or your abdominal muscles."

For anterior pelvic floor muscles: "Imagine you are trying to stop the passage of urine, and tighten the muscles (back and front) for 4 seconds and then release them; repeat 10 times, 6 to 10 times a day." (Can be increased to four times an hour if indicated.)

Instruct person to stop and start the urine stream several times during voiding.

Explain the Relationship of Obesity and Stress Incontinence:

Teach Kegel exercises.

Refer to community programs if weight loss is desired.

Instruct to void every 2 hours and avoid prolonged periods of standing.

Explain the Relationship of Decreased Estrogen Production and Stress Incontinence.

Suggest Vaginal Estrogen Cream.

If There Is No Improvement, Refer to a Urologist for Evaluation of Possible Detrusor Instability or Atony, Mechanical Obstruction, or Neuron Injury.

Maternal Interventions

Teach Woman to Decrease Abdominal Pressure During Pregnancy.

Avoid prolonged periods of standing.
Void at least every 2 hours.
Practice Kegel exercises. (Refer to Generic Interventions.)

Total Incontinence

DEFINITION

Total Incontinence: The state in which an individual experiences continuous unpredictable loss of urine without distention or awareness of bladder fullness.

> ### ✆ AUTHOR'S NOTE
>
> This diagnosis is used only after the other types of incontinence have been ruled out.

DEFINING CHARACTERISTICS
Major (Must Be Present)
Constant flow of urine without distention
Nocturia more than two times during sleep
Incontinence refractory to other treatments

Minor (May Be Present)
Unaware of bladder cues to void
Unaware of incontinence

RELATED FACTORS
Pathophysiologic
Refer to *Impaired Urinary Elimination.*

`NOC` (See Functional Incontinence)

Goals

The person will be continent (specify during day, night, 24 hours).

Indicators

- Identify the cause of incontinence and rationale for treatment.
- Identify daily goal for fluid intake.

`NIC` (See also Functional Incontinence) Environmental Management, Urinary Catheterization, Teaching: Procedural Treatment, Tube Care: Urinary, Urinary Bladder Training

Generic Interventions

Maintain Optimal Hydration.
Increase fluid intake to 2 to 3 L/day, unless contraindicated.
Space fluids every 2 hours.
Decrease fluid intake after 7 p.m., and provide only minimal fluids during the night.
Reduce intake of coffee, tea, dark colas, alcohol, and grapefruit juice because of their diuretic effect.
Avoid large amounts of tomato and orange juice because they tend to make the urine more alkaline.

Maintain Adequate Nutrition to Ensure Bowel Elimination at Least Once Every 3 Days.

Promote Micturition.

Ensure privacy and comfort.
Use toilet facilities, if possible, instead of bedpans.
Provide male with opportunity to stand, if possible.
Assist person on bedpan to flex knees and support back.
Teach postural evacuation (bend forward while sitting on toilet).

Promote Personal Integrity and Provide Motivation to Increase Bladder Control.

Convey to Person that Incontinence Can Be Cured or at Least Controlled to Maintain Dignity.

Expect Person to Be Continent, Not Incontinent (e.g., Encourage Street Clothes, Discourage Use of Bedpans, Protective Pads).

Promote Skin Integrity.

Identify individuals at risk for developing pressure ulcers.
Wash area, rinse, and dry gently after incontinent episode.
Avoid harsh soaps, alcohol products.
Use a no-rinse perineal cleanser.
Select a moisturizer that is occlusive (e.g., lanolin, petroleum).

Assess the Person's Potential for Participation in a Bladder-Retraining Program (Cognition, Willingness to Participate, Desire to Change Behavior).

Provide Individual With Rationale for Plan, and Acquire Informed Consent.

Encourage Individual to Continue Program by Providing Accurate Information Concerning Reasons for Success or Failure.

Assess Voiding Pattern:

Time and amount of fluid intake
Type of fluid
Amount of incontinence
Amount of void, whether it was voluntary or involuntary
Presence of sensation of need to void
Amount of retention
Amount of residual urine
Amount of triggered urine
Identify certain activities that precede voiding (e.g., restlessness, yelling, exercise)

**Schedule Fluid Intake and
Voiding Times.**

**Schedule Intermittent Catheterization
Program, if Indicated.**

**Teach Intermittent Catheterization to
Person and Family for Long-Term
Management of Bladder.**

Explain the reasons for the catheterization program.
Explain the relationship of fluid intake and the frequency
of catheterization.
Explain the importance of emptying the bladder at the prescribed time regardless of circumstances because of the hazards of an overdistended bladder (e.g., circulation contributes to infection, and stasis of urine contributes to bacterial growth).

**Teach Prevention of Urinary
Tract Infections.**

Encourage regular, complete emptying of the bladder.
Ensure adequate fluid intake.
Keep urine acidic; avoid citrus juices, dark colas, and coffee.
Monitor urine pH.

**Teach Individual to Monitor for
Signs and Symptoms of Urinary
Tract Infections:**

Increase in mucus and sediment
Blood in urine (hematuria)
Change in color (from normal straw-colored) or odor
Elevated temperature, chills, and shaking

Changes in urine properties
Suprapubic pain
Painful urination
Urgency
Frequent, small voids or frequent, small incontinences
Increased spasticity in spinal cord-injured individuals
Increase in urine pH
Nausea/vomiting
Lower back or flank pain

**Refer to Community Nurse for
Assistance in Bladder Reconditioning
if Indicated.**

Urge Incontinence

DEFINITION
Urge Incontinence: The state in which an individual experiences an involuntary loss of urine associated with a strong sudden desire to void.

DEFINING CHARACTERISTICS
Major (Must Be Present)
Urgency followed by incontinence

RELATED FACTORS
Pathophysiologic
Related to decreased bladder capacity secondary to:

Infection
Trauma
Urethritis
Neurogenic disorders or
  injury
Parkinsonism

Cerebrovascular accident
Demyelinating diseases
Diabetic neuropathy
Alcoholic neuropathy
Brain injury/tumor/infection

Treatment-Related
Related to decreased bladder capacity secondary to:
Abdominal surgery
Postindwelling catheters

Situational (Personal, Environmental)
Related to irritation of bladder stretch receptors secondary to:
Alcohol   Excess fluid intake
Caffeine

Related to decreased bladder capacity secondary to frequent voiding

Maturational
Child
Related to small bladder capacity

Older Adult
Related to decreased bladder capacity

NOC (Refer to Functional Incontinence)

Goals

The person will report an absence or decreased episodes of incontinence (specify).

Indicators

• Explain causes of incontinence.
• Describe bladder irritants.

NIC (Refer to Functional Incontinence)

Generic Interventions

Explain the Causative or Contributing Factors:
Bladder irritants
    Infection
    Inflammation
    Alcohol, caffeine, or dark cola ingestion
    Concentrated urine

Diminished bladder capacity
    Self-induced deconditioning (frequent, small voids)
    Postindwelling catheter
Overdistended bladder
    Increased urine production (diabetes mellitus, diuretics)
    Intake of alcohol or large quantities of fluids
Uninhibited bladder contractions
    Neurologic disorders (cerebrovascular accident, brain
      tumor/trauma/infection, Parkinson's disease)

**Explain the Risk of Insufficient Fluid
Intake and Its Relation to Infection
and Concentrated Urine.**

**Explain the Relationship between
Incontinence and Intake of Alcohol,
Caffeine, and Dark Colas (Irritants).**

**Determine Amount of Time between
Urge to Void and Need to Void
(Record How Long Person Can Hold
off Urination).**

**For a Person With Difficulty
Prolonging Waiting Time,
Communicate to Personnel the Need
to Respond Rapidly to Request for
Assistance for Toileting (Note on
Care Plan).**

**Teach Person to Increase Waiting
Time by Increasing Bladder Capacity.**

Determine volume of each void.
Ask person to "hold off" urinating as long as possible.
Give positive reinforcement.
Discourage frequent voiding that is result of habit not
    need.
Develop bladder reconditioning program.

**For Uninhibited Bladder Contractions,
Provide an Opportunity to Void on
Awakening, after Meals, Physical
Exercise, Bathing, Drinking Coffee
or Tea, and before Going to Sleep.**

Urge Incontinence, Risk for

DEFINITION

Risk for Urge Incontinence: The state in which an individual is at risk to experience an involuntary loss of urine associated with a strong, sudden desire to void.

RISK FACTORS

Refer to Related Factors in *Urge Incontinence.*

NOC (Refer to Functional Incontinence)

Goals

The person will report continued continence.

Indicators

- Explain causes of incontinence.
- Explain strategies to maintain continence.

NIC (Refer to Functional Incontinence)

Interventions

Refer to *Urge Incontinence.*

DEFINITION

Urinary Retention: The state in which an individual experiences a chronic inability to void followed by involuntary voiding (overflow incontinence).

ⓧ AUTHOR'S NOTE

This diagnosis is not recommended for use with individuals with acute episodes of urinary retention (e.g., fecal impaction, postanesthesia, postdelivery); in these patients, catheterization, treatment of the cause, or surgery (prostatic hypertrophy) cures urinary retention. These situations are collaborative problems: Potential Complication: Acute urinary retention.

DEFINING CHARACTERISTICS
Major (Must Be Present, One or More)
Bladder distention (not related to acute, reversible etiology)
Bladder distention with small, frequent voids or dribbling
 (overflow incontinence)
100 mL or more residual urine

Minor (May Be Present)
The individual states that it feels as though the bladder is
 not empty after voiding.

RELATED FACTORS
Pathophysiologic
Related to sphincter blockage secondary to:
Strictures   Ureterocele
Prostate enlargement   Bladder neck contractures
Perineal swelling

**Related to impaired afferent pathways or inadequacy
secondary to:**
Cord injury/tumor/infection   Multiple sclerosis
Brain injury/tumor/infection   Diabetic neuropathy

Cerebrovascular accident	Alcoholic neuropathy
Demyelinating diseases	Tabes dorsalis

Treatment-Related

Related to bladder outlet obstruction or impaired afferent pathways secondary to drug therapy (iatrogenic):

Antihistamines	Theophylline
Epinephrine	Isoproterenol
Anticholinergics	

Situational (Personal, Environmental)

Related to bladder outlet obstruction secondary to fecal impaction

Related to detrusor inadequacy secondary to deconditioned voiding associated with stress or discomfort

NOC (See Functional Incontinence)

Goals

The person will achieve a state of dryness that is personally satisfactory.

Indicators

- Empty the bladder using Credé's and/or Valsalva's maneuvers with residual urine of less than 50 mL if indicated.
- Void voluntarily.

NIC (See also Functional Incontinence) Urinary Retention Care, Urinary Bladder Training

Generic Interventions

Develop a Bladder Retraining or Reconditioning Program (See *Total Incontinence* for Generic Interventions).

Teach Abdominal Strain and Valsalva's Maneuver, if Indicated.

Lean forward on thighs.

Contract abdominal muscles if possible, and strain or "bear down"; hold breath while straining (Valsalva's maneuver).

Hold strain or breath until urine flow stops; wait 1 minute, and strain again as long as possible.

Continue until no more urine is expelled.

Teach Credé's Maneuver if Indicated.

Place hands flat (or place fist) just below umbilical area.

Place one hand on top of the other.

Press firmly down and in toward the pelvic arch.

Repeat six or seven times until no more urine can be expelled.

Wait a few minutes and repeat to ensure complete emptying.

Teach Anal Stretch Maneuver, if Indicated.

Sit on commode or toilet.

Lean forward on thighs.

Place one gloved hand behind buttocks.

Insert one or two lubricated fingers into the anus to the anal sphincter.

Spread fingers apart, or pull to posterior direction.

Gently stretch the anal sphincter and hold it distended.

Bear down and void.

Take a deep breath and hold it while straining (Valsalva's maneuver).

Relax and repeat the procedure until the bladder is empty.

Instruct Individual to Try All Three Techniques or a Combination of Techniques to Determine Which Is Most Effective in Emptying the Bladder.

Indicate on the Intake and Output Record Which Technique Was Used to Induce Voiding.

Obtain Postvoid Residuals after Attempts at Emptying Bladder; if Residual Urine Volumes Are Greater Than 100 mL, Schedule Intermittent Catheterization Program.

Violence, Risk for

DEFINITION

Risk for Violence: The state in which an individual has been, or is at risk to be, assaultive toward others or the environment.

> ⓧ **AUTHOR'S NOTE**
>
> This diagnosis can be made more specific by adding *Risk for Violence: Self-directed or directed at others.* The author has added *Risk for Suicide* to describe individuals at risk for self-inflicted injuries; thus, the descriptor *self-directed* is not needed. Therefore, the content for *Risk for Violence* will focus exclusively on violence directed at others.

RISK FACTORS

Presence of risk factors (see also Related Factors)

RELATED FACTORS

Pathophysiologic

Related to history of aggressive acts and perception of environment as threatening secondary to: or

Related to history of aggressive acts and delusional thinking secondary to: or

Related to history of aggressive acts and manic excitement secondary to: or

Related to history of aggressive acts and inability to verbalize feelings secondary to: or
Related to history of aggressive acts and psychic overload secondary to:

Temporal lobe epilepsy   Hormonal imbalance
Progressive CNS deterioration   Viral encephalopathy
  (brain tumor)   Mental retardation
Head injury   Minimal brain dysfunction

Related to toxic response to alcohol or drugs
Related to organic brain syndrome

Treatment-Related

Related to toxic reaction to medication

Situational (Personal, Environmental)

Related to history of overt aggressive acts
Related to increase in stressors within a short period
Related to acute agitation
Related to suspiciousness
Related to persecutory delusions
Related to verbal threats of physical assault
Related to low frustration tolerance
Related to poor impulse control
Related to fear of the unknown
Related to response to catastrophic event
Related to response to dysfunctional family throughout developmental stages
Related to dysfunctional communication patterns
Related to drug or alcohol abuse

NOC Abuse Cessation, Abusive Behavior Self-Control, Aggression Control, Impulse Control

Goals

The person will have a decreased number of violent responses.

Indicators

- Demonstrate control of behavior with assistance from others.
- Describe causation and possible preventive measures.
- Explain rationale for interventions.

NIC Abuse Protection Support, Anger Control Assistance, Environmental Management: Violence Prevention, Impulse Control Training, Crisis Intervention, Seclusion, Physical Restraint

Generic Interventions

Acknowledge the Individual's Feelings; Be Genuine and Empathetic.

Tell Individual that You Will Help Control Behavior and Not Let Him or Her Do Anything Destructive.

Set Limits When Individual Presents a Risk to Others. Refer to *Anxiety* for Further Interventions on Limit Setting.

Offer Choices and Options. At Times, It Is Necessary to Give in to Some Demands to Avoid a Power Struggle.

Encourage Individual to Express Anger and Hostility Verbally Instead of "Acting Out."

Remain Calm. If You Are Becoming Upset, Leave the Situation in the Hands of Others, if Possible.

Allow the Acutely Agitated Individual Space that Is Five Times Greater Than that for an Individual Who Is in Control. Do Not Touch the Person Unless You Have a Trusting Relationship. Avoid Physical Entrapment of Individual or Staff.

Do Not Approach a Violent Individual Alone. Often the Presence of Three or Four Staff Members Will Be Enough to Reassure the Individual that You Will Not Let Him or Her Lose Control.

When Assault Is Imminent, Quick, Coordinated Action Is Essential.

Approach Individual in a Calm, Self-Assured Manner to Avoid Communicating Your Anxiety or Fear.

Establish an Environment that Reduces Agitation.

Decrease noise level.
Give short, concise explanations.
Control the number of persons present at one time.
Provide single or semiprivate room.

Establish the Expectation that Person Can Control Behavior, and Continue to Reinforce the Expectation.

Provide Positive Feedback When Person Is Able to Exercise Restraint.

Allow Appropriate Verbal Expressions of Anger. Give Positive Feedback.

Set Limits on Verbal Abuse. Do Not Take Insults Personally. Support Others (Clients, Staff) Who May Be Targets of Abuse.

Plan for Unpredictable Violence.

Assess person's potential for violence and history.
Ensure availability of staff before potential violent behavior (never try to assist person alone when physical restraint is necessary).
Determine who will be in charge of directing personnel to intervene in violent behavior if it occurs.
Ensure protection for oneself (door nearby for withdrawal, pillow to protect face).

Use Seclusion or Restraint, According to Policy.

Remove Individual from Situation if Environment Is Contributing to Aggressive Behavior, Using the Least Amount of Control Needed (e.g., Ask Others to Leave, and Take Individual to Quiet Room).

Reinforce that You Are Going to Help Person Control Self.

Repeatedly Tell the Person What Is Going to Happen before External Control Is Begun.

When Using Seclusion, Institutional Policy Will Provide Specific Guidelines; the Following Are General.

Observe individual at least every 15 minutes.

Search the individual before secluding to remove harmful objects.

Check seclusion room to see that safety is maintained.

Offer fluids and food periodically (in nonbreakable containers).

Have sufficient staff present when approaching an individual to be secluded.

Explain concisely what is going to happen ("You will be placed in a room by yourself until you can better control your behavior."), and give person a chance to cooperate.

Assist person in toileting and personal hygiene (assess ability to be out of seclusion; a urinal or commode may need to be used).

If person is taken out of seclusion, someone must be present continually.

Maintain verbal interaction during seclusion (provides information necessary to assess person's degree of control).

When person is allowed out of seclusion, a staff member needs to be in constant attendance to determine whether person can handle additional stimulation.

Assist Individual in Developing Alternative Coping Strategies When Crisis Has Passed and Learning Can Occur.

Teach Negotiation Skills With Significant Others and Persons in Authority.

Encourage an Increase in Recreational Activities.

Use Group Therapy to Decrease Sense of Aloneness and Increase Communication Skills.

Consult With Person's Therapist or Your Supervisor if Third Parties Need to Be Warned of Danger from the Client (e.g., Police, Potential Victim).

Wandering

DEFINITION

Wandering: A state in which an individual with dementia has meandering, aimless, or repetitive locomotion that exposes him or her to harm.

DEFINING CHARACTERISTIC

Person with dementia who (Algase, 1999; Edgerly & Donovick, 1998):

Ambulates in an aimless, endless manner
Has repetitive locomotion in a circular pattern
Paces repetitively
Exceeds or transgresses environmental limits into hazardous or unauthorized locations
Has spatial disorientation or navigational deficits
Is unable to find what he or she is seeking

RELATED FACTORS
Pathophysiologic

*Related to impaired cerebral function secondary to:
Cerebrovascular accident
Mental retardation
Alzheimer's dementia

Related to physiologic urge (e.g., hunger, thirst, pain, urination, constipation)

Situational (Personal, Environmental)

Related to increased frustration, anxiety, boredom, depression, or agitation
Related to over/understimulating environment
Related to separation from familiar people and places

Maturational
Older Adult
Related to faulty judgments secondary to motor and sensory deficits, medications

---

*This related factor must be present. Other related factors can also be present concurrently.

NOC Safety Behavior: Personal

Goals

The person will not elope or get lost.

Indicators (Person, Family)

- Ambulate safely.
- Identify factors that contribute to wandering behaviors.
- Anticipate wandering behaviors.

NIC Pelvic Control, Environmental Management: Safety, Support Groups, Family Mobilization

Generic Interventions

Assess for Contributing Factors:

Anxiety
Confusion
Frustration
Boredom
Agitation
Separation from familiar people and places
Faulty judgment
Physiologic urge (hunger, thirst, pain, urination, constipation)

Reduce or Eliminate Factors, if Possible.

Physiologic Urges:

Anticipate need for toileting with a schedule.
Schedule times for fluids and food.
Evaluate presence of pain.

Anxiety/Agitation

Refer to *Anxiety* for interventions.

Unfamiliar Environment

Select a familiar picture to exhibit on person's door.
Redirect if lost.

Provide a safe route for walking.

Encourage activities that increase exercise (e.g., sweeping, raking).

Create nature scenes in hallways (Cohen-Mansfield & Werner, 1998).

Mark exit door with big signs.

Make horizontal stripes on exit door or use a cloth panel across the width of door.

Promote a Safe Environment.

Install locks on doors and windows.

Install electronic devices with buzzers on door, property boundaries.

Use pressure-sensitive alarms (doormats, bed sensor, chair sensor).

Provide regular opportunities to walk with a companion or in a safe area.

Notify others about person's wandering behaviors:
  Neighbors
  Police
  Other patients in residence
  Staff
  Community resources

Explain the use of electronic devices.

Instruct them to notify if person is seen wandering.

Have recent photograph and current identification information (age, height, weight, hair color, description of clothes, identifying characteristics).

Contact local Alzheimer's Association for safety programs.

Diagnostic Clusters

CARDIOVASCULAR/HEMATOLOGIC/ PERIPHERAL VASCULAR DISORDERS

CARDIAC CONDITIONS
Angina Pectoris

Nursing Diagnoses*

Anxiety related to chest pain secondary to effects of hypoxia

Fear related to present status and unknown future

Disturbed Sleep Pattern related to treatments and environment

Risk for Constipation related to bed rest, change in lifestyle, and medications

Activity Intolerance related to deconditioning secondary to fear of recurrent angina

Risk for Disturbed Self-Concept related to perceived and/or actual role changes

Risk for Impaired Home Maintenance related to angina or fear of angina

Risk for Interrupted Family Processes related to impaired ability of person to assume role responsibilities

Risk for Ineffective Sexuality Patterns related to fear of angina and altered self-concept

Grieving related to actual or perceived losses secondary to cardiac condition

Risk for Ineffective Therapeutic Regimen Management related to insufficient knowledge of condition, home activities, diet, and medications

---

* List includes nursing diagnoses that may be associated with the medical diagnosis.

Congestive Heart Failure with Pulmonary Edema

Collaborative Problems

†△ PC: Deep vein thrombosis
▲ PC: Severe hypoxia
△ PC: Cardiogenic shock
  PC: Hepatic failure

Nursing Diagnoses

▲ Activity Intolerance related to insufficient oxygen for activities of daily living
△ Imbalanced Nutrition: Less Than Body Requirements related to nausea; anorexia secondary to venous congestion of gastrointestinal tract and fatigue
△ Ineffective Peripheral Tissue Perfusion related to venous congestion secondary to right-sided heart failure
▲ Anxiety related to breathlessness
* Fear related to progressive nature of condition
* Risk for Impaired Home Maintenance related to inability to perform activities of daily living secondary to breathlessness and fatigue
* (Specify) Self-Care Deficit related to dyspnea and fatigue
△ Disturbed Sleep Pattern related to nocturnal dyspnea and inability to assume usual sleep position
▲ Risk for Excessive Fluid Volume: Edema related to decreased renal blood flow secondary to right-sided heart failure
△ Powerlessness related to progressive nature of condition
△ Risk for Ineffective Therapeutic Regimen Management related to insufficient knowledge of low-salt diet, drug therapy (diuretic, digitalis), activity program, and signs and symptoms of complications

---

▲ This diagnosis was reported to be monitored for or managed frequently (75% to 100%).

△ This diagnosis was reported to be monitored for or managed often (50% to 74%).

* This diagnosis was not included in the validation study.

† PCs (potential complications) are collaborative problems, not nursing diagnoses.

Endocarditis, Pericarditis (Rheumatic, Infectious)

See also *Corticosteroid Therapy*. If child, see *Rheumatic Fever*.

Collaborative Problems

PC: Congestive heart failure
PC: Valvular stenosis
PC: Cerebrovascular accident
PC: Emboli (pulmonary, cerebral, renal, splenic, heart)
PC: Cardiac tamponade

Nursing Diagnoses

Activity Intolerance related to insufficient oxygen secondary to decreased cardiac output
Risk for Ineffective Respiratory Function related to decreased respiratory depth secondary to pain
Pain related to friction rub and inflammation process
Risk for Ineffective Therapeutic Regimen Management related to insufficient knowledge of etiology, prevention, antibiotic prophylaxis, and signs and symptoms of complications

Myocardial Infarction (Uncomplicated)

Collaborative Problems

▲ PC: Dysrhythmias
▲ PC: Cardiogenic shock
▲ PC: Thromboembolism
PC: Recurrent myocardial infarction

Nursing Diagnoses

▲ Anxiety related to acute pain secondary to cardiac tissue ischemia
* Fear related to pain, present status, and unknown future

▲ This diagnosis was reported to be monitored for or managed frequently (75% to 100%).

* This diagnosis was not included in the validation study.

* Disturbed Sleep Pattern related to treatments and environment
  Risk for Constipation related to decreased peristalsis secondary to medication effects, decreased activity, and change in diet
▲ Activity Intolerance related to insufficient oxygen for activities of daily living secondary to cardiac tissue ischemia
* Risk for Disturbed Self-Concept related to perceived or actual role changes
  Risk for Impaired Home Maintenance related to angina or fear of angina
▲ Anxiety/Fear (individual, family) related to unfamiliar situation, unpredictable nature of condition, negative effect on lifestyle, possible sexual dysfunction
* Risk for Interrupted Family Processes related to impaired ability of ill person to assume role responsibilities
* Risk for Ineffective Sexuality Patterns related to fear of angina and altered self-concept
△ Grieving related to actual or perceived losses secondary to cardiac condition
△ Risk for Ineffective Therapeutic Regimen Management related to insufficient knowledge of hospital routines, treatments, conditions, medications, diet, activity progression, signs and symptoms of complications, reduction of risks, follow-up care, community resources

HEMATOLOGIC CONDITIONS
Anemia

Collaborative Problems

PC: Bleeding
PC: Cardiac failure
PC: Iron overload (repeated transfusion)

▲ This diagnosis was reported to be monitored for or managed frequently (75% to 100%).

△ This diagnosis was reported to be monitored for or managed often (50% to 74%).

* This diagnosis was not included in the validation study.

Nursing Diagnoses

Activity Intolerance related to impaired oxygen transport secondary to diminished red blood cell count

Risk for Infection related to decreased resistance secondary to tissue hypoxia and/or abnormal white blood cells (neutropenia, leukopenia)

Risk for Injury: Bleeding tendencies related to thrombocytopenia and splenomegaly

Risk for Impaired Oral Mucous Membrane related to gastrointestinal mucosal atrophy

Risk for Ineffective Therapeutic Regimen Management related to insufficient knowledge of condition, nutritional requirements, and drug therapy

Aplastic Anemia

Collaborative Problems

PC: Fatal aplasia
PC: Pancytopenia
PC: Hemorrhage
PC: Hypoxia
PC: Sepsis

Nursing Diagnoses

Activity Intolerance related to insufficient oxygen secondary to diminished red blood cell count

Risk for Infection related to increased susceptibility secondary to leukopenia

Risk for Impaired Oral Mucous Membrane related to tissue hypoxia and vulnerability

Risk for Ineffective Therapeutic Regimen Management related to insufficient knowledge of causes, prevention, and signs and symptoms of complications

Pernicious Anemia

See also *Anemia*.

Nursing Diagnoses

Impaired Oral Mucous Membrane related to sore red tongue secondary to papillary atrophy and inflammatory changes

Diarrhea/Constipation related to gastrointestinal mucosal atrophy

Risk for Imbalanced Nutrition: Less Than Body Requirements related to anorexia secondary to sore mouth

Risk for Ineffective Therapeutic Regimen Management related to insufficient knowledge of chronicity of disease and vitamin B treatment

Disseminated Intravascular Coagulation (DIC)

See also *Underlying Disorders (e.g., Obstetric, Infections, Burns), Anticoagulant Therapy.*

Collaborative Problems

PC: Hemorrhage

PC: Renal failure

PC: Microthrombi (renal, cardiac, pulmonary, cerebral, gastrointestinal)

Nursing Diagnoses

Fear related to treatments, environment, and unpredictable outcome

Interrupted Family Processes related to critical nature of the situation and uncertain prognosis

Anxiety related to insufficient knowledge of causes and treatment

Polycythemia Vera

Collaborative Problems

PC: Thrombus formation

PC: Hemorrhage

PC: Hypertension

PC: Congestive heart failure

PC: Peptic ulcer

PC: Gout

Nursing Diagnoses

Imbalanced Nutrition: Less Than Body Requirements related to anorexia, nausea, and vasocongestion

Activity Intolerance related to insufficient oxygen secondary to pulmonary congestion and tissue hypoxia

Risk for Infection related to hypoxia secondary to vaso-congestion

Risk for Ineffective Therapeutic Regimen Management related to insufficient knowledge of fluid requirements, exercise program, and signs and symptoms of complications

PERIPHERAL VASCULAR CONDITIONS
Deep Vein Thrombosis

See also *Anticoagulant Therapy,* if indicated.

Collaborative Problems

▲ PC: Pulmonary embolism
▲ PC: Chronic leg edema
△ PC: Chronic stasis ulcers

Nursing Diagnoses

Risk for Constipation related to decreased peristalsis secondary to immobility

△ Risk for Ineffective Respiratory Function related to immobility

△ Risk for Impaired Skin Integrity related to chronic ankle edema

▲ Acute Pain related to impaired circulation for ambulation

△ Risk for Ineffective Therapeutic Regimen Management related to insufficient knowledge of prevention of recurrence of deep vein thrombosis and signs and symptoms of complications

Hypertension

Collaborative Problems

PC: Retinal hemorrhage
PC: Cerebrovascular accident

▲ This diagnosis was reported to be monitored for or managed frequently (75% to 100%).

△ This diagnosis was reported to be monitored for or managed often (50% to 74%).

PC: Cerebral hemorrhage
PC: Renal failure

Nursing Diagnoses

Risk for Noncompliance related to negative side effects of prescribed therapy versus the belief that no treatment is needed without the presence of symptoms

Risk for Ineffective Sexuality Patterns related to decreased libido or erectile dysfunction secondary to medication side effects

Risk for Ineffective Therapeutic Regimen Management related to insufficient knowledge of condition, diet restrictions, medications, risk factors, and follow-up care

Varicose Veins

Collaborative Problems

PC: Vascular rupture
PC: Hemorrhage

Nursing Diagnoses

Chronic Pain related to engorgement of veins

Risk for Ineffective Therapeutic Regimen Management related to insufficient knowledge of condition, treatment options, and risk factors

Peripheral Arterial Disease
(Atherosclerosis, Arteriosclerosis)

Collaborative Problems

PC: Stroke (cerebrovascular accident)
PC: Ischemic ulcers
PC: Claudication
PC: Acute arterial thrombosis
PC: Hypertension

Nursing Diagnoses

Risk for Impaired Tissue Integrity related to compromised circulation

Chronic Pain related to muscle ischemia during prolonged activity

Risk for Injury related to decreased sensation secondary to chronic atherosclerosis

Risk for Infection related to compromised circulation

Risk for Injury related to effects of orthostatic hypotension

Activity Intolerance related to claudication

Risk for Ineffective Therapeutic Regimen Management related to insufficient knowledge of condition, management of claudication, risk factors, foot care, and treatment plan

Raynaud's Disease

Collaborative Problems

PC: Acute arterial occlusion
PC: Ischemic ulcers
PC: Gangrene

Nursing Diagnoses

Acute Pain related to ischemia secondary to acute vasospasm

Ineffective Peripheral Tissue Perfusion related to compromised blood flow and vasospasms secondary to cold environment

Risk for Impaired Tissue Integrity: Ischemic ulcers related to vasospasm

Fear related to potential loss of work secondary to work-related aggravating factors

Risk for Ineffective Therapeutic Regimen Management related to insufficient knowledge of condition, risk factors, and self-care

Venous Stasis Ulcers (Postphlebitis Syndrome)

Collaborative Problem

▲ PC: Cellulitis

▲ This diagnosis was reported to be monitored for or managed frequently (75% to 100%).

Nursing Diagnoses

* Ineffective Peripheral Tissue Perfusion related to dependent position of legs
* Risk for Infection related to compromised circulation
▲ Chronic Pain related to ulcers and débridement treatments
△ Risk for Disturbed Body Image related to chronic open wounds and response of others to appearance
△ Risk for Ineffective Therapeutic Regimen Management related to lack of knowledge of condition, prevention of complications, risk factors, and treatment

RESPIRATORY DISORDERS
Adult Respiratory Distress Syndrome

See also *Mechanical Ventilation* (under *Diagnostic and Therapeutic Procedures*).

Collaborative Problems

PC: Electrolyte imbalance
PC: Hypoxemia

Nursing Diagnoses

Anxiety related to implications of condition and critical care setting
Powerlessness related to condition and treatments (ventilator, monitoring)

Chronic Obstructive Pulmonary Disease (Emphysema, Bronchitis)

Collaborative Problems

▲ PC: Hypoxemia
△ PC: Right-sided heart failure

▲ This diagnosis was reported to be monitored for or managed frequently (75% to 100%).

△ This diagnosis was reported to be monitored for or managed often (50% to 74%).

* This diagnosis was not included in the validation study.

Nursing Diagnoses

▲ Ineffective Airway Clearance related to excessive and tenacious secretions

△ Risk for Imbalanced Nutrition: Less Than Body Requirements related to anorexia secondary to dyspnea, halitosis, and fatigue

▲ Activity Intolerance related to insufficient oxygen for activities and fatigue
  Impaired Verbal Communication related to dyspnea

▲ Anxiety related to breathlessness and fear of suffocation

△ Powerlessness related to feeling of loss of control and lifestyle restrictions

△ Disturbed Sleep Pattern related to cough, inability to assume recumbent position, and environmental stimuli

△ Risk for Ineffective Therapeutic Regimen Management related to insufficient knowledge of condition, treatments, prevention of infection, breathing exercises, risk factors, signs and symptoms of complications

Pleural Effusion

See also underlying disorders (*Congestive Heart Disease, Cirrhosis, Malignancy*).

Collaborative Problems

PC: Respiratory failure
PC: Pneumothorax (post-thoracentesis)
PC: Hypoxemia
PC: Hemothorax

Nursing Diagnoses

Activity Intolerance related to insufficient oxygen for activities of daily living
Risk for Imbalanced Nutrition: Less Than Body Requirements related to anorexia secondary to pressure on abdominal structures

---

▲ This diagnosis was reported to be monitored for or managed frequently (75% to 100%).

△ This diagnosis was reported to be monitored for or managed often (50% to 74%).

Impaired Comfort related to accumulation of fluid in
  pleural space
(Specify) Self-Care Deficits related to fatigue and dyspnea

Pneumonia

Collaborative Problems

▲ PC: Respiratory insufficiency
  PC: Septic shock
  PC: Paralytic ileus

Nursing Diagnoses

  Risk for Hyperthermia related to infectious process
▲ Activity Intolerance related to insufficient oxygen for
  activities of daily living
△ Risk for Impaired Oral Mucous Membrane related to
  mouth breathing, frequent expectoration, and decreased
  fluid intake secondary to malaise
* Risk for Deficient Fluid Volume related to increased
  insensible fluid loss secondary to fever and hyperventilation
△ Risk for Imbalanced Nutrition: Less Than Body Requirements related to anorexia, dyspnea, and abdominal distention secondary to air swallowing
▲ Ineffective Airway Clearance related to pain, increased
  tracheobronchial secretions, and fatigue
* Risk for Infection Transmission related to communicable nature of the disease
* Discomfort related to hyperthermia and malaise
* Risk for Impaired Skin Integrity related to prescribed
  bed rest
△ Risk for Ineffective Therapeutic Regimen Management
  related to lack of knowledge of condition, infection
  transmission, prevention of recurrence, diet, signs and
  symptoms of recurrence, and follow-up care

▲ This diagnosis was reported to be monitored for or managed
frequently (75% to 100%).

△ This diagnosis was reported to be monitored for or managed
often (50% to 74%).

* This diagnosis was not included in the validation study.

Pulmonary Embolism

See also *Anticoagulant Therapy*.

Collaborative Problem

PC: Hypoxemia

Nursing Diagnoses

Risk for Impaired Skin Integrity related to immobility and prescribed bed rest

Risk for Ineffective Therapeutic Regimen Management related to insufficient knowledge of anticoagulant therapy and signs and symptoms of complications

METABOLIC/ENDOCRINE DISORDERS
Addison's Disease

Collaborative Problems

PC: Addisonian crisis (shock)

PC: Electrolyte imbalances (sodium, potassium)

PC: Hypoglycemia

Nursing Diagnoses

Risk for Imbalanced Nutrition: Less Than Body Requirements related to anorexia and nausea

Risk for Deficient Fluid Volume related to excessive loss of sodium and water secondary to polyuria

Diarrhea related to increased excretion of sodium and water

Risk for Disturbed Self-Concept related to appearance changes secondary to increased skin pigmentation and decreased axillary and pubic hair (female)

Risk for Injury related to postural hypotension secondary to fluid/electrolyte imbalances

Risk for Ineffective Therapeutic Regimen Management related to insufficient knowledge of disease, signs and symptoms of complications, risks for crisis (infection, diarrhea, decreased sodium intake, diaphoresis), overexertion, dietary management, identification (card, medallion), emergency kit, and pharmacologic management

Aldosteronism, Primary

Collaborative Problems

PC: Hypokalemia
PC: Alkalosis
PC: Hypertension
PC: Hypernatremia

Nursing Diagnoses

Impaired Comfort related to excessive urine excretion and polydipsia

Risk for Deficient Fluid Volume related to excessive urinary excretion

Risk for Ineffective Therapeutic Regimen Management related to insufficient knowledge of condition, surgical treatment, and effects of corticosteroid therapy

Cirrhosis (Laënnec's Disease)

See also *Substance Abuse,* if indicated.

Collaborative Problems

▲ PC: Hemorrhage
△ PC: Hypokalemia
△ PC: Portal systemic encephalopathy
* PC: Negative nitrogen balance
▲ PC: Drug toxicity (opiates, short-acting barbiturates, major tranquilizers)
△ PC: Renal failure
* PC: Anemia
* PC: Esophageal varices

Nursing Diagnoses

▲ Pain related to liver enlargement and ascites
△ Diarrhea related to excessive secretion of fats in stool secondary to liver dysfunction

───────

▲ This diagnosis was reported to be monitored for or managed frequently (75% to 100%).

△ This diagnosis was reported to be monitored for or managed often (50% to 74%).

* This diagnosis was not included in the validation study.

* Risk for Injury related to decreased prothrombin production and synthesis of substances used in blood
coagulation

▲ Imbalanced Nutrition: Less Than Body Requirements
related to anorexia, impaired protein, fat, glucose
metabolism, and impaired storage of vitamins
(A, C, K, D, E)

* Risk for Ineffective Respiratory Function related to
pressure on diaphragm secondary to ascites

* Risk for Disturbed Self-Concept related to appearance
changes (jaundice, ascites)

△ Risk for Infection related to leukopenia secondary to
enlarged, overactive spleen and hypoproteinemia

△ Impaired Comfort: Pruritus related to accumulation of
bilirubin pigment and bile salts on skin

▲ Excess Fluid Volume related to portal hypertension,
lowered plasma colloidal osmotic pressure, and sodium
retention

△ Risk for Ineffective Therapeutic Regimen Management
related to insufficient knowledge of pharmacologic
contraindications, nutritional requirements, signs
and symptoms of complications, and risks of
alcohol ingestion

Cushing's Syndrome

Collaborative Problems

PC: Hypertension
PC: Congestive heart failure
PC: Psychosis
PC: Electrolyte imbalance (sodium, potassium)

Nursing Diagnoses

Disturbed Self-Concept related to physical changes secondary to disease process (moon face, thinning of hair,
truncal obesity, virilism)

▲ This diagnosis was reported to be monitored for or managed
frequently (75% to 100%).

△ This diagnosis was reported to be monitored for or managed
often (50% to 74%).

* This diagnosis was not included in the validation study.

Risk for Infection related to excessive protein catabolism
   and depressed leukocytic phagocytosis secondary to
   hyperglycemia
Risk for Injury: Fractures related to osteoporosis
Risk for Impaired Skin Integrity related to loss of tissue,
   edema, and dryness
Ineffective Sexuality Patterns related to loss of libido and
   cessation of menses (female) secondary to excessive
   adrenocorticotropic hormone production
Risk for Ineffective Therapeutic Regimen Management related to insufficient knowledge of disease and diet
   therapy (high protein, low cholesterol, low sodium)

Diabetes Mellitus

Collaborative Problems
Acute Complications:
▲ PC: Ketoacidosis (DKA)
△ PC: Hyperosmolar hyperglycemic nonketotic coma
   (HHNR)
▲ PC: Hypoglycemia
▲ PC: Infections

Chronic Complications:
   Macrovascular
▲ PC: Cardiac artery disease
▲ PC: Peripheral vascular disease
   Microvascular
△ PC: Retinopathy
▲ PC: Neuropathy
△ PC: Nephropathy

Nursing Diagnoses
△ Risk for Injury related to decreased tactile sensation,
   diminished visual acuity, and hypoglycemia

▲ This diagnosis was reported to be monitored for or managed
frequently (75% to 100%).

△ This diagnosis was reported to be monitored for or managed
often (50% to 74%).

△ Fear (client, family) related to diagnosis of diabetes, potential complications of diabetes, insulin injection, negative effect on lifestyle

△ Risk for Ineffective Coping (client, family) related to chronic disease, complex self-care regimen, and uncertain future

▲ Imbalanced Nutrition: More Than Body Requirements related to intake in excess of activity expenditures, lack of knowledge, and ineffective coping

Risk for Ineffective Sexuality Patterns (male) related to erectile problems secondary to peripheral neuropathy or psychological conflicts

Risk for Ineffective Sexuality Patterns (female) related to frequent genitourinary problems and physical and psychological stressors of diabetes

△ Powerlessness related to the future development of complications of diabetes (blindness, amputations, kidney failure, painful neuropathy)

* Social Isolation related to visual impairment/blindness

△ Risk for Noncompliance related to the complexity and chronicity of the prescribed regimen

△ Risk for Ineffective Therapeutic Regimen Management related to insufficient knowledge of condition, self-monitoring of blood glucose, medications, American Diabetes Association exchange diet, treatment of hypo-glycemia, weight control, sick day care, exercise pro-gram, foot care, signs and symptoms of complications, and community resources

Hepatitis (Viral)

Collaborative Problems

* PC: Hepatic failure
* PC: Coma
* PC: Subacute hepatic necrosis

▲ This diagnosis was reported to be monitored for or managed frequently (75% to 100%).

△ This diagnosis was reported to be monitored for or managed often (50% to 74%).

* This diagnosis was not included in the validation study.

* PC: Fulminant hepatitis
△ PC: Portal systemic encephalopathy
△ PC: Hypokalemia
△ PC: Hemorrhage
△ PC: Drug toxicity
△ PC: Renal failure
△ PC: Progressive liver degeneration

Nursing Diagnoses

* Fatigue related to reduced metabolism by liver
▲ Risk for Infection Transmission related to contagious nature of virus type A and type B
▲ Imbalanced Nutrition: Less Than Body Requirements related to anorexia, epigastric distress, and nausea
* Risk for Deficient Fluid Volume related to lack of desire to drink
△ Impaired Comfort related to accumulation of bilirubin pigment and bile salts
* Risk for Injury related to reduced prothrombin synthesis and reduced vitamin K absorption
△ Pain related to swelling of inflamed liver
* Deficient Diversional Activity related to the monotony of confinement and isolation precautions
△ Risk for Ineffective Therapeutic Regimen Management related to insufficient knowledge of condition, rest requirements, precautions to prevent transmission, nutritional requirements, and contraindications

Hyperthyroidism
(Thyrotoxicosis, Graves' Disease)

Collaborative Problems

PC: Thyroid storm
PC: Cardiac dysrhythmias

▲ This diagnosis was reported to be monitored for or managed frequently (75% to 100%).

△ This diagnosis was reported to be monitored for or managed often (50% to 74%).

* This diagnosis was not included in the validation study.

Nursing Diagnoses

Imbalanced Nutrition: Less Than Body Requirements related to intake less than metabolic needs secondary to excessive metabolic rate

Activity Intolerance related to fatigue and exhaustion secondary to excessive metabolic rate

Diarrhea related to increased peristalsis secondary to excessive metabolic rate

Impaired Comfort related to heat intolerance and profuse diaphoresis

Risk for Impaired Tissue Integrity: Corneal related to inability to close eyelids secondary to exophthalmos

Risk for Injury related to tremors

Risk for Hyperthermia related to lack of metabolic compensatory mechanism secondary to hyperthyroidism

Risk for Ineffective Therapeutic Regimen Management related to insufficient knowledge of condition, treatment regimen, pharmacologic therapy, eye care, dietary management, and signs and symptoms of complications

Hypothyroidism (Myxedema)

Collaborative Problems

PC: Atherosclerotic heart disease
PC: Normochromic, normocytic anemia
PC: Acute organic psychosis
PC: Myxedemic coma
PC: Metabolic
PC: Hematologic

Nursing Diagnoses

Imbalanced Nutrition: More Than Body Requirements related to intake greater than metabolic needs secondary to slowed metabolic rate

Activity Intolerance related to insufficient oxygen secondary to slowed metabolic rate

Constipation related to decreased peristaltic action secondary to decreased metabolic rate and decreased physical activity

Impaired Skin Integrity related to edema and dryness secondary to decreased metabolic rate and infiltration of fluid into interstitial tissues

Impaired Comfort related to cold intolerance secondary to decreased metabolic rate

Risk for Impaired Social Interactions related to listlessness and depression

Risk for Ineffective Therapeutic Regimen Management related to insufficient knowledge of condition, treatment regimen, dietary management, signs and symptoms of complications, pharmacologic therapy, and contraindications

Obesity

Nursing Diagnoses

Ineffective Health Maintenance related to imbalance between caloric intake and energy expenditure

Ineffective Coping related to increased food consumption secondary to response to external stressors

Chronic Low Self-Esteem related to feelings of self-degradation and the response of others to the condition

Pancreatitis

Collaborative Problems

△ PC: Hypovolemia/shock
* PC: Hemorrhagic pancreatitis
* PC: Respiratory failure
* PC: Pleural effusion
△ PC: Hypocalcemia
▲ PC: Hyperglycemia
△ PC: Delirium tremens

Nursing Diagnoses

▲ Acute Pain related to nasogastric suction, distention of pancreatic capsule, and local peritonitis
Risk for Deficient Fluid Volume related to decreased intake secondary to nausea and vomiting

---

▲ This diagnosis was reported to be monitored for or managed frequently (75% to 100%).

△ This diagnosis was reported to be monitored for or managed often (50% to 74%).

* This diagnosis was not included in the validation study.

▲ Imbalanced Nutrition: Less Than Body Requirements related to vomiting, anorexia, and impaired digestion secondary to decreased pancreatic enzymes

△ Diarrhea related to excessive excretion of fats in stools secondary to insufficient pancreatic enzymes

△ Ineffective Denial related to acknowledgment of alcohol abuse or dependency

△ Risk for Ineffective Therapeutic Regimen Management related to insufficient knowledge of disease process, treatments, contraindications, dietary management, and follow-up care

GASTROINTESTINAL DISORDERS
Esophageal Disorders
(Esophagitis, Hiatal Hernia)

Collaborative Problems

PC: Hemorrhage
PC: Gastric ulcers

Nursing Diagnoses

Risk for Imbalanced Nutrition: Less Than Body Requirements related to anorexia, heartburn, and dysphagia

Impaired Comfort: Heartburn related to regurgitation and eructation

Risk for Ineffective Therapeutic Regimen Management related to insufficient knowledge of condition, dietary management, hazards of alcohol and tobacco, positioning after meals, pharmacologic therapy, and weight reduction (if indicated)

Gastroenteritis

Collaborative Problem

PC: Fluid/electrolyte imbalance

▲ This diagnosis was reported to be monitored for or managed frequently (75% to 100%).

△ This diagnosis was reported to be monitored for or managed often (50% to 74%).

Nursing Diagnoses

Risk for Deficient Fluid Volume related to vomiting and
   diarrhea
Acute Pain related to abdominal cramping, diarrhea, and
   vomiting secondary to vascular dilatation and hyper-
   peristalsis
Risk for Ineffective Therapeutic Regimen Management
   related to insufficient knowledge of condition, dietary
   restrictions, and signs and symptoms of complications

Hemorrhoids/Anal Fissure (Nonsurgical)

Collaborative Problems

PC: Bleeding
PC: Bowel strangulation
PC: Thrombosis

Nursing Diagnoses

Acute Pain related to pressure on defecation
Risk for Constipation related to fear of pain on defecation
Risk for Ineffective Therapeutic Regimen Management
   related to insufficient knowledge of condition, bowel
   routine, diet instructions, exercise program, and
   perianal care

Inflammatory Bowel Disease
(Diverticulosis, Diverticulitis,
Regional Enteritis, Ulcerative Colitis)

Collaborative Problems

▲ PC: Gastrointestinal bleeding
* PC: Anal fissure
* PC: Perianal abscess, fissure, fistula
▲ PC: Fluid/electrolyte imbalances
   PC: Toxic megacolon
▲ PC: Anemia

▲ This diagnosis was reported to be monitored for or managed
frequently (75% to 100%).

* This diagnosis was not included in the validation study.

▲ PC: Intestinal obstruction
  PC: Urolithiasis
△ PC: Fistula/fissure/abscess

Nursing Diagnoses

▲ Chronic Pain related to intestinal inflammatory process
▲ Diarrhea related to intestinal inflammatory process
* Constipation related to inadequate dietary intake of fiber
* Risk for Impaired Skin Integrity (Perianal) related to diarrhea and chemical irritants
△ Risk for Ineffective Coping related to chronicity of condition and lack of definitive treatment
▲ Imbalanced Nutrition: Less Than Body Requirements related to dietary restrictions, nausea, diarrhea, and abdominal cramping associated with eating or painful ulcers of the oral mucous membrane
△ Risk for Ineffective Therapeutic Regimen Management related to insufficient knowledge of condition, diagnostic tests, prognosis, treatment, and signs and symptoms of complications

Peptic Ulcer Disease

Collaborative Problems

▲ PC: Hemorrhage
▲ PC: Perforation
△ PC: Pyloric obstruction

Nursing Diagnoses

▲ Acute/Chronic Pain related to lesions secondary to increased gastric secretions
▲ Constipation/Diarrhea related to effects of medications on bowel function
△ Risk for Ineffective Therapeutic Regimen Management related to insufficient knowledge of disease process,

▲ This diagnosis was reported to be monitored for or managed frequently (75% to 100%).

△ This diagnosis was reported to be monitored for or managed often (50% to 74%).

* This diagnosis was not included in the validation study.

contraindications, signs and symptoms of complications, and treatment regimen

RENAL/URINARY TRACT DISORDERS
Neurogenic Bladder

Collaborative Problems

PC: Renal calculi
PC: Autonomic dysreflexia

Nursing Diagnoses

Risk for Impaired Skin Integrity related to constant irritation from urine

Risk for Infection related to retention of urine or introduction of urinary catheter

Risk for Social Isolation related to embarrassment from wetting self in front of others and fear of odor from urine

Urinary Retention related to chronically overfilled bladder with loss of sensation of bladder distention *or*

Reflex Urinary Incontinence related to absence of sensation to void and loss of ability to inhibit bladder contraction *or*

Urge Incontinence related to disruption of the inhibitory efferent impulses secondary to brain or spinal cord dysfunction

Risk for Dysreflexia related to reflex stimulation of sympathetic nervous system secondary to loss of autonomic control

Risk for Ineffective Therapeutic Regimen Management related to insufficient knowledge of etiology of incontinence, management, bladder retraining programs, signs and symptoms of complications, and community resources

Renal Failure (Acute)

Collaborative Problems

▲ PC: Fluid overload
▲ PC: Metabolic acidosis
▲ PC: Electrolyte imbalances

▲ This diagnosis was reported to be monitored for or managed frequently (75% to 100%).

Nursing Diagnoses

△ Imbalanced Nutrition: Less Than Body Requirements related to anorexia, nausea, vomiting, loss of taste, loss of smell, stomatitis, and unpalatable diet
▲ Risk for Infection related to invasive procedures
* Anxiety related to present status and unknown prognosis
* Risk for Ineffective Therapeutic Regimen Management related to insufficient knowledge of condition, dietary restriction, daily recording, pharmacologic therapy, signs and symptoms of complications, follow-up visits, and community resources

Renal Failure (Chronic, Uremia)

See also *Peritoneal Dialysis* and *Hemodialysis,* if indicated.

Collaborative Problems

▲ PC: Fluid/electrolyte imbalance
△ PC: Gastrointestinal bleeding
  PC: Hyperparathyroidism
  PC: Pathologic fractures
* PC: Malnutrition
▲ PC: Anemia
▲ PC: Fluid overload
△ PC: Hypoalbuminemia
△ PC: Polyneuropathy
△ PC: Congestive heart failure
* PC: Pulmonary edema
△ PC: Metabolic acidosis
△ PC: Pleural effusion
  PC: Pericarditis, cardiac tamponade

Nursing Diagnoses

△ Imbalanced Nutrition: Less Than Body Requirements related to anorexia, nausea/vomiting, loss of taste/smell, stomatitis, and unpalatable diet

---

▲ This diagnosis was reported to be monitored for or managed frequently (75% to 100%).

△ This diagnosis was reported to be monitored for or managed often (50% to 74%).

* This diagnosis was not included in the validation study.

Ineffective Sexuality Patterns related to decreased libido, impotence, amenorrhea, sterility, fatigue
* Disturbed Self-Concept related to effects of limitation on achievement of developmental tasks
* Risk for Caregiver Role Strain related to long-term care needs secondary to disability and treatment requirements
* Discomfort related to (examples) fatigue, headaches, fluid retention, anemia
* Fatigue related to insufficient oxygenation secondary to anemia
△ Impaired Comfort: Pruritus related to calcium phosphate or urate crystals on skin
▲ Risk for Infection related to invasive procedures
△ Powerlessness related to progressively disabling nature of illness
▲ Risk for Ineffective Therapeutic Regimen Management related to insufficient knowledge of condition, dietary restriction, daily recording, pharmacologic therapy, signs and symptoms of complications, follow-up visits, and community resources

Urinary Tract Infections (Cystitis, Pyelonephritis, Glomerulonephritis)

See also *Acute Renal Failure.*

Nursing Diagnoses

Chronic Pain related to inflammation and tissue trauma
Impaired Comfort related to inflammation and infection
Risk for Imbalanced Nutrition: Less Than Body Requirements related to anorexia secondary to malaise
Risk for Ineffective Coping related to the chronicity of the condition
Risk for Ineffective Therapeutic Regimen Management related to insufficient knowledge of prevention of recur-

---

▲ This diagnosis was reported to be monitored for or managed frequently (75% to 100%).

△ This diagnosis was reported to be monitored for or managed often (50% to 74%).

* This diagnosis was not included in the validation study.

rence (adequate fluid intake, frequent voiding, hygiene measures [post-toileting], and voiding after sexual activity), signs and symptoms of recurrence, and pharmacologic therapy

Urolithiasis (Renal Calculi)

Collaborative Problems

△ PC: Pyelonephritis
▲ PC: Renal insufficiency

Nursing Diagnoses

▲ Acute Pain related to inflammation secondary to irritation of calculi and smooth muscle spasms
* Diarrhea related to renointestinal reflexes
△ Risk for Ineffective Therapeutic Regimen Management related to insufficient knowledge of prevention of recurrence, dietary restrictions, and fluid requirements

NEUROLOGIC DISORDERS
Brain Tumor

Because this disorder can cause alterations varying from minimal to profound, the following possible nursing diagnoses reflect individuals with varying degrees of involvement.

See also *Surgery (General, Cranial); Cancer.*

Collaborative Problems

PC: Increased intracranial pressure
PC: Paralysis
PC: Hyperthermia
PC: Motor losses
PC: Sensory losses
PC: Cognitive losses

▲ This diagnosis was reported to be monitored for or managed frequently (75% to 100%).

△ This diagnosis was reported to be monitored for or managed often (50% to 74%).

* This diagnosis was not included in the validation study.

Nursing Diagnoses

Risk for Injury related to gait disorders, vertigo, or visual disturbances, secondary to compression/displacement of brain tissue

Anxiety related to implications of condition and uncertain future

(Specify) Self-Care Deficit related to inability to perform/ difficulty in performing activities of daily living secondary to sensory–motor impairments

Imbalanced Nutrition: Less Than Body Requirements related to dysphagia and fatigue

Grieving related to actual/perceived loss of function and uncertain future

Impaired Physical Mobility related to sensory–motor impairment

Acute Pain: Headache related to compression/displacement of brain tissue and increased intracranial pressure

Interrupted Family Processes related to the nature of the condition, role disturbances, and uncertain future

Disturbed Self-Concept related to interruption in achieving/ failure to achieve developmental tasks (childhood, adolescence, young adulthood, middle age)

Risk for Deficient Fluid Volume related to vomiting secondary to increased intracranial pressure

Risk for Injury related to impaired/uncontrolled sensory–motor function

Cerebrovascular Accident

Because this disorder can cause alterations varying from minimal to profound, the following possible nursing diagnoses reflect individuals with varying degrees of involvement.

Collaborative Problems

▲ PC: Increased intracranial pressure
▲ PC: Pneumonia
▲ PC: Atelectasis

▲ This diagnosis was reported to be monitored for or managed frequently (75% to 100%).

Nursing Diagnoses

* Disturbed Sensory Perception: (specify) related to hypoxia and compression or displacement of brain tissue

▲ Impaired Physical Mobility related to decreased motor function of (specify) secondary to damage to upper motor neurons

▲ Impaired Communication related to dysarthria or aphasia

▲ Risk for Injury related to visual field, motor, or perception deficits

* Activity Intolerance related to deconditioning secondary to fatigue and weakness

* Disuse Syndrome

△ Total Incontinence related to loss of bladder tone, loss of sphincter control, or inability to perceive bladder cues

▲ Self-Care Deficit related to impaired physical mobility or confusion

▲ Impaired Swallowing related to muscle paralysis or paresis secondary to damage to upper motor neurons

△ Grieving (Family, Individual) related to loss of function and inability to meet role responsibilities

△ Risk for Impaired Social Interactions related to difficulty communicating and embarrassment regarding disabilities

△ Risk for Deficient Fluid Volume related to dysphagia, difficulty in obtaining fluids secondary to weakness or motor deficits

△ Risk for Impaired Home Maintenance related to altered ability to maintain self at home secondary to sensory/motor/cognitive deficits and lack of knowledge by caregivers of home care, reality orientation, bowel/bladder program, skin care, signs and symptoms of complications, and community resources

▲ Functional Urinary Incontinence related to inability or difficulty in reaching toilet secondary to decreased mobility or motivation

---

▲ This diagnosis was reported to be monitored for or managed frequently (75% to 100%).

△ This diagnosis was reported to be monitored for or managed often (50% to 74%).

* This diagnosis was not included in the validation study.

△ Unilateral Neglect related to (specify site) secondary to
   right hemispheric brain damage
* Risk for Caregiver Role Strain related to complex care
   requirements secondary to (specify sensory or motor
   deficits)
△ Risk for Disturbed Self-Concept related to effects of prolonged debilitating condition on achieving developmental tasks and lifestyle
* Risk for Ineffective Therapeutic Regimen Management
   related to insufficient knowledge of condition, pharmacologic therapy, self-care activities of daily living, home
   care, speech therapy, exercise program, community
   resources, self-help groups, and signs and symptoms
   of complications
* Wandering related to impaired cerebral function secondary to cerebrovascular accident

Nervous System Disorders (Degenerative, Demyelinating, Inflammatory, Myasthenia Gravis, Multiple Sclerosis, Muscular Dystrophy, Parkinson's Disease, Guillain-Barré Syndrome, Amyotrophic Lateral Sclerosis)

Because the responses associated with these disorders can
range from minimal to profound, the following possible diagnoses reflect individuals with varying degrees of involvement.

Collaborative Problems

PC: Renal failure
PC: Pneumonia
PC: Atelectasis

Nursing Diagnoses

Risk for Disturbed Self-Concept related to the effects of
   prolonged debilitating condition on lifestyle and on
   achieving developmental tasks
Risk for Injury related to visual disturbances, unsteady
   gait, sensory losses, weakness, or uncontrolled movements

△ This diagnosis was reported to be monitored for or managed
often (50% to 74%).

* This diagnosis was not included in the validation study.

Impaired Verbal Communication related to dysarthrias secondary to ataxia of muscles of speech

Risk for Imbalanced Nutrition: Less Than Body Requirements related to dysphagia/chewing difficulties secondary to cranial nerve impairment

Activity Intolerance related to fatigue and difficulty in performing activities of daily living

Disuse Syndrome

Impaired Physical Mobility related to effects of muscle rigidity, tremors, and slowness of movement on activities of daily living

Impaired Swallowing related to cerebellar lesions

Fatigue related to extremity weakness, spasticity, fear of injury, and stressors

Urinary Retention related to sensory/motor deficits

Chronic Sorrow (Client, Family) related to nature of disease and uncertain prognosis

Ineffective Sexuality Patterns (female) related to loss of libido, fatigue, and decreased perineal sensation

Interrupted Family Processes related to nature of disorder, role disturbances, and uncertain future

Risk for Deficient Diversional Activity related to inability to perform usual job-related/recreational activities

Risk for Social Isolation related to mobility difficulties and associated embarrassment

Impaired Home Maintenance related to inability to care for/difficulty in caring for self/home secondary to disability or unavailable or inadequate caregiver

Parental Role Conflict related to disruptions secondary to disability

Caregiver Role Strain related to continuous, multiple care needs

(Specify) Self-Care Deficits related to (examples) headaches, muscular spasms, joint pain, fatigue, paresis/paralysis

Powerlessness related to the unpredictable nature of the condition (i.e., remissions/exacerbations)

Incontinence: (specify) related to poor sphincter control and spastic bladder

Ineffective Airway Clearance related to impaired ability to cough

Risk for Ineffective Therapeutic Regimen Management related to insufficient knowledge of condition, treatments, prevention of infection, stress management, aggravating factors, signs and symptoms of complications, and community resources

Presenile Dementia (Alzheimer's Disease, Huntington's Disease)

See also *Nervous System Disorders* (pp. 538–539).*

Nursing Diagnoses

Risk for Injury related to lack of awareness of environmental hazards

Chronic Confusion related to inability to evaluate reality secondary to cerebral neuron degeneration

Impaired Physical Mobility related to gait instability

Risk for Interrupted Family Processes related to effects of condition on relationships, role responsibilities, and finances

Impaired Home Maintenance related to inability to care for/difficulty in caring for self/home or inadequate or unavailable caregiver

Unilateral Neglect related to (specify site) secondary to neurologic pathology

(Specify) Self-Care Deficit related to (specify)

Decisional Conflict related to placement of person in a care facility

Caregiver Role Strain related to multiple care needs and insufficient resources

Wandering related to impaired cerebral function secondary to Alzheimer's dementia

Seizure Disorders (Epilepsy)

If the client is a child, see also *Developmental Problems / Needs.*

Nursing Diagnoses

* Risk for Injury related to uncontrolled tonic-clonic movements during seizure episode

▲ Risk for Ineffective Airway Clearance related to relaxation of tongue and gag reflexes secondary to disruption in muscle innervation

Risk for Social Isolation related to fear of embarrassment secondary to having a seizure in public

---

▲ This diagnosis was reported to be monitored for or managed frequently (75% to 100%).

* This diagnosis was not included in the validation study.

* Risk for Delayed Growth and Development related to interruption in achieving/failure to achieve developmental tasks (adolescence, young adulthood, middle age)
* Risk for Impaired Oral Mucous Membrane related to effects of drug therapy on oral tissue
* Fear related to unpredictable nature of seizures and embarrassment
△ Risk for Ineffective Therapeutic Regimen Management related to insufficient knowledge of condition, medication, activity, care during seizures, environmental hazards, and community resources

Spinal Cord Injury†

Collaborative Problems

△ PC: Electrolyte imbalance
* PC: Spinal shock
△ PC: Hemorrhage
* PC: Respiratory complications
△ PC: Paralytic ileus
* PC: Sepsis
* PC: Hydronephrosis
△ PC: Gastrointestinal bleeding
▲ PC: Thrombophlebitis
* PC: Postural hypotension
△ PC: Fracture dislocation
△ PC: Cardiovascular
▲ PC: Hypoxemia
▲ PC: Urinary retention
△ PC: Renal insufficiency

Nursing Diagnoses

▲ Self-Care Deficit related to sensory/motor deficits secondary to level of spinal cord injury

---

▲ This diagnosis was reported to be monitored for or managed frequently (75% to 100%).

△ This diagnosis was reported to be monitored for or managed often (50% to 74%).

* This diagnosis was not included in the validation study.

† PCs (potential complications) are collaborative problems, not nursing diagnoses.

* Impaired Verbal Communication related to impaired ability to speak secondary to tracheostomy
* Fear related to possible abandonment by others, changes in role responsibilities, effects of injury on lifestyle, multiple tests and procedures, or separation from support systems
△ Interrupted Family Processes related to adjustment requirements, role disturbances, and uncertain future
* Risk for Aspiration related to inability to cough secondary to level of injury
△ Risk for Impaired Home Maintenance related to insufficient knowledge of the effects of altered skin, bowel, bladder, respiratory, thermoregulation, and sexual function and their management, signs and symptoms of complications, follow-up care, and community resources
▲ Anxiety related to perceived effects of injury on lifestyle and unknown future
▲ Chronic Grieving related to loss of body function and its effects on lifestyle
* Risk for Social Isolation (individual/family) related to disability or requirements for the caregiver(s)
* Risk for Caregiver Role Strain related to continuous, multiple care needs, inadequate resources, and coping mechanisms
△ Risk for Disturbed Self-Concept related to effects of disability on achieving developmental tasks and lifestyle
* Risk for Deficient Fluid Volume related to difficulty obtaining liquids
* Risk for Imbalanced Nutrition: More Than Body Requirements related to imbalance of intake versus activity expenditures
* Risk for Imbalanced Nutrition: Less Than Body Requirements related to anorexia and increased metabolic requirements
* Risk for Deficient Diversional Activity related to effects of limitations on ability to participate in recreational activities

---

▲ This diagnosis was reported to be monitored for or managed frequently (75% to 100%).

△ This diagnosis was reported to be monitored for or managed often (50% to 74%).

* This diagnosis was not included in the validation study.

* Reflex Urinary Incontinence or Urinary Retention related to bladder atony secondary to sensory–motor deficits
* Disuse Syndrome
* Risk for Injury related to impaired ability to control movements and sensory–motor deficits
* Risk for Infection related to urinary stasis, repeated catheterizations, and invasive procedures (skeletal tongs, tracheostomy, venous lines, surgical sites)
△ Risk for Ineffective Sexuality Patterns related to physiologic, sensory, and psychological effects of disability on sexuality or function
△ Bowel Incontinence: Reflex related to lack of voluntary sphincter control secondary to spinal cord injury of the 11th thoracic vertebra (T_{11})
△ Bowel Incontinence: Areflexia related to lack of voluntary sphincter control secondary to spinal cord injury involving sacral reflex arc (S_2–S_4)
△ Risk for Dysreflexia related to reflex stimulation of sympathetic nervous system secondary to loss of autonomic control
* Risk for Ineffective Therapeutic Regimen Management related to insufficient knowledge of condition, treatment regimen, rehabilitation, and assistance devices

Unconscious Individual

See also *Mechanical Ventilation,* if indicated.

Collaborative Problems

* PC: Respiratory insufficiency
▲ PC: Pneumonia
▲ PC: Atelectasis
▲ PC: Fluid/electrolyte imbalance
* PC: Negative nitrogen balance
* PC: Bladder distention
* PC: Seizures

▲ This diagnosis was reported to be monitored for or managed frequently (75% to 100%).

△ This diagnosis was reported to be monitored for or managed often (50% to 74%).

* This diagnosis was not included in the validation study.

* PC: Stress ulcers
* PC: Increased intracranial pressure
△ PC: Sepsis
▲ PC: Thrombophlebitis
* PC: Renal calculi
△ PC: Urinary tract infection

Nursing Diagnoses

* Risk for Infection related to immobility and invasive devices (tracheostomy, Foley catheter, venous lines)
* Risk for Impaired Tissue Integrity: Corneal related to corneal drying secondary to open eyes and lower tear production
* Family Anxiety/Fear related to present state of individual and uncertain prognosis
* Risk for Impaired Oral Mucous Membrane related to inability to perform own mouth care and pooling of secretions
▲ Total Incontinence related to unconscious state
△ Disuse Syndrome
△ Powerlessness (family) related to feelings of loss of control and restrictions on lifestyle
▲ Risk for Ineffective Airway Clearance related to stasis of secretions secondary to inadequate cough and decreased mobility

SENSORY DISORDERS
Ophthalmic Disorders (Cataracts, Detached Retina, Glaucoma, Inflammations)
See also *Cataract Extractions; Scleral Buckle/Vitrectomy.*

Collaborative Problem

PC: Increased intraocular pressure

▲ This diagnosis was reported to be monitored for or managed frequently (75% to 100%).

△ This diagnosis was reported to be monitored for or managed often (50% to 74%).

* This diagnosis was not included in the validation study.

Nursing Diagnoses

Risk for Injury related to visual limitations

Acute Pain related to (examples) inflammation (lid, lacrimal structures, conjunctiva, uveal tract, retina, cornea, sclera), infection, increased intraocular pressure, ocular tumors

Risk for Noncompliance related to negative side effects of prescribed therapy versus the belief that no treatment is needed without the presence of symptoms

Risk for Social Isolation related to fear of injury or embarrassment outside home environment

Risk for Impaired Home Maintenance related to impaired ability to perform activities of daily living secondary to impaired vision

(Specify) Self-Care Deficit related to impaired vision

Anxiety related to actual or possible vision loss and perceived impact of chronic illness on lifestyle

Risk for Disturbed Self-Concept related to effects of visual limitations

Risk for Ineffective Therapeutic Regimen Management related to insufficient knowledge of condition, eye care, medications, safety measures, activity restrictions, and follow-up care

Otic Disorders
(Infections, Mastoiditis, Trauma)

Nursing Diagnoses

Risk for Injury related to disturbances of balance and impaired ability to detect environmental hazards

Impaired Verbal Communication related to difficulty understanding others secondary to impaired hearing

Risk for Impaired Social Interactions related to difficulty in participating in conversations

Social Isolation related to the lack of contact with others secondary to fear and embarrassment of hearing losses

Acute Pain related to inflammation, infection, tinnitus, or vertigo

Fear related to actual or possible loss of hearing

Risk for Ineffective Therapeutic Regimen Management related to insufficient knowledge of condition, medications, prevention of recurrence, hazards (swimming, air travel, showers), signs and symptoms of complications, and hearing aids

INTEGUMENTARY DISORDERS
Dermatologic Disorders
(Dermatitis, Psoriasis, Eczema)

Nursing Diagnoses

Impaired Skin Integrity related to lesions and inflammatory response

Pruritus related to dermal eruptions

Risk for Impaired Social Interaction related to fear of
embarrassment and negative reactions of others

Risk for Disturbed Self-Concept related to appearance and
response of others

Risk for Ineffective Therapeutic Regimen Management
related to insufficient knowledge of condition, topical
agents, and contraindications

Pressure Ulcers†

Collaborative Problem

△ PC: Sepsis

Nursing Diagnoses

▲ Risk for Infection related to exposure of ulcer base to
fecal/urinary drainage

▲ Impaired Tissue Integrity related to mechanical destruction of tissue secondary to pressure, shear, and friction

* Impaired Home Maintenance related to complexity of
care or unavailable caregiver

▲ Imbalanced Nutrition: Less Than Body Requirements
related to anorexia secondary to (specify)

▲ Impaired Physical Mobility related to imposed restrictions, deconditioned status, loss of motor control, or
altered mental status

▲ This diagnosis was reported to be monitored for or managed
frequently (75% to 100%).

△ This diagnosis was reported to be monitored for or managed
often (50% to 74%).

* This diagnosis was not included in the validation study.

† PCs (potential complications) are collaborative problems, not
nursing diagnoses.

* Excess Fluid Volume: Edema related to (specify)
* Total Urinary Incontinence related to (specify)
△ Risk for Ineffective Therapeutic Regimen Management related to insufficient knowledge of etiology, prevention, treatment, and home care

Skin Infections (Impetigo, Herpes Zoster, Fungal Infections)

Herpes Zoster

Collaborative Problems

PC: Postherpetic neuralgia
PC: Keratitis
PC: Uveitis
PC: Corneal ulceration
PC: Blindness

Nursing Diagnoses

Impaired Skin Integrity related to lesions and pruritus
Impaired Comfort related to dermal eruptions and pruritus
Risk for Infection Transmission related to contagious nature of the organism
Risk for Ineffective Therapeutic Regimen Management related to insufficient knowledge of condition (causes, course), prevention, treatment, and skin care

Thermal Injuries (Burns, Severe Hypothermia)

Acute Period

Collaborative Problems

▲ PC: Hypovolemic shock
△ PC: Hypervolemia
* PC: Fluid overload

▲ This diagnosis was reported to be monitored for or managed frequently (75% to 100%).

△ This diagnosis was reported to be monitored for or managed often (50% to 74%).

* This diagnosis was not included in the validation study.

* PC: Anemia
△ PC: Negative nitrogen balance
▲ PC: Electrolyte imbalance
△ PC: Metabolic acidosis
▲ PC: Respiratory
△ PC: Thromboembolism
▲ PC: Sepsis
* PC: Emboli
▲ PC: Graft rejection/infection
* PC: Hypothermia
* PC: Hypokalemia/hyperkalemia
△ PC: Curling's ulcer
△ PC: Paralytic ileus
* PC: Convulsive disorders
* PC: Stress diabetes
  PC: Adrenocortical insufficiency
* PC: Pneumonia
△ PC: Renal insufficiency
* PC: Compartmental syndrome
* PC: Adrenal insufficiency

Nursing Diagnoses

▲ Risk for Infection related to loss of protective layer secondary to thermal injury
▲ Imbalanced Nutrition: Less Than Body Requirements related to increased caloric requirement secondary to thermal injury and inability to ingest sufficient quantities to meet increased requirements
* Impaired Physical Mobility related to acute pain secondary to thermal injury and treatments
△ (Specify) Self-Care Deficit related to impaired range-of-motion ability secondary to pain
* Fear related to painful procedures and possibility of death
* Risk for Social Isolation related to infection control measures and separation from family and support systems

---

▲ This diagnosis was reported to be monitored for or managed frequently (75% to 100%).

△ This diagnosis was reported to be monitored for or managed often (50% to 74%).

* This diagnosis was not included in the validation study.

△ Disuse Syndrome

* Disturbed Sleep Pattern related to position restrictions, pain, and treatment interruptions

* Risk for Disturbed Sensory Perception related to (examples) excessive environmental stimuli, stress, imposed immobility, sleep deprivation, protective isolation

▲ Grieving (family, individual) related to actual or perceived impact of injury on life, appearance, relationships, lifestyle

▲ Anxiety related to sudden injury, treatments, uncertainty of outcome, and pain

* Anxiety related to pain secondary to thermal injury treatments and immobility

▲ Acute Pain related to thermal injury treatments and immobility

Postacute Period

If individual is a child, see also *Developmental Problems / Needs.*

Collaborative Problem

PC: Same as in acute period

Nursing Diagnoses

△ Deficient Diversional Activity related to monotony of confinement

* Risk for Social Isolation related to embarrassment and response of others to injury

* Powerlessness related to inability to control situation

△ Risk for Disturbed Self-Concept related to effects of thermal injury on achieving developmental tasks (child, adolescent, adult)

* Fear related to uncertain future and effects of injury on lifestyle, relationships, occupation

* Impaired Home Maintenance related to long-term requirements of treatments

---

▲ This diagnosis was reported to be monitored for or managed frequently (75% to 100%).

△ This diagnosis was reported to be monitored for or managed often (50% to 74%).

* This diagnosis was not included in the validation study.

△ Risk for Ineffective Therapeutic Regimen Management
related to insufficient knowledge of exercise program,
wound care, nutritional requirements, pain management, signs and symptoms of complications, and burn
prevention and follow-up care

MUSCULOSKELETAL/CONNECTIVE TISSUE DISORDERS
Fractured Jaw

Nursing Diagnoses

Risk for Aspiration related to inadequate cough secondary
to pain and fixative devices

Impaired Oral Mucous Membrane related to difficulty in
performing oral hygiene secondary to fixation devices

Impaired Verbal Communication related to fixation devices

Acute Pain related to tissue trauma and fixation device

Risk for Imbalanced Nutrition: Less Than Body Requirements related to inability to ingest solid food secondary
to fixation devices

Risk for Ineffective Therapeutic Regimen Management
related to insufficient knowledge of mouth care, nutritional requirements, signs and symptoms of infection,
and procedure for emergency wire cutting (e.g., vomiting)

Fractures
See also *Casts.*

Collaborative Problems

▲ PC: Neurovascular compromise
▲ PC: Fat embolism
▲ PC: Hemorrhage/hematoma formation
* PC: Osteomyelitis
* PC: Compartmental syndrome
* PC: Contracture
▲ PC: Thromboemboli

▲ This diagnosis was reported to be monitored for or managed
frequently (75% to 100%).

△ This diagnosis was reported to be monitored for or managed
often (50% to 74%).

* This diagnosis was not included in the validation study.

Nursing Diagnoses

* Acute Pain related to tissue trauma and immobility
▲ Impaired Physical Mobility related to tissue trauma secondary to fracture
* Disuse Syndrome
* Risk for Infection related to invasive fixation devices
▲ Self-Care Deficit (specify) related to limitation of movement secondary to fracture
* Deficient Diversional Activity related to boredom of confinement secondary to immobilization devices
* Risk for Impaired Home Maintenance related to (examples) fixation device, impaired physical mobility, unavailable support system
* Interrupted Family Processes related to difficulty of ill person in assuming role responsibilities secondary to limited motion
△ Risk for Ineffective Therapeutic Regimen Management related to insufficient knowledge of condition, signs and symptoms of complications, activity restrictions

Low Back Pain

Collaborative Problems

PC: Pulposus
PC: Herniated nucleus pulposus

Nursing Diagnoses

Pain related to (examples) acute lumbosacral strain, weak muscles, osteoarthritis of spine, unstable lumbosacral ligaments, spinal stenosis, intervertebral disk problem
Impaired Physical Mobility related to decreased mobility and flexibility secondary to muscle spasm
Risk for Ineffective Coping related to effects of chronic pain on lifestyle

---

▲ This diagnosis was reported to be monitored for or managed frequently (75% to 100%).

△ This diagnosis was reported to be monitored for or managed often (50% to 74%).

* This diagnosis was not included in the validation study.

Risk for Interrupted Family Processes related to impaired
   ability to meet role responsibilities (financial, home, social)
Risk for Ineffective Therapeutic Regimen Management
   related to insufficient knowledge of condition, exercise
   program, noninvasive pain relief methods (relaxation,
   imagery), proper posture and body mechanics, and risk
   factors (smoking, inactivity, overweight)

Osteoporosis

Collaborative Problems

PC: Fractures
PC: Kyphosis
PC: Paralytic ileus

Nursing Diagnoses

Pain related to muscle spasm and fractures
Ineffective Health Maintenance related to insufficient daily
   physical activity
Imbalanced Nutrition: Less Than Body Requirements
   related to inadequate dietary intake of calcium, protein,
   and vitamin D
Impaired Physical Mobility related to limited range of
   motion secondary to skeletal changes
Fear related to unpredictable nature of condition
Risk for Ineffective Therapeutic Regimen Management
   related to insufficient knowledge of condition, risk
   factors, nutritional therapy, and prevention

Inflammatory Joint Disease

Collaborative Problems

PC: Septic arthritis
PC: Sjögren's syndrome
PC: Neuropathy
PC: Anemia, leukopenia

Nursing Diagnoses

Chronic Pain related to local and systemic inflammatory
   lesions

(Specify) Self-Care Deficit related to loss of motion, muscle weakness, pain, stiffness, or fatigue

Powerlessness related to physical and psychological changes imposed by the disease

Ineffective Coping related to the stress imposed by unpredictable exacerbations

(Specify) Self-Care Deficit related to limitations secondary to disease process

Fatigue related to effects of chronic inflammatory process

Risk for Impaired Oral Mucous Membrane related to effects of medications or Sjögren's syndrome

Impaired Home Maintenance related to impaired ability to perform household responsibilities secondary to limited mobility and pain

Disturbed Sleep Pattern related to pain or secondary to fibrositis

Impaired Physical Mobility related to pain and limited joint motion

Ineffective Sexuality Patterns related to pain, fatigue, difficulty in assuming positions, and lack of adequate lubrication (female) secondary to disease process

Risk for Social Isolation related to ambulation difficulties and fatigue

Interrupted Family Processes related to difficulty/inability of ill person to assume role responsibilities secondary to fatigue and limited motion

Risk for Ineffective Therapeutic Regimen Management related to insufficient knowledge of condition, pharmacologic therapy, home care, stress management, and quackery

INFECTIOUS/IMMUNODEFICIENT DISORDERS
Lupus Erythematosus (Systemic)

See also *Rheumatic Diseases; Corticosteroid Therapy.*

Collaborative Problems

PC: Polymyositis
PC: Vasculitis
PC: Hematologic problem
PC: Raynaud's disease
PC: Renal failure secondary to corticosteroid therapy
PC: Pericarditis
PC: Pleuritis

Nursing Diagnoses

Powerlessness related to unpredictable course of disease

Ineffective Coping related to unpredictable course and altered appearance

Risk for Social Isolation related to embarrassment and the response of others to appearance

Risk for Disturbed Self-Concept related to inability to achieve developmental tasks secondary to disabling condition and changes in appearance

Risk for Injury related to increased dermal vulnerability secondary to disease process

Fatigue related to decreased mobility and effects of chronic inflammation

Risk for Ineffective Therapeutic Regimen Management related to insufficient knowledge of condition, rest versus activity requirements, pharmacologic therapy, signs and symptoms of complications, risk factors, and community resources

Meningitis/Encephalitis

Collaborative Problems

PC: Fluid/electrolyte imbalance

PC: Cerebral edema

PC: Adrenal damage

PC: Circulatory collapse

PC: Hemorrhage

PC: Seizures

PC: Sepsis

PC: Alkalosis

PC: Increased intracranial pressure

Nursing Diagnoses

Risk for Infection Transmission related to contagious nature of organism

Acute Pain related to headache, fever, neck pain secondary to meningeal irritation

Activity Intolerance related to fatigue and malaise secondary to infection

Risk for Impaired Skin Integrity related to immobility, dehydration, and diaphoresis

Risk for Impaired Oral Mucous Membrane related to dehydration and impaired ability to perform mouth care

Risk for Imbalanced Nutrition: Less Than Body Requirements related to anorexia, fatigue, nausea, and vomiting
Risk for Ineffective Respiratory Function related to immobility and pain
Risk for Injury related to restlessness and disorientation
secondary to meningeal irritation
Interrupted Family Processes related to critical nature of
situation and uncertain prognosis
Anxiety related to treatments, environment, and risk of
death
Risk for Ineffective Therapeutic Regimen Management
related to insufficient knowledge of condition, treatments,
pharmacologic therapy, rest/activity balance, signs and
symptoms of complications, follow-up care, and prevention of recurrence

Sexually Transmitted Infections/Diseases

Nursing Diagnoses

Risk for Infection Transmission related to lack of knowledge of the contagious nature of the disease and reports
of high-risk behaviors
Fear related to nature of the condition and its implications
for lifestyle
Acute Pain related to inflammatory process
Social Isolation related to fear of transmitting disease to
others
Risk for Ineffective Therapeutic Regimen Management
related to insufficient knowledge of condition, modes of
transmission, consequences of repeated infections, and
prevention of recurrences

Acquired Immunodeficiency Syndrome (AIDS) (Adult)
See also *End-Stage Cancer.*

Collaborative Problems

* PC: Encephalopathy
▲ PC: Sepsis

▲ This diagnosis was reported to be monitored for or managed
frequently (75% to 100%).

* This diagnosis was not included in the validation study.

* PC: Gastrointestinal bleeding
* PC: *Pneumocystis carinii* pneumonia
* PC: Meningitis
* PC: Esophagitis
* PC: Electrolyte imbalances
▲ PC: Opportunistic infections
△ PC: Myelosuppression

Nursing Diagnoses

* Chronic Pain related to headache, fever secondary to inflammation of cerebral tissue
▲ Fatigue related to effects of disease, stress, chronic infections, and nutritional deficiency
* Risk for Impaired Skin Integrity related to perineal and anal tissue excoriation secondary to diarrhea and chronic genital candidal or herpes lesions
* Imbalanced Nutrition: Less Than Body Requirements related to chronic diarrhea, gastrointestinal malabsorption, fatigue, anorexia, or oral/esophageal lesions
▲ Risk for Infection Transmission related to contagious nature of blood and body secretions
△ Social Isolation related to fear of rejection or actual rejection of others secondary to fear
* Hopelessness related to nature of the condition and poor prognosis
△ Powerlessness related to unpredictable nature of condition
▲ Interrupted Family Processes related to the nature of the AIDS condition, role disturbance, and uncertain future
△ Anxiety related to perceived effects of illness on lifestyle and unknown future
△ Chronic Sorrow related to loss of body function and its effects on lifestyle
▲ Risk for Infection related to increased susceptibility secondary to compromised immune system

---

▲ This diagnosis was reported to be monitored for or managed frequently (75% to 100%).

△ This diagnosis was reported to be monitored for or managed often (50% to 74%).

* This diagnosis was not included in the validation study.

▲ Risk for Impaired Oral Mucous Membrane related to compromised immune system
* Risk for Caregiver Role Strain related to multiple needs of ill person and chronicity
△ Risk for Ineffective Therapeutic Regimen Management related to insufficient knowledge of condition, medications, home care, infection control, and community resources

NEOPLASTIC DISORDERS
Cancer

Cancer: Initial Diagnosis
See also specific types.

Nursing Diagnoses

▲ Anxiety related to unfamiliar hospital environment, uncertainty about outcomes, feelings of helplessness and hopelessness, and insufficient knowledge about cancer and treatment
▲ Grieving related to potential loss of body function and the perceived losses associated with cancer on lifestyle
* Powerlessness related to uncertainty about prognosis and outcome of cancer treatment
▲ Interrupted Family Processes related to fears associated with recent cancer diagnosis, disruptions associated with treatments, financial problems, and uncertain future
△ Decisional Conflict related to treatment modality choices
△ Risk for Disturbed Self-Concept related to changes in lifestyle, role responsibilities, and appearance
△ Risk for Social Isolation related to fear of rejection or actual rejection secondary to fear
△ Risk for Spiritual Distress related to conflicts centering on the meaning of life, cancer, spiritual beliefs, and death

----

▲ This diagnosis was reported to be monitored for or managed frequently (75% to 100%).

△ This diagnosis was reported to be monitored for or managed often (50% to 74%).

* This diagnosis was not included in the validation study.

* Risk for Ineffective Therapeutic Regimen Management related to insufficient knowledge of cancer, cancer treatment options, diagnostic tests, effects of treatment, treatment plan, and support services

Cancer: General (Applies to Malignancies in Varied Sites and Stages)

Nursing Diagnoses

Impaired Oral Mucous Membranes related to (examples) disease process, therapy, radiation, chemotherapy, inadequate oral hygiene, and altered nutritional/hydration status

Risk for Ineffective Sexuality Patterns related to (examples) fear, grieving, changes in body image, anatomic changes, pain, fatigue (treatments, disease), or change in role responsibilities

Acute/Chronic Pain related to disease process and treatments

Diarrhea related to (examples) disease process, chemotherapy, radiation, and medications

Constipation related to (examples) disease process, chemotherapy, radiation therapy, immobility, dietary intake, and medications

Disturbed Self-Concept related to (examples) anatomic changes, role disturbances, uncertain future, disruption of lifestyle

(Specify) Self-Care Deficit related to fatigue, pain, or depression

Risk for Infection related to altered immune system

Imbalanced Nutrition: Less Than Body Requirements related to anorexia, fatigue, nausea, and vomiting secondary to disease process and treatments

Risk for Injury related to disorientation, weakness, sensory/perceptual deterioration, or skeletal/muscle deterioration

Disuse Syndrome

Risk for Deficient Fluid Volume related to (examples) altered ability/desire to obtain fluids, weakness, vomiting, diarrhea, depression, and fatigue

---

* This diagnosis was not included in the validation study.

Risk for Impaired Home Maintenance related to (examples) lack of knowledge, lack of resources (support system, equipment, finances), motor deficits, sensory deficits, cognitive deficits, and emotional deficits

Risk for Impaired Social Interactions related to fear of rejection or actual rejection of others after diagnosis

Powerlessness related to inability to control situation

Interrupted Family Processes related to (examples) stress of diagnosis/treatments, role disturbances, and uncertain future

Grieving (Family, Individual) related to actual, perceived, or anticipated losses associated with diagnosis

Risk for Ineffective Therapeutic Regimen Management related to insufficient knowledge of disease, misconceptions, treatments, home care, and support agencies

Cancer: End-Stage

See also specific types.

Collaborative Problems

PC: Hypercalcemia
PC: Intracerebral metastasis
PC: Malignant effusions
PC: Narcotic toxicity
PC: Pathologic fractures
PC: Spinal cord compression
PC: Superior vena cava syndrome
PC: Negative nitrogen imbalance
PC: Myelosuppression

Nursing Diagnoses

See also *Cancer (General).*

Imbalanced Nutrition: Less Than Body Requirements related to decreased oral intake, increased metabolic demands of tumor, and altered lipid metabolism

Impaired Comfort related to pruritus secondary to dry skin and biliary obstruction

Ineffective Airway Clearance related to inability to cough up secretions secondary to weakness, increased viscosity, and pain

Impaired Physical Mobility related to pain, sedation, weakness, fatigue, and edema

(Specify) Self-Care Deficit related to fatigue, weakness,
  sedation, pain, or decreased sensory/perceptual capacity
Activity Intolerance related to hypoxia, fatigue, malnutrition, and decreased mobility
Grieving related to terminal illness, impending death,
  functional losses, and withdrawal of, or from, others
Hopelessness related to overwhelming functional losses or
  impending death
Disturbed Self-Concept related to dependence on others to
  meet basic needs and decrease in functional ability
Powerlessness related to change from curative status to
  palliative status
Caregiver Role Strain related to multiple care needs and
  concern about ability to manage home care
Risk for Spiritual Distress related to fear of death, overwhelming grief, belief system conflicts, and unresolved
  conflicts
Death Anxiety related to effects of disease process and
  inadequate pain-relief measures
Risk for Impaired Home Maintenance related to insufficient knowledge of home care, pain management, signs
  and symptoms of complications, and community
  resources available

Colorectal Cancer

See also *Cancer (General).*

Nursing Diagnoses

Risk for Ineffective Sexuality Patterns (Male) related to
  inability to have or sustain an erection secondary to
  surgical procedure on perineal structures
Risk for Ineffective Therapeutic Regimen Management related to insufficient knowledge of ostomy care, supplies,
  dietary management, signs and symptoms of complications, and community services

General Surgery

Preoperative Period

Nursing Diagnoses

Fear related to surgical experience, loss of control, and
  unpredictable outcome

Anxiety related to preoperative procedures (surgical permit, diagnostic studies, Foley catheter, diet and fluid
  restrictions, medications, skin preparation, waiting area
  for family) and postoperative procedures (disposition
  [recovery room, intensive care unit], medications for pain,
  coughing/turning/leg exercises, tube/drain placement,
  nothing by mouth [NPO]/diet restrictions, bed rest)

Postoperative Period

Collaborative Problems

†PC: Urinary retention
PC: Hemorrhage
PC: Hypovolemia/shock
PC: Renal failure
PC: Pneumonia (stasis)
PC: Peritonitis
PC: Thrombophlebitis
PC: Paralytic ileus
PC: Evisceration
PC: Dehiscence

Nursing Diagnoses

Risk for Infection related to site for bacterial invasion
Risk for Ineffective Respiratory Function related to
  postanesthesia state, postoperative immobility, and pain
Acute Pain related to incision, flatus, and immobility

---

†PCs (potential complications) are collaborative problems, not
nursing diagnoses.

Risk for Constipation related to decreased peristalsis secondary to the effects of anesthesia, immobility, and pain medication

Risk for Imbalanced Nutrition: Less Than Body Requirements related to increased protein/vitamin requirements for wound healing and decreased intake secondary to pain, nausea, vomiting, and diet restrictions

Risk for Ineffective Therapeutic Regimen Management related to insufficient knowledge of home care, incisional care, signs and symptoms of complications, activity restriction, and follow-up care

Amputation (Lower Extremity)

Preoperative Period
See also *Surgery (General).*

Nursing Diagnoses

▲ Anxiety related to insufficient knowledge of postoperative routines, postoperative sensations, and crutch-walking techniques

Postoperative Period

Collaborative Problems

▲ PC: Edema of stump
▲ PC: Hemorrhage
▲ PC: Hematoma site

Nursing Diagnoses

* Disuse Syndrome
▲ Grieving related to loss of limb and its effects on lifestyle
▲ Acute/Chronic Pain related to phantom limb sensations secondary to peripheral nerve stimulation or abnormal impulses to central nervous system
▲ Risk for Injury related to altered gait and hazards of assistive devices

---

▲ This diagnosis was reported to be monitored for or managed frequently (75% to 100%).

* This diagnosis was not included in the validation study.

△ Risk for Impaired Home Maintenance related to archi-
tectural barriers

△ Risk for Disturbed Body Image related to perceived negative effects of amputation and response of others to
appearance

▲ Risk for Contractures related to impaired movement
secondary to pain

△ Risk for Ineffective Therapeutic Regimen Management
related to insufficient knowledge of activities of daily
living adaptations, stump care, prosthesis care, gait
training, and follow-up care

Aneurysm Resection (Abdominal Aortic)

See also *Surgery (General)*.

Preoperative Period

Collaborative Problems

▲ PC: Rupture of aneurysm

Postoperative Period

Collaborative Problems

▲ PC: Distal vessel thrombosis or emboli
▲ PC: Renal failure
△ PC: Mesenteric ischemia/thrombosis
△ PC: Spinal cord ischemia

Nursing Diagnoses

▲ Risk for Infection related to location of surgical incision
Risk for Ineffective Sexuality Patterns (male) related to
possible loss of ejaculate and erections secondary to
surgery

△ Risk for Ineffective Therapeutic Regimen Management
related to insufficient knowledge of home care, activity
restrictions, signs and symptoms of complications, and
follow-up care

▲ This diagnosis was reported to be monitored for or managed
frequently (75% to 100%).

△ This diagnosis was reported to be monitored for or managed
often (50% to 74%).

Anorectal Surgery
See also *Surgery (General)*.

Preoperative Period
See also *Hemorrhoids / Anal Fissure*.

Postoperative Period

Collaborative Problems

PC: Hemorrhage
PC: Urinary retention

Nursing Diagnoses

Risk for Constipation related to fear of pain
Risk for Infection related to surgical incision and fecal contamination
Risk for Ineffective Therapeutic Regimen Management related to insufficient knowledge of wound care, prevention of recurrence, nutritional requirements (diet, fluid), exercise program, and signs and symptoms of complications

Arterial Bypass Graft of Lower Extremity (Aortic, Iliac, Femoral, Popliteal)
See also *Surgery (General); Anticoagulant Therapy*.

Postoperative Period

Collaborative Problems

▲ PC: Thrombosis of graft
△ PC: Compartmental syndrome
  PC: Lymphocele
▲ PC: Disruption of anastomosis

Nursing Diagnoses

▲ Risk for Infection related to location of surgical incision
▲ Acute Pain related to increased tissue perfusion to previous ischemic tissue

---

▲ This diagnosis was reported to be monitored for or managed frequently (75% to 100%).

△ This diagnosis was reported to be monitored for or managed often (50% to 74%).

△ Risk for Impaired Tissue Integrity related to immobility and vulnerability of heels

△ Risk for Ineffective Therapeutic Regimen Management related to insufficient knowledge of wound care, signs and symptoms of complications, activity restrictions, and follow-up care

Arthroplasty (Total Hip, Knee, or Ankle Replacement)

See also *Surgery (General)*.

Postoperative Period

Collaborative Problems

▲ PC: Fat emboli
* PC: Hemorrhage/hematoma formation
* PC: Infection
▲ PC: Dislocation of joint
* PC: Stress fractures
▲ PC: Neurovascular compromise
* PC: Synovial herniation
▲ PC: Thromboemboli
▲ PC: Sepsis

Nursing Diagnoses

▲ Risk for Impaired Skin Integrity related to immobility and incision
* Activity Intolerance related to fatigue, pain, and impaired gait
* Impaired Home Maintenance related to postoperative flexion restrictions
▲ Risk for Constipation related to activity restriction
▲ Risk for Injury related to altered gait and assistive devices
△ Risk for Ineffective Therapeutic Regimen Management related to insufficient knowledge of activity restrictions,

---

▲ This diagnosis was reported to be monitored for or managed frequently (75% to 100%).

△ This diagnosis was reported to be monitored for or managed often (50% to 74%).

* This diagnosis was not included in the validation study.

use of supportive devices, rehabilitative program, follow-up care, apparel restrictions, signs of complications, supportive services, and prevention of infection

Arthroscopy, Arthrotomy, Meniscectomy, Bunionectomy

See also *Surgery (General)*.

Postoperative Period

Collaborative Problems

PC: Hematoma formation
PC: Neurovascular impairments
PC: Hemorrhage
PC: Effusion

Nursing Diagnoses

Risk for Ineffective Therapeutic Regimen Management related to insufficient knowledge of home care, incision care, activity restrictions, signs of complications, and follow-up care

Carotid Endarterectomy

See also *Surgery (General)*.

Preoperative Period

Nursing Diagnoses

△ Anxiety related to anticipated surgery and unfamiliarity with preoperative and postoperative routines and postoperative sensations

Postoperative Period

Collaborative Problems

▲ PC: Thrombosis
▲ PC: Hypotension

▲ This diagnosis was reported to be monitored for or managed frequently (75% to 100%).

△ This diagnosis was reported to be monitored for or managed often (50% to 74%).

▲ PC: Hypertension
▲ PC: Hemorrhage
▲ PC: Cerebral infarction
  PC: Cranial nerve impairment
▲ PC: Facial
▲ PC: Hypoglossal
▲ PC: Glossopharyngeal
△ PC: Vagus
△ PC: Local nerve impairment (peri-incisional numbness of skin)
▲ PC: Respiratory obstruction

Nursing Diagnoses

△ Risk for Injury related to syncope secondary to vascular insufficiency
△ Risk for Ineffective Therapeutic Regimen Management related to insufficient knowledge of home care, signs and symptoms of complications, risk factors, activity restrictions, and follow-up care

Cataract Extraction

Postoperative Period

Collaborative Problem

▲ PC: Hemorrhage

Nursing Diagnoses

△ Acute Pain related to surgical procedure
▲ Risk for Infection related to increased susceptibility secondary to surgical interruption of eye surface
▲ Risk for Injury related to visual limitations, presence in unfamiliar environment, limited mobility, and postoperative presence of eye patch
  Risk for Social Isolation related to altered visual acuity and fear of falling

---

▲ This diagnosis was reported to be monitored for or managed frequently (75% to 100%).

△ This diagnosis was reported to be monitored for or managed often (50% to 74%).

△ Risk for Impaired Home Maintenance related to inability to perform activities of daily living secondary to activity restrictions and visual limitations
▲ Risk for Ineffective Therapeutic Regimen Management related to insufficient knowledge of activities permitted and restricted, medications, complications, and follow-up care

Cesarean Section
See *Surgery (General); Postpartum Period.*

Cholecystectomy
See also *Surgery (General).*

Postoperative Period

Collaborative Problem
PC: Peritonitis

Nursing Diagnoses
Risk for Ineffective Respiratory Function related to high abdominal incision and splinting secondary to pain
Risk for Impaired Oral Mucous Membrane related to NPO state and mouth breathing secondary to nasogastric intubation

Colostomy
See also *Surgery (General).*

Postoperative Period

Collaborative Problems
▲ PC: Peristomal ulceration/herniation
▲ PC: Stomal necrosis, retraction, prolapse, stenosis, obstruction

---

▲ This diagnosis was reported to be monitored for or managed frequently (75% to 100%).

△ This diagnosis was reported to be monitored for or managed often (50% to 74%).

Nursing Diagnoses

△ Grieving related to implications of cancer diagnosis

▲ Risk for Disturbed Self-Concept related to effects of ostomy on body image and lifestyle

△ Risk for Ineffective Sexuality Patterns related to perceived negative impact of ostomy on sexual functioning and attractiveness

Risk for Sexual Dysfunction related to physiologic impotence secondary to damaged sympathetic nerves (male) or inadequate vaginal lubrication (female)

△ Risk for Social Isolation related to anxiety about possible odor and leakage from appliance

▲ Risk for Ineffective Therapeutic Regimen Management related to insufficient knowledge of stoma pouching procedure, colostomy irrigation, peristomal skin care, perineal wound care, and incorporation of ostomy care into activities of daily living

Corneal Transplant (Penetrating Keratoplasty)

See also *Surgery (General)*.

Postoperative Period

Collaborative Problems

PC: Endophthalmitis

▲ PC: Increased intraocular pressure

PC: Epithelial defects

PC: Graft failure

Nursing Diagnoses

△ Risk for Infection related to nonintact ocular tissue

▲ Acute Pain related to surgical procedure

▲ Risk for Ineffective Therapeutic Regimen Management related to insufficient knowledge of eye care, resumption

---

▲ This diagnosis was reported to be monitored for or managed frequently (75% to 100%).

△ This diagnosis was reported to be monitored for or managed often (50% to 74%).

of activities, medications/medication administration, signs and symptoms of complications, and long-term follow-up care

Coronary Artery Bypass Graft (CABG)

See also *Surgery (General)*.

Postoperative Period

Collaborative Problems

▲ PC: Cardiovascular insufficiency
▲ PC: Respiratory insufficiency
▲ PC: Renal insufficiency

Nursing Diagnoses

▲ Acute Pain related to surgical incisions, chest tubes, and immobility secondary to lengthy surgery
  Impaired Physical Mobility related to surgical incisions, chest tubes, and fatigue
△ Fear related to transfer from intensive environment of the critical care unit and potential for complications
  Impaired Verbal Communication related to endotracheal tube (temporary)
△ Interrupted Family Processes related to disruption of family life, fear of outcome (death, disability), and stressful environment (intensive care unit)
△ Risk for Disturbed Self-Concept related to the symbolic meaning of the heart and changes in lifestyle
△ Risk for Ineffective Therapeutic Regimen Management related to insufficient knowledge of incisional care, pain management (angina, incisions), signs and symptoms of complications, condition, pharmacologic care, risk factors, restrictions, stress management techniques, and follow-up care

Cranial Surgery

See also *Surgery (General); Brain Tumor* for preoperative and postoperative care.

▲ This diagnosis was reported to be monitored for or managed frequently (75% to 100%).

△ This diagnosis was reported to be monitored for or managed often (50% to 74%).

Postoperative Period

Collaborative Problems

- ▲ PC: Increased intracranial pressure
- ▲ PC: Cerebral/cerebellar dysfunction
- * PC: Hypoxemia
- ▲ PC: Seizures
- ▲ PC: Brain hemorrhage, hematomas
- ▲ PC: Cranial nerve dysfunctions
- * PC: Cardiac dysrhythmias
- ▲ PC: Fluid/electrolyte imbalances
- △ PC: Meningitis/encephalitis
- ▲ PC: Sensory–motor losses
- ▲ PC: Hypothermia/hyperthermia
- △ PC: Antidiuretic hormone secretion disorders
- ▲ PC: Cerebrospinal fluid leaks
- ▲ PC: Hygromas
- * PC: Brain shifts/herniations
- * PC: Hydrocephalus
- * PC: Gastrointestinal bleeding

Nursing Diagnoses

- ▲ Acute Pain related to compression/displacement of brain tissue and increased intracranial pressure
- △ Risk for Impaired Corneal Tissue Integrity related to inadequate lubrication secondary to tissue edema
- △ Risk for Ineffective Therapeutic Regimen Management related to insufficient knowledge of wound care, signs and symptoms of complications, restrictions, and follow-up care

Dilatation and Curettage

See also *Surgery (General)—Preoperative and Postoperative.*

Postoperative Period

Collaborative Problems

PC: Hemorrhage

▲ This diagnosis was reported to be monitored for or managed frequently (75% to 100%).

△ This diagnosis was reported to be monitored for or managed often (50% to 74%).

* This diagnosis was not included in the validation study.

Nursing Diagnoses

Risk for Ineffective Therapeutic Regimen Management
related to insufficient knowledge of condition, home care,
signs and symptoms of complications, and activity
restrictions.

Enucleation

Postoperative Period

Collaborative Problems

▲ PC: Hemorrhage
  PC: Abscess

Nursing Diagnoses

△ Risk for Injury related to visual limitations and presence in unfamiliar environment
△ Grieving related to loss of eye and its effects on
  lifestyle
△ Risk for Disturbed Self-Concept related to effects of
  change in appearance on lifestyle
△ Risk for Social Isolation related to changes in body
  image and altered vision
△ Risk for Impaired Home Maintenance related to inability to perform activities of daily living secondary to
  change in visual abilities
△ Risk for Ineffective Therapeutic Regimen Management
  related to insufficient knowledge of activities permitted,
  self-care activities, medications, complications, and
  plans for follow-up care

Fractured Hip and Femur

See also *Surgery (General).*

▲ This diagnosis was reported to be monitored for or managed
frequently (75% to 100%).

△ This diagnosis was reported to be monitored for or managed
often (50% to 74%).

Postoperative Period

Collaborative Problems

- ▲ PC: Hemorrhage/shock
- ▲ PC: Pulmonary embolism
- ▲ PC: Sepsis
- ▲ PC: Fat emboli
- ▲ PC: Compartmental syndrome
- △ PC: Peroneal nerve palsy
- ▲ PC: Displacement of hip joint
- ▲ PC: Venous stasis/thrombosis
-   PC: Avascular necrosis of femoral head

Nursing Diagnoses

- ▲ (Specify) Self-Care Deficit related to prescribed activity restriction
- ▲ Disuse syndrome
- △ Fear related to anticipated postoperative dependence
- △ Risk for Disturbed Sensory Perceptions related to increased age, pain, and immobility
- △ Risk for Ineffective Therapeutic Regimen Management related to insufficient knowledge of activity restrictions, assistive devices, home care, follow-up care, and supportive services

Hysterectomy (Vaginal, Abdominal)

See also *Surgery (General)*.

Postoperative Period

Collaborative Problems

- ▲ PC: Vaginal bleeding
- * PC: Urinary retention (postcatheter removal)
- * PC: Fistula formation

▲ This diagnosis was reported to be monitored for or managed frequently (75% to 100%).

△ This diagnosis was reported to be monitored for or managed often (50% to 74%).

* This diagnosis was not included in the validation study.

▲ PC: Deep vein thrombosis
▲ PC: Trauma (ureter, bladder, rectum)

Nursing Diagnoses

* Risk for Infection related to surgical intervention and presence of urinary catheter
▲ Risk for Disturbed Self-Concept related to significance of loss
* Grieving related to loss of body part and childbearing ability
△ Risk for Ineffective Therapeutic Regimen Management related to insufficient knowledge of perineal/incisional care, signs of complications, activity restrictions, loss of menses, hormone therapy, and follow-up care

Ileostomy

Postoperative Period

Collaborative Problems

▲ PC: Peristomal ulceration/herniation
▲ PC: Stomal necrosis, retraction, prolapse, stenosis, obstruction
▲ PC: Fluid and electrolyte imbalances
PC: Pouchitis

Nursing Diagnoses

▲ Risk for Disturbed Self-Concept related to effects of ostomy on body image
△ Risk for Ineffective Sexuality Patterns related to perceived negative impact of ostomy on sexual functioning and attractiveness
△ Risk for Social Isolation related to anxiety about possible odor and leakage from appliance

---

▲ This diagnosis was reported to be monitored for or managed frequently (75% to 100%).

△ This diagnosis was reported to be monitored for or managed often (50% to 74%).

* This diagnosis was not included in the validation study.

△ Risk for Ineffective Therapeutic Regimen Management related to insufficient knowledge of stoma pouching procedure, peristomal skin care, perineal wound care, and incorporation of ostomy care into activities of daily living

△ Risk for Ineffective Therapeutic Regimen Management related to insufficient knowledge of care of ileoanal reservoir

Risk for Ineffective Therapeutic Regimen Management related to insufficient knowledge of intermittent intubation of Kock continent ileostomy

Laminectomy

See also *Surgery (General)*.

Postoperative Period

Collaborative Problems

▲ PC: Neurosensory impairments
* PC: Bowel/bladder dysfunction
▲ PC: Paralytic ileus
* PC: Cord edema
* PC: Skeletal misalignment
△ PC: Cerebrospinal fistula
* PC: Hematoma
▲ PC: Urinary retention

Nursing Diagnoses

* Risk for Injury related to vertigo secondary to postural hypotension
▲ Acute Pain related to muscle spasms (back, thigh) secondary to surgical trauma
* (Specify) Self-Care Deficit related to activity restrictions
▲ Risk for Ineffective Therapeutic Regimen Management related to insufficient knowledge of home care, brace care, activity restrictions, and exercise program

---

▲ This diagnosis was reported to be monitored for or managed frequently (75% to 100%).

△ This diagnosis was reported to be monitored for or managed often (50% to 74%).

* This diagnosis was not included in the validation study.

Mastectomy

See also *Cancer (General); Surgery (General).*

Postoperative Period

Collaborative Problems

▲ PC: Neurovascular compromise

Nursing Diagnoses

▲ Risk for Impaired Physical Mobility (shoulder, arm) related to lymphedema, nerve/muscle damage, and pain
▲ Risk for Injury related to compromised lymph, motor, and sensory function in affected arm
▲ Grieving related to loss of breast and change in appearance
▲ Risk for Ineffective Therapeutic Regimen Management related to insufficient knowledge of wound care, exercises, breast prosthesis, signs and symptoms of complications, hand/arm precautions, community resources, and follow-up care

Ophthalmic Surgery

See also *Surgery (General).*

Postoperative Period

Collaborative Problems

△ PC: Wound dehiscence/evisceration
△ PC: Increased intraocular pressure
△ PC: Retinal detachment
  PC: Dislocation of lens implant
  PC: Choroidal hemorrhage
  PC: Endophthalmitis
  PC: Hyphema
  PC: Hypopyon
△ PC: Blindness

▲ This diagnosis was reported to be monitored for or managed frequently (75% to 100%).

△ This diagnosis was reported to be monitored for or managed often (50% to 74%).

Nursing Diagnoses

△ Risk for Infection related to increased susceptibility secondary to surgical trauma

▲ Risk for Injury related to visual limitations, presence in unfamiliar environment, and presence of postoperative eye patches

▲ Feeding, Bathing/Hygiene Self-Care Deficit related to activity restrictions, visual impairment, or presence of eye patch(es)

▲ Risk for Disturbed Sensory Perceptions related to insufficient input secondary to impaired vision or presence of unilateral/bilateral eye patches

△ Risk for Ineffective Therapeutic Regimen Management related to insufficient knowledge of activities permitted and restricted, medications, complications, and follow-up care

Otic Surgery (Stapedectomy, Tympanoplasty, Myringotomy, Tympanic Mastoidectomy)

See also *Surgery (General)*.

Postoperative Period

Collaborative Problems

PC: Hemorrhage
PC: Facial paralysis
PC: Infection
PC: Impaired hearing/deafness

Nursing Diagnoses

Impaired Communication related to decreased hearing
Risk for Social Isolation related to embarrassment of not being able to hear in a social setting
Risk for Injury related to vertigo

▲ This diagnosis was reported to be monitored for or managed frequently (75% to 100%).

△ This diagnosis was reported to be monitored for or managed often (50% to 74%).

Risk for Ineffective Therapeutic Regimen Management
related to insufficient knowledge of signs and symptoms
of complications (facial nerve injury, vertigo, tinnitus,
gait disturbances, and ear discharge), ear care, contraindications, and follow-up care

Radical Neck Dissection (Laryngectomy)

See also *Surgery (General); Cancer (General); Tracheostomy.*

Postoperative Period

Collaborative Problems

* * PC: Hypoxemia
* ▲ PC: Flap rejection
* ▲ PC: Hemorrhage
* ▲ PC: Carotid artery rupture
* * PC: Cranial nerve injury
* * PC: Infection

Nursing Diagnoses

* ▲ Risk for Impaired Physical Mobility: Shoulder, head
  related to removal of muscles, nerves, flap graft reconstruction, and surgical trauma
* ▲ Risk for Disturbed Self-Concept related to change in
  appearance
* ▲ Risk for Ineffective Therapeutic Regimen Management
  related to insufficient knowledge of wound care, signs and
  symptoms of complications, exercises, and follow-up care

Radical Vulvectomy

See also *Surgery (General); Anticoagulant Therapy.*

Postoperative Period

Collaborative Problems

* ▲ PC: Hemorrhage/shock
* ▲ PC: Urinary retention

▲ This diagnosis was reported to be monitored for or managed
frequently (75% to 100%).

* This diagnosis was not included in the validation study.

▲ PC: Sepsis
△ PC: Pulmonary embolism
▲ PC: Thrombophlebitis

Nursing Diagnoses

▲ Acute Pain related to effects of surgery and immobility
▲ Grieving related to loss of body function and its effects on lifestyle
△ Risk for Ineffective Sexuality Patterns related to negative impact of surgery on sexual functioning and attractiveness
△ Risk for Ineffective Therapeutic Regimen Management related to insufficient knowledge of home care, wound care, self-catheterization, and follow-up care

Renal Surgery (General, Percutaneous Nephrostomy/Extracorporeal Renal Surgery, Nephrectomy)

See also *Surgery (General)*.

Collaborative Problems

▲ PC: Hemorrhage
▲ PC: Shock
▲ PC: Paralytic ileus
* PC: Pneumothorax
* PC: Fistulae
▲ PC: Renal insufficiency
△ PC: Pyelonephritis
△ PC: Ureteral stent dislodgement
△ PC: Pneumothorax secondary to thoracic approach

Nursing Diagnoses

△ Impaired Physical Mobility related to distention of renal capsule and incision

---

▲ This diagnosis was reported to be monitored for or managed frequently (75% to 100%).

△ This diagnosis was reported to be monitored for or managed often (50% to 74%).

* This diagnosis was not included in the validation study.

▲ Risk for Ineffective Respiratory Function related to pain on breathing and coughing secondary to location of incision

▲ Risk for Ineffective Therapeutic Regimen Management related to insufficient knowledge of hydration requirements, nephrostomy care, and signs and symptoms of complications

Renal Transplant

See also *Corticosteroid Therapy; Surgery (General).*

Collaborative Problems

▲ PC: Hemodynamic instability
▲ PC: Hypervolemia/hypovolemia
▲ PC: Hypertension/hypotension
▲ PC: Renal insufficiency (donor kidney). Examples:
  Ischemic damage before implantation
  Hematoma
  Rupture of anastomosis
  Bleeding at anastomosis
  Renal vein thrombosis
  Renal artery stenosis
  Blockage of ureter (kinks, clots)
  Kinking of ureter, renal artery
▲ PC: Rejection of donor tissue
▲ PC: Excessive immunosuppression
▲ PC: Electrolyte imbalances (potassium, phosphate)
▲ PC: Deep vein thrombosis
▲ PC: Sepsis

Nursing Diagnoses

▲ Risk for Infection related to altered immune system secondary to medications
▲ Risk for Impaired Oral Mucous Membrane related to increased susceptibility to infection secondary to immunosuppression

---

▲ This diagnosis was reported to be monitored for or managed frequently (75% to 100%).

△ Risk for Disturbed Self-Concept related to transplant experience and potential for rejection

▲ Fear related to possibility of rejection and death

▲ Risk for Noncompliance related to complexity of treatment regimen (diet, medications, record-keeping, weight, blood pressure, urine testing) and euphoria (post-transplant)

▲ Risk for Ineffective Therapeutic Regimen Management related to insufficient knowledge of prevention of infection, activity progression, dietary management, daily recording (intake, output, weights, urine testing, blood pressure, temperature), pharmacologic therapy, daily urine testing (protein), signs and symptoms of rejection/ infection, avoidance of pregnancy, follow-up care, and community resources

Thoracic Surgery

See also *Surgery (General); Mechanical Ventilation.*

Postoperative Period

Collaborative Problems

* PC: Atelectasis
* PC: Pneumonia
▲ PC: Respiratory insufficiency
▲ PC: Pneumothorax, hemothorax
* PC: Hemorrhage
▲ PC: Pulmonary embolism
▲ PC: Subcutaneous emphysema
△ PC: Mediastinal shift
▲ PC: Acute pulmonary edema
△ PC: Thrombophlebitis

▲ This diagnosis was reported to be monitored for or managed frequently (75% to 100%).

△ This diagnosis was reported to be monitored for or managed often (50% to 74%).

* This diagnosis was not included in the validation study.

Nursing Diagnoses

▲ Acute Pain related to surgical incision, chest tube sites, and immobility secondary to lengthy surgery

▲ Ineffective Airway Clearance related to increased secretions and diminished cough secondary to pain and fatigue

Activity Intolerance related to reduction in exercise capacity secondary to loss of alveolar ventilation

▲ Impaired Physical Mobility related to restricted arm and shoulder movement secondary to pain and muscle dissection and imposed position restrictions

Grieving related to loss of body part and its perceived effects on lifestyle

* Risk for Ineffective Therapeutic Regimen Management related to insufficient knowledge of condition, pain management, shoulder/arm exercises, incisional care, breathing exercises, splinting, prevention of infection, nutritional needs, rest versus activity, respiratory toilet, and follow-up care

Tonsillectomy
See also *Surgery (General)*.

Collaborative Problems
PC: Airway obstruction
PC: Aspiration
PC: Bleeding

Nursing Diagnoses
Risk for Deficient Fluid Volume related to decreased fluid intake secondary to pain on swallowing

Risk for Imbalanced Nutrition: Less Than Body Requirements related to decreased intake secondary to pain on swallowing

Risk for Ineffective Therapeutic Regimen Management related to insufficient knowledge of rest requirements,

---

▲ This diagnosis was reported to be monitored for or managed frequently (75% to 100%).

* This diagnosis was not included in the validation study.

nutritional needs, signs and symptoms of complications, pain management, positioning, and activity restrictions

Transurethral Resection (Prostate [Benign Hypertrophy or Cancer], Bladder Tumor)

See also *Surgery (General)*.

Postoperative Period

Collaborative Problems

PC: Oliguria/anuria
PC: Hemorrhage
PC: Perforated bladder (intraoperative)
PC: Hyponatremia
PC: Sepsis
PC: Occlusion of drainage devices
PC: Prostatectomy
PC: Clot formation

Nursing Diagnoses

Acute Pain related to bladder spasms, clot retention, or back and leg pain
Risk for Ineffective Therapeutic Regimen Management related to insufficient knowledge of fluid requirements, activity restrictions, catheter care, urinary control, follow-up, and signs and symptoms of complications

Urostomy

See also *Surgery (General)*.

Postoperative Period

Collaborative Problems

△ PC: Internal urine leakage
▲ PC: Urinary tract infection

▲ This diagnosis was reported to be monitored for or managed frequently (75% to 100%).

△ This diagnosis was reported to be monitored for or managed often (50% to 74%).

▲ PC: Peristomal ulceration/herniation
▲ PC: Stomal necrosis, retraction, prolapse, stenosis, obstruction

Nursing Diagnoses

△ Risk for Disturbed Self-Concept related to effects of ostomy on body image
Risk for Ineffective Sexuality Patterns related to perceived negative impact of ostomy on sexual functioning and attractiveness
Risk for Ineffective Sexuality Patterns related to erectile dysfunction (male) or inadequate vaginal lubrication (female)
△ Risk for Social Isolation related to anxiety about possible odor and leakage from appliance
▲ Risk for Ineffective Therapeutic Regimen Management related to insufficient knowledge of stoma pouching procedure, colostomy irrigation, peristomal skin care, perineal wound care, incorporation of ostomy care into activities of daily living
△ Risk for Ineffective Therapeutic Regimen Management related to insufficient knowledge of intermittent self-catheterization of Kock continent urostomy

▲ This diagnosis was reported to be monitored for or managed frequently (75% to 100%).

△ This diagnosis was reported to be monitored for or managed often (50% to 74%).

OBSTETRIC CONDITIONS
Prenatal Period (General)

Nursing Diagnoses

Nausea related to elevated estrogen levels, decreased blood sugar, or decreased gastric motility and pressure on cardiac sphincter from enlarged uterus

Constipation related to decreased gastric motility and pressure of uterus on lower colon

Activity Intolerance related to fatigue and dyspnea secondary to pressure of enlarging uterus on diaphragm and increased blood volume

Risk for Impaired Oral Mucous Membranes related to hyperemic gums secondary to estrogen and progesterone levels

Risk for Injury related to syncope/hypotension secondary to peripheral venous pooling

Risk for Ineffective Health Maintenance related to insufficient knowledge of (examples) effects of pregnancy on body systems (cardiovascular, integumentary, gastrointestinal, urinary, pulmonary, musculoskeletal), psychosocial domain, sexuality/sexual function, family unit (spouse, children), fetal growth and development, nutritional requirements, hazards of smoking, excessive alcohol intake, drug abuse, excessive caffeine intake, excessive weight gain, signs and symptoms of complications (vaginal bleeding, cramping, gestational diabetes, excessive edema, preeclampsia), preparation for childbirth (classes, printed references)

Abortion, Induced
Preprocedure Period

Nursing Diagnoses

Anxiety related to significance of decision, procedure, and postprocedure care

Postprocedure Period

Collaborative Problems

PC: Hemorrhage
PC: Infection

Nursing Diagnoses

Risk for Ineffective Coping related to unresolved emotional responses (guilt) to societal, moral, religious, and familial opposition

Risk for Interrupted Family Processes related to effects of procedure on relationships (disagreement about decisions, previous conflicts [personal, marital], or adolescent identity problems)

Risk for Ineffective Health Maintenance related to insufficient knowledge of self-care (hygiene, breast care), nutritional needs, expected bleeding, cramping, signs and symptoms of complications, resumption of sexual activity, contraception, sex education as indicated, comfort measures, expected emotional responses, follow-up appointment, and community resources

Abortion, Spontaneous

Nursing Diagnoses

Fear related to possibility of subsequent abortions
Grieving related to loss of pregnancy

Extrauterine Pregnancy
(Ectopic Pregnancy)

Collaborative Problems

PC: Hemorrhage
PC: Shock
PC: Sepsis
PC: Acute pain

Nursing Diagnoses

Grieving related to loss of fetus
Fear related to possibility of not being able to carry subsequent pregnancies

Hyperemesis Gravidarum

Collaborative Problems

PC: Negative nitrogen balance

Nursing Diagnoses

Risk for Imbalanced Nutrition: Less Than Body Requirements related to loss of nutrients and fluid secondary to vomiting

Pregnancy-Induced Hypertension

See also *Prenatal Period; Postpartum Period.*

Collaborative Problems

PC: Malignant hypertension
PC: Seizures
PC: Proteinuria
PC: Visual disturbances
PC: Coma
PC: Renal failure
PC: Cerebral edema
PC: Fetal compromise

Nursing Diagnoses

Fear related to the effects of condition on self, pregnancy, and infant
Risk for Injury related to vertigo, visual disturbances, or seizures
Risk for Ineffective Therapeutic Regimen Management related to insufficient knowledge of dietary restrictions, signs and symptoms of complications, conservation of energy, pharmacologic therapy, and comfort measures for headaches and backaches

Pregnant Adolescent

See also *General Prenatal, Intrapartum Period,* and *Postpartum Period.*

Prenatal

Collaborative Problems

PC: Pregnancy-induced hypertension

Nursing Diagnoses

Interrupted Family Processes related to stressors associated with adolescent pregnancy and future implications for family

Risk for Imbalanced Nutrition: Less Than Body Requirements related to maternal growth needs and lower nutritional stores secondary to adolescence

Disturbed Self-Concept related to pregnancy-associated body changes and conflict with adolescent and parenting roles

Risk for Social Isolation related to negative response of peer group to pregnancy

Risk for Urinary Tract Infection related to insufficient knowledge of prevention of infection and increased vulnerability secondary to effects of pregnancy on renal and ureter anatomy

Postpartum

Nursing Diagnoses

Risk for Impaired Parenting related to conflicting developmental task of adolescence and parenthood

Decisional Conflict related to caregiver of infant, adoption options, or living arrangements

Uterine Bleeding During Pregnancy (Placenta Previa, Abruptio Placentae, Uterine Rupture, Nonmalignant Lesions, Hydatidiform Mole)

See also *Postpartum Period.*

Collaborative Problems

PC: Hemorrhage
PC: Shock
PC: Disseminated intravascular coagulation
PC: Renal failure
PC: Fetal death
PC: Anemia
PC: Sepsis

Nursing Diagnoses

Fear related to effects of bleeding on pregnancy and infant

Impaired Physical Mobility related to increased bleeding in response to activity

Grieving related to anticipated possible loss of pregnancy and loss of expected child

Fear related to possibility of subsequent future complications of pregnancy

Intrapartum Period (General)

Collaborative Problems

PC: Hemorrhage (placenta previa, abruptio placentae)

PC: Fetal distress

PC: Hypertension

PC: Uterine rupture

PC: Dystocia

Nursing Diagnoses

Acute Pain related to uterine contractions during labor

Fear related to unpredictability of uterine contractions and possibility of having an impaired baby

Anxiety related to insufficient knowledge of relaxation/breathing exercises, positioning and procedures (preparations [bowel, skin], frequent assessments, anesthesia [regional, inhalation])

Postpartum Period

General Postpartum Period

Collaborative Problems

PC: Hemorrhage

PC: Uterine atony

PC: Retained placental fragments

PC: Lacerations

PC: Hematomas

PC: Urinary retention

Nursing Diagnoses

Risk for Infection related to bacterial invasion secondary to trauma during labor, delivery, and episiotomy

Risk for Ineffective Breastfeeding related to inexperience or engorged breasts

Acute Pain related to trauma to perineum during labor and delivery, hemorrhoids, engorged breasts, and involution of uterus

Risk for Constipation related to decreased intestinal peristalsis (postdelivery) and decreased activity

Risk for Impaired Parenting related to (examples) inexperience, feelings of incompetence, powerlessness, unwanted child, disappointment with child, or lack of role models

Stress Incontinence related to tissue trauma during delivery

Risk for Situational Low Self-Esteem related to changes that persist after delivery (skin, weight, lifestyle)

Risk for Ineffective Health Maintenance related to insufficient knowledge of postpartum routines, hygiene (breast, perineum), exercises, sexual counseling (contraception), nutritional requirements (infant, maternal), infant care, stresses of parenthood, adaptation of father, sibling, parent–infant bonding, postpartum emotional responses, sleep/rest requirements, household management, community resources, management of discomforts (breast, perineum), and signs and symptoms of complications

Mastitis (Lactational)

Collaborative Problems

PC: Abscess

Nursing Diagnoses

Acute Pain related to inflammation of breast tissue

Risk for Ineffective Breastfeeding related to interruption secondary to inflammation

Risk for Ineffective Health Maintenance related to insufficient knowledge of need for breast support, breast hygiene, breastfeeding restrictions, and signs and symptoms of abscess formation

Fetal/Newborn Death

Nursing Diagnoses

Interrupted Family Processes related to emotional trauma of loss on each family member

Grieving related to loss of infant

Fear related to the possibility of future fetal deaths

Concomitant Medical Conditions (Cardiac Disease [Prenatal, Postpartum], Diabetes [Prenatal, Postpartum])

Cardiac Disease
See also *Cardiac Disorders; Prenatal Period; Postpartum Period.*

Collaborative Problems

PC: Congestive heart failure

PC: Pregnancy-induced hypertension (preeclampsia, eclampsia)

PC: Valvular damage

Nursing Diagnoses

Fear related to effects of condition on self, pregnancy, and infant

Activity Intolerance related to increased metabolic requirements (pregnancy) in presence of compromised cardiac function

Impaired Home Maintenance related to impaired ability to perform role responsibilities during and after pregnancy

Risk for Interrupted Family Processes related to disruption of activity restrictions and fears of effects on lifestyle

Risk for Ineffective Therapeutic Regimen Management related to insufficient knowledge of dietary requirements, prevention of infection, conservation of energy, signs and symptoms of complications, and community resources

Diabetes (Prenatal)
See also *Prenatal Period; Diabetes Mellitus; Postpartum Period.*

Collaborative Problems

PC: Hypoglycemia/hyperglycemia
PC: Hydramnios
PC: Acidosis
PC: Pregnancy-induced hypertension

Nursing Diagnoses

Risk for Impaired Skin Integrity related to excessive skin stretching secondary to hydramnios

Risk for Vaginal Infection related to susceptibility to monilial infection

Acute Pain related to cerebral edema or hyperirritability

Risk for Ineffective Therapeutic Regimen Management related to insufficient knowledge of effects of pregnancy on diabetes, effects of diabetes on pregnancy, nutritional requirements, insulin requirements, signs and symptoms of complications, and need for frequent blood/urine samples

Diabetes (Postpartum)
See also *Postpartum Period (General).*

Collaborative Problems

PC: Hypoglycemia
PC: Hyperglycemia
PC: Hemorrhage (secondary to uterine atony from excessive amniotic fluid)
PC: Pregnancy-induced hypertension

Nursing Diagnoses

Anxiety related to separation from infant secondary to the special care needs of infant

Risk for Infection of perineal area related to depleted host defenses and depressed leukocytic phagocytosis secondary to hyperglycemia

Risk for Ineffective Therapeutic Regimen Management related to insufficient knowledge of risks of future pregnancies, birth control methods, types contraindicated, and special care requirements for infant

GYNECOLOGIC CONDITIONS

Endometriosis

Collaborative Problems

PC: Hypermenorrhea
PC: Polymenorrhea

Nursing Diagnoses

Chronic Pain related to response of displaced endometrial
tissue (abdominal, peritoneal) to cyclic ovarian hormonal
stimulation
Ineffective Sexuality Patterns related to painful intercourse or infertility
Anxiety related to unpredictable nature of disease
Risk for Ineffective Therapeutic Regimen Management
related to insufficient knowledge of condition, myths,
pharmacologic therapy, and potential for pregnancy

Pelvic Inflammatory Disease

Collaborative Problems

PC: Septicemia
PC: Abscess formation
PC: Pneumonia
PC: Pulmonary embolism

Nursing Diagnoses

Acute Pain related to malaise, increased temperature
secondary to infectious process
Risk for Deficient Fluid Volume related to inadequate
intake, fatigue, pain, and fluid losses secondary to
elevated temperature
Chronic Pain related to inflammatory process
Risk for Ineffective Coping: Depression related to chronicity of condition and lack of definitive diagnosis/treatment
Risk for Ineffective Therapeutic Regimen Management
related to insufficient knowledge of condition, nutritional
requirements, signs and symptoms of complications, prevention of sexually transmitted diseases, and sleep/rest
requirements

Neonate, Normal

Collaborative Problems

PC: Hypothermia
PC: Hypoglycemia
PC: Hyperbilirubinemia
PC: Bradycardia

Nursing Diagnoses

Risk for Infection related to vulnerability of infant, lack of normal flora, environmental hazards, and open wound (umbilical cord, circumcision)

Risk for Ineffective Airway Clearance related to oropharynx secretions

Risk for Impaired Skin Integrity related to susceptibility to nosocomial infection and lack of normal skin flora

Ineffective Thermoregulation related to newborn extrauterine transition

Risk for Ineffective Therapeutic Regimen Management related to insufficient knowledge of (specify) (see *Postpartum Period*)

Neonate, Premature

See also *Family of High-Risk Neonate.*

Collaborative Problems

PC: Cold stress
PC: Apnea
PC: Bradycardia
PC: Hypoglycemia
PC: Acidosis
PC: Hypocalcemia
PC: Sepsis
PC: Seizures
PC: Pneumonia
PC: Hyperbilirubinemia

Nursing Diagnoses

Risk for Constipation related to decreased intestinal motility and immobility

Risk for Aspiration related to immobility and increased secretions

Risk for Infection related to vulnerability of infant, lack of normal flora, environmental hazards, and open wounds (umbilical cord, circumcision)

Risk for Impaired Skin Integrity related to susceptibility to nosocomial infection (lack of normal skin flora)

Ineffective Thermoregulation related to newborn transition to extrauterine environment

Ineffective Infant Feeding Pattern related to lethargy secondary to prematurity

Risk for Sudden Infant Death Syndrome related to increased vulnerability secondary to prematurity

Neonate, Postmature (Small for Gestational Age [SGA], Large for Gestational Age [LGA])

Collaborative Problems

PC: Asphyxia at birth
PC: Meconium aspiration
PC: Hypoglycemia
PC: Polycythemia (SGA)
PC: Edema (generalized, cerebral)
PC: Central nervous system depression
PC: Renal tubular necrosis
PC: Impaired intestinal absorption
PC: Birth injuries (LGA)

Nursing Diagnoses

Risk for Impaired Skin Integrity related to absence of protective vernix and prolonged exposure to amniotic fluid (LGA)

Ineffective Infant Feeding Pattern related to lethargy

Neonate With Special Problem (Congenital Infections—Cytomegalovirus, Rubella, Toxoplasmosis, Syphilis, Herpes)

See also *High-Risk Neonate; Family of High-Risk Neonate; Developmental Problems/Needs* under *Pediatric Disorders.*

Collaborative Problems

PC: Hyperbilirubinemia
PC: Hepatosplenomegaly
PC: Anemia
PC: Hydrocephalus
PC: Microcephaly
PC: Mental retardation
PC: Congenital heart disease (rubella)
PC: Cataracts (rubella)
PC: Retinitis
PC: Thrombocytopenic purpura (rubella)
PC: Sensory–motor deafness (cytomegalovirus)
PC: Periostitis (syphilis)
PC: Seizures

Nursing Diagnoses

Risk for Infection Transmission related to contagious
    nature of organism
Risk for Injury related to uncontrolled tonic-clonic
    movements

Neonate With Meningomyelocele

See also *Normal Neonate; Family of High-Risk Neonate.*

Collaborative Problems

PC: Hydrocephalus
PC: Neurovascular insufficiency (below lesion)

Nursing Diagnoses

Risk for Trauma related to vulnerability of meningo-
    myelocele
Constipation/Bowel Incontinence related to effects of
    spinal cord disorder on anal sphincter
Urinary Retention related to effects of spinal cord injury
    on bladder function
Risk for Impaired Skin Integrity related to inability to
    move lower extremities

Neonate With Congenital Heart Disease (Preoperative)

See also *Normal Neonate; Family of High-Risk Neonate.*

Collaborative Problems

PC: Congestive heart failure
PC: Dysrhythmias
PC: Decreased cardiac output

Nursing Diagnoses

Risk for Ineffective Infant Feeding Pattern related to
   difficulty breathing and fatigue

Neonate of a Diabetic Mother
See also *Neonate, Normal; Family of High-Risk Neonate.*

Collaborative Problems

PC: Hypoglycemia
PC: Hypocalcemia
PC: Polycythemia
PC: Hyperbilirubinemia
PC: Sepsis
PC: Acidosis
PC: Birth injury (macrosomia)
PC: Hyaline membrane disease
PC: Respiratory distress syndrome
PC: Venous thrombosis

Nursing Diagnoses

Risk for Deficient Fluid Volume related to increased
   urinary excretion and osmotic diuresis

High-Risk Neonate
See also *Family of High-Risk Neonate.*

Collaborative Problems

PC: Hypoxemia
PC: Shock
PC: Respiratory distress
PC: Seizures
PC: Hypotension
PC: Septicemia

Nursing Diagnoses

Disorganized Infant Behavior related to immature central
nervous system and excess stimulation

Risk for Infection related to vulnerability of infant, lack of
normal flora, environmental hazards, open wounds
(umbilical cord, circumcision), and invasive lines

Ineffective Infant Feeding Pattern related to (specify)

Risk for Ineffective Respiratory Function related to
increased oropharyngeal secretions

Risk for Impaired Skin Integrity related to susceptibility to
nosocomial infection secondary to lack of normal skin flora

Ineffective Thermoregulation related to newborn transition
to extrauterine environment

Family of High-Risk Neonate

Nursing Diagnoses

Chronic Sorrow related to realization of possible present or
future loss for family or child

Interrupted Family Processes related to effect of extended
hospitalization on family (role responsibilities, finances)

Anxiety related to unpredictable prognosis

Risk for Impaired Parenting related to inadequate bonding
secondary to parent–child separation or failure to accept
impaired child

Hyperbilirubinemia (Rh Incompatibility, ABO Incompatibility)

See also *Family of High-Risk Neonate; Neonate, Normal.*

Collaborative Problems

PC: Anemia
PC: Jaundice
PC: Kernicterus
PC: Hepatosplenomegaly
PC: Hydrops fetalis (cardiac failure, hypoxia, anasarca,
and pericardial, pleural, and peritoneal effusions)
PC: Renal failure (phototherapy complications,
hyperthermia/hypothermia, dehydration, priapism,
"bronze baby" syndrome)

Nursing Diagnoses

Risk for Impaired Corneal Tissue Integrity related to exposure to phototherapy light and continuous wearing of eye pads

Risk for Impaired Skin Integrity related to diarrhea, urinary excretions of bilirubin, and exposure to phototherapy light

Neonate of Narcotic-Addicted Mother

See also *Family of High-Risk Neonate; Neonate, Normal; Substance Abuse for Mother.*

Collaborative Problems

PC: Hyperirritability/seizures
PC: Withdrawal
PC: Hypocalcemia
PC: Hypoglycemia
PC: Sepsis
PC: Dehydration
PC: Electrolyte imbalances

Nursing Diagnoses

Risk for Impaired Skin Integrity related to generalized diaphoresis and marked rigidity

Diarrhea related to increased peristalsis secondary to hyperirritability

Disturbed Sleep Pattern related to hyperirritability

Risk for Injury related to frantic sucking of fists

Risk for Injury related to uncontrolled tremors or tonic-clonic movements

Disturbed Sensory Perceptions related to hypersensitivity to environmental stimuli

Ineffective Infant Feeding Pattern related to lethargy

Risk for Sudden Infant Death Syndrome related to increased vulnerability secondary to maternal drug use

Respiratory Distress Syndrome

See also *High-Risk Neonate; Mechanical Ventilation.*

Collaborative Problems

PC: Hypoxemia
PC: Atelectasis
PC: Acidosis
PC: Sepsis
PC: Hyperthermia

Nursing Diagnoses

Activity Intolerance related to insufficient oxygenation of tissues secondary to impaired respirations

Risk for Infection related to vulnerability of infant, lack of normal flora, environmental hazards (personnel, other newborns, parents), and open wounds (umbilical cord, circumcision)

Risk for Impaired Skin Integrity related to susceptibility to nosocomial infection and lack of normal skin flora

Sepsis (Septicemia)

See also *Neonate, Normal; Family of High-Risk Neonate; High-Risk Neonate.*

Collaborative Problems

PC: Anemia
PC: Respiratory distress
PC: Hypothermia/hyperthermia
PC: Hypotension
PC: Edema
PC: Seizures
PC: Hepatosplenomegaly
PC: Hemorrhage
PC: Jaundice
PC: Meningitis
PC: Pyarthrosis

Nursing Diagnoses

Risk for Impaired Skin Integrity related to edema and immobility

Diarrhea related to intestinal irritation secondary to infecting organism

Risk for Injury related to uncontrolled tonic-clonic movements and hematopoietic insufficiency

Developmental Problems/Needs Related to
Chronic Illness (e.g., Permanent Disability,
Multiple Handicaps, Developmental
Disability [Mental/Physical],
Life-Threatening Illness)

Nursing Diagnoses

Chronic Sorrow (parental) related to anticipated losses secondary to condition

Interrupted Family Processes related to adjustment requirements for situation: (examples) time, energy (emotional, physical), financial, and physical care

Risk for Impaired Home Maintenance related to inadequate resources, housing, or impaired caregiver(s)

Risk for Parental Role Conflict related to separations secondary to frequent hospitalizations

Risk for Social Isolation (child/family) related to the disability and the requirements of the caregiver(s)

Risk for Impaired Parenting related to abuse, rejection, overprotection secondary to inadequate resources or coping mechanisms

Decisional Conflict related to illness, health care interventions, and parent–child separation

(Specify) Self-Care Deficit related to illness limitations or hospitalization

Risk for Delayed Growth and Development related to impaired ability to achieve developmental tasks

---

* For additional pediatric medical diagnoses, see the adult diagnoses and Developmental Problems/Needs, for example:

Diabetes mellitus	Neoplastic disorders
Anorexia nervosa	Fractures
(psychiatric disorders)	Congestive heart failure
Spinal cord injury	Pneumonia
Head trauma	

Caregiver Role Strain related to multiple ongoing care
needs secondary to restrictions imposed by disease,
disability, or treatments

Anxiety/School Phobia

Nursing Diagnoses

Anxiety related to altered self-esteem, change in environment, fear of separation, and negative responses (peers,
family)

Ineffective Coping related to inadequate problem-solving
skills and denial of problem

Disturbed Self-Esteem related to negative peer responses,
perceived mental deficits, and unrealistic expectations in
performance

Acquired Immunodeficiency
Syndrome (Child)

See also *Acquired Immunodeficiency Syndrome (Adult);
Developmental Problems/Needs Related to Chronic Illness.*

Nursing Diagnoses

Risk for Infection Transmission related to exposure to stool
and other secretions during diaper changes or failure of
child to follow handwashing procedure after toileting

Imbalanced Nutrition: Less Than Body Requirements
related to lactose intolerance, need for double the usual
recommended daily allowance, anorexia secondary to oral
lesions, and malaise

Delayed Growth and Development related to decreased
muscle tone secondary to encephalopathy

Impaired Physical Mobility related to hypotonia or hyper-
tonia secondary to cortical atrophy

Interrupted Family Processes related to the impact of the
child's condition on role responsibilities, siblings, and
finances and negative responses of relatives, friends, and
community

Risk for Ineffective Therapeutic Regimen Management
related to insufficient knowledge of modes of transmission, risks of live virus vaccines, avoidance of infections,
school attendance, and community resources

Asthma

See also *Developmental Problems/Needs.*

Collaborative Problems

PC: Hypoxemia
PC: Corticosteroid therapy
PC: Respiratory acidosis

Nursing Diagnoses

Ineffective Airway Clearance related to bronchospasm and
  increased pulmonary secretions
Fear related to breathlessness and recurrences
Risk for Ineffective Therapeutic Regimen Management
  related to insufficient knowledge of condition, environmental hazards (smoking, allergens, weather), prevention
  of infection, breathing/relaxation exercises, signs and
  symptoms of complications, pharmacologic therapy, fluid
  requirements, behavioral modification, and daily diary
  recording of peak flaws

Attention Deficit Disorder
(Hootman, 1993)

Collaborative Problems

PC: Adverse effects of central nervous system stimulants

Nursing Diagnoses

Activity Intolerance related to delayed physical, emotional,
  or mental capacity and fatigue
Ineffective Coping related to fatigue and delayed
  development
Delayed Growth and Development related to delayed
  maturation secondary to genetic, physical, and mental
  disability
Risk for Injury related to motor deficits and hyperactivity
Disturbed Self-Esteem related to lack of success in school
  and negative peer interactions
Impaired Social Interaction related to delayed social
  development and poor peer acceptance

Celiac Disease

See also *Developmental Problems/Needs.*

Collaborative Problems

PC: Severe malnutrition/dehydration
PC: Anemia
PC: Altered blood coagulation
PC: Osteoporosis
PC: Electrolyte imbalances
PC: Metabolic acidosis
PC: Shock
PC: Delayed growth

Nursing Diagnoses

Risk for Imbalanced Nutrition: Less Than Body Requirements related to malabsorption, dietary restrictions, and anorexia

Diarrhea related to decreased absorption in small intestines secondary to damaged villi resulting from toxins from undigested gliadin

Risk for Deficient Fluid Volume related to fluid loss in diarrhea

Risk for Ineffective Therapeutic Regimen Management related to insufficient knowledge of dietary management, restrictions, and requirements

Cerebral Palsy*

See also *Developmental Problems/Needs.*

Collaborative Problems

PC: Contractures
PC: Seizures
PC: Respiratory infections

---

* Because disabilities associated with cerebral palsy can be varied (hemiparesis, quadriparesis, diplegia, monoplegia, triplegia, paraplegia), the nurse will have to specify clearly the child's limitations in the diagnostic statements.

Nursing Diagnoses

Risk for Injury related to inability to control movements

Risk for Imbalanced Nutrition: Less Than Body Requirements related to sucking difficulties (infant) and dysphagia

(Specify) Self-Care Deficit related to sensory–motor impairments

Impaired Verbal Communication related to impaired ability to speak words related to facial muscle involvement

Risk for Deficient Fluid Volume related to difficulty obtaining or swallowing liquids

Risk for Deficient Diversional Activity related to effects of limitations on ability to participate in recreational activities

Risk for Ineffective Therapeutic Regimen Management related to insufficient knowledge of disease, pharmacologic regimen, activity program, education, community services, and orthopedic appliances

Child Abuse (Battered Child Syndrome, Child Neglect)

See also *Fractures, Burns; Failure to Thrive.*

Collaborative Problems

PC: Failure to thrive
PC: Malnutrition

Nursing Diagnoses

Ineffective Family Coping: Disabling related to presence of factors that contribute to child abuse: (examples) lack of or unavailability of extended family, economic problems (inflation, unemployment); lack of role model as a child, high-risk children (unwanted, of undesired gender or appearance, physically or mentally handicapped, hyperactive, terminally ill); and high-risk parents (single, adolescent, emotionally disturbed, alcoholic, drug-addicted, or physically ill)

Ineffective Coping (child abuser) related to (examples) history of abuse by own parents and lack of warmth and affection from them, social isolation (few friends or outlets for tensions), marked lack of self-esteem with low tolerance for criticism, emotional immaturity and dependency, distrust of others, inability to admit need for help, high expectations for/of child (perceiving child as a source of emotional gratification), and unrealistic desire for child to give pleasure

Ineffective Coping (nonabusing parent) related to passive and compliant response to abuse

Fear related to possibility of placement in a shelter or foster home

Parental Fear related to responses of others, possible loss of child, and criminal prosecution

Risk for Imbalanced Nutrition: Less Than Body Requirements related to inadequate intake secondary to lack of knowledge or neglect

Risk for Ineffective Therapeutic Regimen Management related to insufficient knowledge of parenting skills (discipline, expectations), constructive stress management, signs and symptoms of abuse, high-risk groups, child protection laws, and community services

Cleft Lip and Palate

See also *Developmental Problems/Needs; Surgery (General).*

Preoperative Period

Nursing Diagnoses

Risk for Imbalanced Nutrition: Less Than Body Requirements related to impaired sucking secondary to cleft lip

Postoperative Period

Collaborative Problems

PC: Respiratory distress
PC: Failure to thrive (organic)

Nursing Diagnoses

Impaired Physical Mobility related to restricted activity secondary to use of restraints

Risk for Impaired Verbal Communication related to impaired muscle development, insufficient palate function, faulty dentition, or hearing loss

Risk for Aspiration related to impaired sucking

Risk for Ineffective Therapeutic Regimen Management
related to insufficient knowledge of condition, feeding and
suctioning techniques, surgical site care, risks for otitis
media (dental/oral problems), and referral to speech
therapist

Communicable Diseases

See also *Developmental Problems / Needs.*

Nursing Diagnoses

Acute Pain related to pruritus, fatigue, malaise, sore
throat, and elevated temperature
Risk for Infection Transmission related to contagious agents
Risk for Deficient Fluid Volume related to increased fluid
loss secondary to elevated temperature or insufficient
oral intake secondary to malaise
Risk for Imbalanced Nutrition: Less Than Body Requirements related to anorexia and sore throat or pain on
chewing (mumps)
Risk for Ineffective Airway Clearance related to increased
mucus production (whooping cough)
Risk for Ineffective Therapeutic Regimen Management
related to insufficient knowledge of condition, transmission, prevention, immunizations, and skin care

Congenital Heart Disease

See also *Developmental Problems / Needs Related to Chronic
Illness.*

Collaborative Problems

PC: Congestive heart failure
PC: Pneumonia
PC: Hypoxemia
PC: Cerebral thrombosis
PC: Digoxin toxicity

Nursing Diagnoses

Activity Intolerance related to insufficient oxygenation
secondary to heart defects
Risk for Imbalanced Nutrition: Less Than Body Requirements related to inadequate sucking, fatigue, and dyspnea

Risk for Ineffective Therapeutic Regimen Management related to insufficient knowledge of condition, prevention of infection, signs and symptoms of complications, digoxin therapy, nutrition requirements, and community services

Convulsive Disorders
See also *Developmental Problems/Needs; Mental Disabilities,* if indicated.

Collaborative Problems

PC: Respiratory arrest

Nursing Diagnoses

Risk for Injury related to uncontrolled movements of seizure activity

Anxiety related to embarrassment and fear of seizure episodes

Risk for Ineffective Coping related to restrictions, parental overprotection, and parental indulgence

Risk for Ineffective Therapeutic Regimen Management related to insufficient knowledge of condition/cause, pharmacologic therapy, treatment during seizures, and environmental hazards (water, driving, heights)

Craniocerebral Trauma

Collaborative Problems

PC: Increased intracranial pressure
PC: Hemorrhage
PC: Tentorial herniation
PC: Cranial nerve dysfunction

Nursing Diagnoses

Acute Pain related to compression/displacement of cerebral tissue

Risk for Injury related to uncontrolled tonic-clonic movements during seizure episode or somnolence

Risk for Ineffective Therapeutic Regimen Management related to insufficient knowledge of condition, signs and symptoms of complications, post-traumatic syndrome, activity restrictions, and follow-up care

Cystic Fibrosis

See also *Developmental Problems/Needs.*

Collaborative Problems

PC: Bronchopneumonia, atelectasis
PC: Paralytic ileus

Nursing Diagnoses

Ineffective Airway Clearance related to mucopurulent secretions

Risk for Imbalanced Nutrition: Less Than Body Requirements related to need for increased calories and protein secondary to impaired intestinal absorption, loss of fat, and fat-soluble vitamins in stools

Constipation/Diarrhea related to excessive or insufficient pancreatic enzyme replacement

Activity Intolerance related to impaired oxygen transport secondary to mucopurulent secretions

Risk for Ineffective Therapeutic Regimen Management related to insufficient knowledge of condition (genetic transmission), risk of infection, pharmacologic therapy (side effects, ototoxicity, renal toxicity), equipment, nutritional therapy, salt replacement requirements, breathing exercises, postural drainage, exercise program, and community resources (Cystic Fibrosis Foundation)

Down Syndrome

See also *Developmental Problems/Needs; Mental Disabilities,* if indicated.

Nursing Diagnoses

Risk for Ineffective Respiratory Function related to decreased respiratory expansion secondary to decreased muscle tone, inadequate mucus drainage, and mouth breathing

Risk for Impaired Skin Integrity related to rough, dry skin surface, and flaccid extremities

Risk for Constipation related to decreased gastric motility

Risk for Imbalanced Nutrition: More Than Body Requirements related to increased caloric consumption secondary
to boredom in the presence of limited physical activity
and decreased metabolic rate

(Specify) Self-Care Deficit related to physical limitations

Ineffective Infant Feeding Pattern related to neurologic
impairment

Risk for Ineffective Therapeutic Regimen Management
related to insufficient knowledge of condition, home care,
education, and community services

Dysmenorrhea

Nursing Diagnoses

Acute Pain related to insufficient knowledge of comfort
measures, menstrual physiology, and nutritional
management

Failure to Thrive (Nonorganic)

See also *Developmental Problems / Needs.*

Collaborative Problems

PC: Metabolic dysfunction
PC: Dehydration

Nursing Diagnoses

Imbalanced Nutrition: Less Than Body Requirements
related to inadequate intake secondary to lack of emotional and sensory stimulation or lack of knowledge of
caregiver

Disturbed Sensory Perceptions related to history of insufficient sensory input from primary caregiver

Disturbed Sleep Pattern related to anxiety and apprehension secondary to parental deprivation

Impaired Parenting related to (examples) insufficient
knowledge of parenting skills, impaired caregiver,
impaired child, lack of support system, lack of role model,
relationship problems, unrealistic expectations for child,
unmet psychological needs

Impaired Home Maintenance related to difficulty of caregiver with maintaining a safe home environment

Risk for Ineffective Therapeutic Regimen Management
related to insufficient knowledge of growth and development requirements, feeding guidelines, risk for child
abuse, parenting skills, and community agencies

Glomerular Disorders (Glomerulonephritis: Acute, Chronic; Nephrotic Syndrome: Congenital, Secondary, Idiopathic)

See also *Developmental Problems/Needs; Corticosteroid Therapy.*

Collaborative Problems

PC: Anasarca (generalized edema)
PC: Hypertension
PC: Azotemia
PC: Sepsis
PC: Malnutrition
PC: Ascites
PC: Pleural effusion
PC: Hypoalbuminemia

Nursing Diagnoses

Risk for Infection related to increased susceptibility during
edematous phase and lowered resistance secondary to
corticosteroid therapy
Risk for Impaired Skin Integrity related to (examples)
immobility, lowered resistance, edema, or frequent
application of collection bags
Imbalanced Nutrition: Less Than Body Requirements
related to dietary restrictions, anorexia secondary to
fatigue, malaise, and pressure on abdominal structures
(edema)
Fatigue related to circulatory toxins, fluid, and electrolytic
imbalance
Deficient Diversional Activity related to hospitalization
and impaired ability to perform usual activities
Risk for Ineffective Therapeutic Regimen Management
related to insufficient knowledge of condition, etiology,
course, treatments, signs and symptoms of complications,
pharmacologic therapy, nutritional/fluid requirements,
prevention of infection, home care, follow-up care, and
community services

Hemophilia

See also *Developmental Problems / Needs.*

Collaborative Problems

PC: Hemorrhage

Nursing Diagnoses

Acute/Chronic Pain related to joint swelling and limitations secondary to hemarthrosis

Risk for Impaired Physical Mobility related to joint swelling and limitations secondary to hemarthrosis

Risk for Impaired Oral Mucous Membranes related to trauma from coarse food and insufficient dental hygiene

Risk for Ineffective Therapeutic Regimen Management related to insufficient knowledge of condition, contraindications (e.g., aspirin), genetic transmission, environmental hazards, and emergency treatment to control bleeding

Hydrocephalus

See also *Developmental Problems / Needs Related to Chronic Illness.*

Collaborative Problems

PC: Increased intracranial pressure
PC: Sepsis (postshunt procedure)

Nursing Diagnoses

Risk for Impaired Skin Integrity related to impaired ability to move head secondary to size

Risk for Injury related to inability to support large head and strain on neck

Risk for Imbalanced Nutrition: Less Than Body Requirements related to vomiting secondary to cerebral compression and irritability

Risk for Ineffective Therapeutic Regimen Management related to insufficient knowledge of condition, home care, signs and symptoms of infection, increased intracranial pressure, and emergency treatment of shunt

Infectious Mononucleosis (Adolescent)

Collaborative Problems

PC: Enlarged spleen
PC: Hepatic dysfunction

Nursing Diagnoses

Activity Intolerance related to fatigue secondary to infectious process

Acute Pain related to sore throat, malaise, and headaches

Risk for Imbalanced Nutrition: Less Than Body Requirements related to sore throat and malaise

Risk for Infection Transmission related to contagious condition

Risk for Ineffective Therapeutic Regimen Management related to insufficient knowledge of condition, communicable nature, diet therapy, risks of alcohol ingestion (with hepatic dysfunction), signs and symptoms of complications (hepatic, splenic, neurologic, hematologic), and activity restrictions

Legg-Calvé-Perthes Disease

See also *Developmental Problems/Needs.*

Collaborative Problems

PC: Permanently deformed femoral head

Nursing Diagnoses

Acute/Chronic Pain related to joint dysfunction

Risk for Impaired Skin Integrity related to immobilization devices (casts, braces)

(Specify) Self-Care Deficit related to pain and immobilization devices

Risk for Ineffective Therapeutic Regimen Management related to insufficient knowledge of disease, weight-bearing restrictions, application/maintenance of devices, and pain management at home

Leukemia

See also *Chemotherapy; Radiation Therapy; Cancer (General); Developmental Problems/Needs.*

Collaborative Problems

PC: Hepatosplenomegaly
PC: Increased intracranial edema
PC: Metastasis (brain, lungs, kidneys, gastrointestinal tract, spleen, liver)
PC: Hypermetabolism
PC: Hemorrhage
PC: Dehydration
PC: Myelosuppression
PC: Lymphadenopathy
PC: Central nervous system involvement
PC: Electrolyte imbalance

Nursing Diagnoses

Risk for Infection related to increased susceptibility secondary to leukemic process and side effects of chemotherapy
Risk for Social Isolation related to effects of disease and treatments on appearance and embarrassment
Risk for Injury related to bleeding tendencies secondary to leukemic process and side effects of chemotherapy
Powerlessness related to inability to control situation
Risk for Delayed Growth and Development related to impaired ability to achieve developmental tasks secondary to limitations of disease and treatments
Risk for Ineffective Therapeutic Regimen Management related to insufficient knowledge of disease process, treatment, signs and symptoms of complications, reduction of risk factors, and community resources

Meningitis (Bacterial)

See also *Developmental Problems/Needs.*

Collaborative Problems

PC: Peripheral circulatory collapse
PC: Disseminated intravascular coagulation

PC: Increased intracranial pressure/hydrocephalus
PC: Visual/auditory nerve palsies
PC: Paresis (hemiparesis, quadriparesis)
PC: Subdural effusions
PC: Respiratory distress
PC: Seizures
PC: Fluid/electrolyte imbalances

Nursing Diagnoses

Risk for Injury related to seizure activity secondary to infectious process

Acute Pain related to nuchal rigidity, muscle aches, immobility, and increased sensitivity to external stimuli secondary to infectious process

Impaired Physical Mobility related to intravenous infusion, nuchal rigidity, and restraining devices

Risk for Impaired Skin Integrity related to immobility

Risk for Ineffective Therapeutic Regimen Management related to insufficient knowledge of condition, antibiotic therapy, and diagnostic procedures

Meningomyelocele

See also *Developmental Problems/Needs.*

Collaborative Problems

PC: Hydrocephalus/shunt infections
PC: Increased intracranial pressure
PC: Urinary tract infections

Nursing Diagnoses

Reflex Urinary Incontinence related to sensory–motor dysfunction

Risk for Infection related to vulnerability of meningomyelocele sac

Risk for Impaired Skin Integrity related to sensory–motor impairments and orthopedic appliances

(Specify) Self-Care Deficit related to sensory–motor impairments

Impaired Physical Mobility related to lower limb impairments

Parental Grieving related to birth of infant with defects

Risk for Ineffective Therapeutic Regimen Management related to insufficient knowledge of condition, home care, orthopedic appliances, self-catheterization, activity program, and community services

Mental Disabilities

See also *Developmental Problems/Needs.*

Nursing Diagnoses

(Specify) Self-Care Deficit related to sensory–motor deficits

Impaired Communication related to impaired receptive skills or impaired expressive skills

Risk for Social Isolation (family, child) related to fear and embarrassment of child's behavior/appearance

Risk for Ineffective Therapeutic Regimen Management related to insufficient knowledge of condition, child's potential, home care, and community services

Muscular Dystrophy

See also *Developmental Problems/Needs.*

Collaborative Problems

PC: Seizures

PC: Respiratory infections

PC: Metabolic failure

Nursing Diagnoses

Risk for Injury related to inability to control movements

Risk for Imbalanced Nutrition: Less Than Body Requirements related to sucking difficulties (infant) and dysphagia

Ineffective Infant Feeding Pattern related to muscle weakness and impaired coordination

(Specify) Self-Care Deficit related to sensory–motor impairments

Impaired Verbal Communication related to impaired ability to speak secondary to facial muscle involvement

Risk for Impaired Physical Mobility related to muscle weakness

Risk for Imbalanced Nutrition: More Than Body Requirements related to increased caloric consumption in pres-

ence of decreased metabolic needs secondary to limited
physical activity

Chronic Sorrow (parental) related to progressive, terminal
nature of disease

Impaired Swallowing related to sensory–motor deficits

Risk for Hopelessness related to progressive nature of
disease

Risk for Deficient Diversional Activity related to effects of
limitations on ability to participate in recreational
activities

Risk for Ineffective Therapeutic Regimen Management
related to insufficient knowledge of disease, pharmacologic regimen, activity program, education, and
community services

Obesity
See also *Developmental Problems/Needs.*

Nursing Diagnoses

Ineffective Coping related to increased food consumption in
response to stressors

Ineffective Health Maintenance related to the need for
exercise program, nutrition counseling, and behavioral
modification

Disturbed Self-Concept related to feelings of self-degradation
and response of others (peers, family, others) to obesity

Interrupted Family Processes related to responses to and
effects of weight loss therapy on parent–child relationship

Risk for Impaired Social Interaction related to inability to
initiate and maintain relationships secondary to feelings
of embarrassment and negative responses of others

Risk for Ineffective Therapeutic Regimen Management
related to insufficient knowledge of condition, etiology,
course, risks, therapies available, destructive versus
constructive eating patterns, and self-help groups

Osteomyelitis
See also *Developmental Problems/Needs.*

Collaborative Problems

PC: Infective emboli

PC: Side effects of antibiotic therapy (hematologic, renal,
hepatic)

Nursing Diagnoses

Acute Pain related to swelling, hyperthermia, and infectious process of bone

Deficient Diversional Activity related to impaired mobility and long-term hospitalization

Risk for Imbalanced Nutrition: Less Than Body Requirements related to anorexia secondary to infectious process

Risk for Constipation related to immobility

Risk for Impaired Skin Integrity related to mechanical irritation of cast/splint

Risk for Injury: Pathologic fractures related to disease process

Risk for Ineffective Therapeutic Regimen Management related to insufficient knowledge of condition, wound care, activity restrictions, signs and symptoms of complications, pharmacologic therapy, and follow-up care

Parasitic Disorders

See also *Developmental Problems/Needs.*

Nursing Diagnoses

Risk for Imbalanced Nutrition: Less Than Body Requirements related to anorexia, nausea, vomiting, and deprivation of host nutrients by parasites

Impaired Skin Integrity related to pruritus secondary to emergence of parasites (pinworms) onto perianal skin, lytic necrosis, and tissue digestion

Diarrhea related to parasitic irritation to intestinal mucosa

Acute Pain related to parasitic invasion of small intestines

Risk for Infection Transmission related to contagious nature of parasites

Risk for Ineffective Therapeutic Regimen Management related to insufficient knowledge of condition, mode of transmission, and prevention of reinfection

Pediculosis (Hootman, 1993)

Nursing Diagnoses

Risk for Infection related to lesions

Impaired Comfort: Pruritus related to lesions

Risk for Infection Transmission related to insufficient knowledge of modes of transmission, treatment, and prevention

Risk for Ineffective Therapeutic Regimen Management
related to insufficient resources, low prioritization of
problem, or repeated infections

Poisoning

See also *Dialysis,* if indicated; *Unconscious Individual.*

Collaborative Problems

PC: Respiratory alkalosis
PC: Metabolic acidosis
PC: Hemorrhage
PC: Fluid/electrolyte imbalance
PC: Burns (acid/alkaline)
PC: Aspiration
PC: Blindness

Nursing Diagnoses

Acute Pain related to heat production secondary to poisoning (e.g., salicylate)
Fear related to invasive nature of treatments (gastric
lavage, dialysis)
Anxiety (parental) related to uncertainty of situation and
feelings of guilt
Risk for Ineffective Therapeutic Regimen Management
related to insufficient knowledge of condition, treatments,
home treatment of accidental poisoning, and poison
prevention (storage, teaching, poisonous plants, locks)

Respiratory Tract Infection (Lower)

See also *Developmental Problems/Needs; Adult Pneumonia.*

Collaborative Problems

PC: Hyperthermia
PC: Respiratory insufficiency
PC: Septic shock
PC: Paralytic ileus

Nursing Diagnoses

Acute Pain related to hyperthermia, malaise, and respiratory distress

Risk for Imbalanced Nutrition: Less Than Body Requirements related to anorexia secondary to dyspnea and
malaise

Anxiety related to breathlessness and apprehension

Risk for Deficient Fluid Volume related to insufficient
intake secondary to dyspnea and malaise

Risk for Ineffective Therapeutic Regimen Management
related to insufficient knowledge of condition, prevention
of recurrence, and treatment

Rheumatic Fever

See also *Developmental Problems/Needs.*

Collaborative Problems

PC: Endocarditis

Nursing Diagnoses

Deficient Diversional Activity related to prescribed bed rest

Imbalanced Nutrition: Less Than Body Requirements
related to anorexia and malaise

Acute Pain related to arthralgia

Risk for Injury related to choreic movements

Risk for Noncompliance related to difficulty maintaining
preventive drug therapy when illness is resolved

Risk for Ineffective Therapeutic Regimen Management
related to insufficient knowledge of condition, signs and
symptoms of complications, long-term antibiotic therapy,
prevention of recurrence, and risk factors (surgery,
e.g., dental)

Rheumatoid Arthritis (Juvenile)

See also *Developmental Problems/Needs; Corticosteroid
Therapy.*

Collaborative Problems

PC: Pericarditis
PC: Iridocyclitis

Nursing Diagnoses

Impaired Physical Mobility related to pain and restricted
joint movement

Acute Pain related to swollen, inflamed joints and restricted movement

Fatigue related to chronic inflammatory process

Risk for Ineffective Therapeutic Regimen Management related to insufficient knowledge of condition, pharmacologic therapy, exercise program, rest versus activity, myths, and community resources

Reye's Syndrome

See also *Unconscious Individual,* if indicated.

Collaborative Problems

PC: Renal failure
PC: Increased intracranial pressure
PC: Fluid/electrolyte imbalance
PC: Hepatic failure
PC: Shock
PC: Seizures
PC: Coma
PC: Respiratory distress
PC: Diabetes insipidus

Nursing Diagnoses

Parental Anxiety related to diagnosis and uncertain prognosis

Risk for Injury related to uncontrolled tonic-clonic movements

Risk for Infection related to invasive monitoring procedures

Acute Pain related to hyperpyrexia and malaise secondary to disease process

Fear related to separation from family, sensory bombardment (intensive care, treatments), and unfamiliar experiences

Interrupted Family Processes related to critical nature of syndrome, hospitalization of child, and separation of family members

Grieving related to actual, anticipated, or possible death of child

Risk for Impaired Skin Integrity related to immobility

Risk for Ineffective Therapeutic Regimen Management related to insufficient knowledge of condition, treatment, and complications

Scoliosis

See also *Developmental Problems / Needs.*

Nursing Diagnoses

Impaired Physical Mobility related to restricted movement secondary to braces

Risk for Impaired Skin Integrity related to mechanical irritation of brace

Risk for Noncompliance related to chronicity and complexity of treatment regimen

Risk for Falls related to restricted range of motion

Risk for Ineffective Therapeutic Regimen Management related to insufficient knowledge of condition, treatment, exercises, environmental hazards, care of appliances, follow-up care, and community services

Sickle Cell Anemia

See also *Developmental Problems / Needs* if the individual is a child.

Collaborative Problems

PC: Sickling crisis of transfusion therapy

PC: Thrombosis and infarction

PC: Cholelithiasis

Nursing Diagnoses

Ineffective Peripheral Tissue Perfusion related to viscous blood and occlusion of microcirculation

Acute Pain related to viscous blood and tissue hypoxia

(Specify) Self-Care Deficit related to pain and immobility of exacerbations

Risk for Ineffective Therapeutic Regimen Management related to insufficient knowledge of hazards, signs and symptoms of complications, fluid requirements, and hereditary factors

Tonsillitis

See also *Tonsillectomy,* if indicated.

Collaborative Problems

PC: Otitis media
PC: Rheumatic fever (β-hemolytic streptococci)

Nursing Diagnoses

Risk for Deficient Fluid Volume related to inadequate fluid
intake secondary to pain
Risk for Ineffective Therapeutic Regimen Management
related to insufficient knowledge of condition, treatments,
nutritional/fluid requirements, and signs and symptoms
of complications

Wilms' Tumor

See also *Developmental Problems/Needs; Nephrectomy; Cancer (General).*

Collaborative Problems

PC: Metastases to liver, lung, bone, brain
PC: Sepsis
PC: Tumor rupture

Nursing Diagnoses

Anxiety related to (examples) age-related concerns (separation, strangers, pain), response of others to visible signs
(alopecia), and uncertain future
Parental Anxiety related to (examples) unknown prognosis, painful procedures, treatments (chemotherapy), and
feelings of inadequacy
Grieving related to actual, anticipated, or possible death of
child
Spiritual Distress related to nature of disease and its possible disturbances in belief systems
Risk for Ineffective Therapeutic Regimen Management
related to insufficient knowledge of condition, prognosis,
treatments (side effects), home care, nutritional requirements, follow-up care, and community services

Mental Health Disorders

Affective Disorders (Depression)

Nursing Diagnoses

Dressing/Grooming Self-Care Deficit related to decreased interest in body, inability to make decisions, and feelings of worthlessness

Ineffective Coping related to internal conflicts (guilt, low self-esteem) or feelings of rejection

Social Isolation related to inability to initiate activities to reduce isolation secondary to low energy levels

Dysfunctional Grieving related to unresolved grief, prolonged denial, and repression

Chronic Low Self-Esteem related to feelings of worthlessness and failure secondary to (specify)

Ineffective Family Coping related to marital discord and role conflicts secondary to effects of chronic depression

Powerlessness related to unrealistic negative beliefs about self-worth or abilities

Disturbed Thought Processes related to negative cognitive set (overgeneralizing, polarized thinking, selected abstraction, arbitrary inference)

Ineffective Sexuality Patterns related to decreased sex drive, loss of interest and pleasure

Deficient Diversional Activity related to a loss of interest or pleasure in usual activities and low energy levels

Impaired Home Maintenance related to inability to make decisions or concentrate

Risk for Self-Harm related to feelings of hopelessness and loneliness

Disturbed Sleep Pattern related to difficulty falling asleep or early morning awakening secondary to emotional stress

Constipation related to sedentary lifestyle, insufficient exercise, or inadequate diet

Risk for Imbalanced Nutrition: More Than Body Requirements related to increased intake versus decreased activity expenditures secondary to boredom and frustration

Risk for Imbalanced Nutrition: Less Than Body Requirements related to anorexia secondary to emotional stress
Risk for Ineffective Therapeutic Regimen Management
related to insufficient knowledge of condition, behavior
modification, therapy options (pharmacologic,
electroshock), and community resources

Anorexia Nervosa

Collaborative Problems

PC: Anemia
PC: Hypotension
PC: Dysrhythmias
PC: Amenorrhea

Nursing Diagnoses

Imbalanced Nutrition: Less Than Body Requirements related to exercise in excess of caloric intake, refusal to
eat, self-induced vomiting following eating, or laxative
abuse
Disturbed Self-Concept related to inaccurate perception of
self as obese
Risk for Deficient Fluid Volume related to vomiting and
excessive weight loss
Disturbed Sleep Pattern related to fears and anxiety concerning weight status
Activity Intolerance related to fatigue secondary to
malnutrition
Ineffective Coping related to self-induced vomiting, denial
of hunger, and insufficient food intake secondary to feelings of loss of control and inaccurate perceptions of body
states
Ineffective Family Coping related to marital discord and
its effect on family members
Constipation related to insufficient food and fluid intake
Impaired Social Interactions related to inability to form
relationships with others or fear of trusting relationships
with others
Fear related to implications of a maturing body and
dissatisfaction with relationships with others

Anxiety and Adjustment Disorders (Phobias, Anxiety States, Traumatic Stress Disorders, Adjustment Reactions)

See also *Substance Abuse Disorders,* if indicated.

Nursing Diagnoses

Impaired Social Interactions related to effects of behavior and actions on forming and maintaining relationships

Anxiety related to irrational thoughts or guilt

Ineffective Coping related to inadequate psychological resources to adapt to a traumatic event

Disturbed Sleep Pattern related to recurrent nightmares

Ineffective Coping related to altered ability to manage stressors constructively secondary to (examples) physical illness, marital discord, business crisis, natural disasters, or developmental crisis

Risk for Ineffective Therapeutic Regimen Management related to insufficient knowledge of condition, pharmacologic therapy, and legal system regarding violence

Bipolar Disorder (Mania)

Nursing Diagnoses

Defensive Coping related to exaggerated sense of self-importance and abilities secondary to feelings of inadequacy and inferiority

Impaired Social Interaction related to overt hostility, over-confidence, or manipulation of others

Risk for Violence: Directed at others related to impaired reality testing, impaired judgment, or inability to control behavior

Disturbed Sleep Pattern related to hyperactivity

Disturbed Thought Processes related to flight of ideas, delusions, or hallucinations

Impaired Verbal Communication related to pressured speech and hyperactivity

Risk for Deficient Fluid Volume related to altered sodium excretion secondary to lithium therapy

Noncompliance related to feelings of no longer requiring medication

Risk for Ineffective Therapeutic Regimen Management related to insufficient knowledge of condition, pharmacologic therapy, and follow-up care

**Childhood Behavioral Disorders
(Attention Deficit Disorders,
Learning Disabilities)**

Nursing Diagnoses

Impaired Social Interactions related to inattention,
impulsivity, or hyperactivity

Chronic Sorrow (parental) related to anticipated losses
secondary to condition

Interrupted Family Processes related to adjustment
requirements for situation: (examples) time, energy,
money, physical care, and prognosis

Risk for Violence related to history of aggressive acts and
(specify)

Risk for Impaired Home Maintenance related to inadequate
resources, inadequate housing, or impaired caregivers

Risk for Social Isolation (child, family) related to disability
and requirements for caregivers

Risk for Impaired Parenting related to inadequate
resources or inadequate coping mechanisms

Disturbed Self-Concept related to effects of limitations on
achievement of developmental tasks

Obsessive–Compulsive Disorder

Nursing Diagnoses

(Specify) Self-Care Deficit related to ritualistic obsessions
interfering with performance of activities of daily living

Noncompliance related to poor concentration and poor
impulse control secondary to obsessive thought patterns

Social Isolation related to fear of vulnerability associated
with need for closeness and embarrassment about ritualistic behavior

Anxiety related to the perceived threat of actual or anticipated events

Paranoid Disorders

Nursing Diagnoses

Impaired Social Interactions related to feelings of mistrust
and suspicion of others

Ineffective Denial related to inability to accept own feelings
  and responsibility for actions secondary to low self-esteem
Risk for Imbalanced Nutrition: Less Than Body Requirements related to reluctance to eat secondary to fear of
  poisoning
Impaired Thought Processes related to inability to
  evaluate reality secondary to feelings of mistrust
Social Isolation related to fear and mistrust of situations
  and others

Personality Disorders

Examples:

Schizoid	Histrionic
Antisocial	Passive–aggressive
Borderline	Paranoid
Narcissistic	Schizotypal
Avoidant	Dependent
Compulsive	

Nursing Diagnoses

Ineffective Coping related to subordinating one's needs to
  decisions of others
Ineffective Coping:
  Inappropriate intense anger
  Poor impulse control
  Marked mood shifts
  Habitual disregard for social norms related to altered
    ability to meet responsibilities (role, social) secondary to
    (specify)
Impaired Social Interaction related to inability to maintain
  enduring attachments secondary to (specify)
Ineffective Coping related to resistance (procrastination,
  stubbornness, intentional inefficiency) in responses to
  responsibilities (role, social)

Schizophrenic Disorders

Nursing Diagnoses

Risk for Violence: Self-directed or directed at others related
  to responding to delusional thoughts or hallucinations

Impaired Verbal Communication related to incoherent/
illogical speech pattern and side effects of medications

Impaired Social Interactions related to preoccupation with
egocentric and illogical ideas and extreme suspiciousness

Impaired Home Maintenance related to impaired judgment, inability to self-initiate activity, and loss of skills
over long course of illness

Somatoform Disorders (Somatization, Hypochondriasis, Conversion Reactions)

See also *Affective Disorders,* if indicated.

Nursing Diagnoses

Impaired Social Interaction related to effects of multiple
somatic complaints and complaining on relationships

Ineffective Coping related to unrealistic fear of having a
disease despite reassurance to contrary

Ineffective Coping: Depression related to belief of not get-
ting proper care or sufficient response from others for
complaints

Ineffective Family Coping related to chronicity of illness

Noncompliance related to impaired judgments and thought
disturbances

Dressing/Grooming Self-Care Deficit related to loss of
skills and lack of interest in body and appearance

Deficient Diversional Activity related to apathy, inability
to initiate goal-directed activities, and loss of skills

Disturbed Self-Concept related to feelings of worthlessness
and lack of ego boundaries

Risk for Ineffective Therapeutic Regimen Management
related to insufficient knowledge of condition, pharmacologic therapy, tardive dyskinesia, occupational skills,
and follow-up care

Substance Abuse Disorders

Collaborative Problems

PC: Delirium tremens
PC: Autonomic hyperactivity
PC: Seizures
PC: Alcohol hallucinosis

PC: Hypertension (alcohol, opiates, heroin)
PC: Sepsis (intravenous drug use)

Nursing Diagnoses

Imbalanced Nutrition: Less Than Body Requirements related to anorexia

Risk for Deficient Fluid Volume related to abnormal fluid loss secondary to vomiting and diarrhea

Risk for Injury related to disorientation, tremors, or impaired judgment

Risk for Self-Harm related to disorientation, tremors, or impaired judgment

Risk for Violence related to (examples) impulsive behavior, disorientation, tremors, or impaired judgment

Disturbed Sleep Pattern related to irritability, tremors, and nightmares

Anxiety related to loss of control, memory losses, and fear of withdrawal

Ineffective Coping: Anger, dependence, or denial related to inability to manage stressors constructively without drugs/alcohol

Disturbed Self-Concept related to guilt, mistrust, or ambivalence

Impaired Social Interaction related to (examples) emotional immaturity, irritability, high anxiety, impulsive behavior, or aggressive responses

Social Isolation related to loss of work or withdrawal from others

Ineffective Sexuality Patterns related to impotence/loss of libido secondary to altered self-concept and substance abuse

Ineffective Family Coping related to disruption in marital dyad and inconsistent limit setting

Risk for Ineffective Therapeutic Regimen Management related to insufficient knowledge of condition, treatments available, high-risk situations, and community resources

Diagnostic and Therapeutic Procedures

Angioplasty (Percutaneous, Transluminal, Coronary, Peripheral)

Preprocedure Period

Nursing Diagnoses

▲ Anxiety/Fear (individual, family) related to health status, angioplasty procedure, routines, outcome, and possible need for cardiac surgery

Postprocedure Period

Collaborative Problems

▲ PC: Dysrhythmias
▲ PC: Acute coronary occlusion (clot, spasm, collapse)
▲ PC: Myocardial infarction
▲ PC: Arterial dissection or rupture
▲ PC: Hemorrhage/hematoma at angioplasty site
* PC: Paresthesia distal to site
* PC: Arterial thrombosis
* PC: Embolization (peripheral)

Nursing Diagnoses

▲ Impaired Physical Mobility related to prescribed bed rest and restricted movement of involved extremity
▲ Risk for Ineffective Therapeutic Regimen Management related to insufficient knowledge of care of insertion site, discharge activities, diet, medications, signs and symptoms of complications, exercises, and follow-up care

Anticoagulant Therapy

Collaborative Problem

▲ PC: Hemorrhage

▲ This diagnosis was reported to be monitored for or managed frequently (75% to 100%).

* This diagnosis was not included in the validation study.

Nursing Diagnosis

△ Risk for Ineffective Therapeutic Regimen Management related to insufficient knowledge of administration schedule, identification card/band, contraindications, and signs and symptoms of bleeding

Arteriogram

Preprocedure Period

Nursing Diagnosis

△ Fear related to potential negative findings of arteriogram and insufficient knowledge of routines and expected sensations

Postprocedure Period

Collaborative Problems

- ▲ PC: Hematoma
- ▲ PC: Hemorrhage
- * PC: Stroke
- ▲ PC: Thrombosis (arterial site)
- △ PC: Urinary retention
- △ PC: Renal failure
- ▲ PC: Paresthesia
- ▲ PC: Embolism
- ▲ PC: Allergic reaction

Nursing Diagnosis

▲ Risk for Ineffective Therapeutic Regimen Management related to insufficient knowledge of activity restrictions and signs and symptoms of complications

---

▲ This diagnosis was reported to be monitored for or managed frequently (75% to 100%).

△ This diagnosis was reported to be monitored for or managed often (50% to 74%).

* This diagnosis was not included in the validation study.

Cardiac Catheterization

Postprocedure Period

Collaborative Problems

- ▲ PC: Systemic (allergic reaction)
- ▲ PC: Cardiac (dysrhythmias, myocardial infarction, pulmonary edema)
- * PC: CVA
- ▲ PC: Circulatory (hematoma formation or hemorrhage at entry site, hypovolemia, thromboembolic phenomenon)

Nursing Diagnoses

- * Acute Pain related to tissue trauma and prescribed postprocedure immobilization
- △ Risk for Ineffective Therapeutic Regimen Management related to insufficient knowledge of site care, signs and symptoms of complications, and follow-up care

Casts

Collaborative Problems

- * PC: Pressure (edema, mechanical)
- ▲ PC: Compartmental syndrome
- * PC: Ulcer formation
- ▲ PC: Infection

Nursing Diagnoses

- * Risk for Injury related to hazards of crutch-walking and impaired mobility secondary to cast
- ▲ Risk for Impaired Skin Integrity related to pressure of cast on skin surface

---

▲ This diagnosis was reported to be monitored for or managed frequently (75% to 100%).

△ This diagnosis was reported to be monitored for or managed often (50% to 74%).

* This diagnosis was not included in the validation study.

△ Risk for Impaired Home Maintenance related to the restrictions imposed by cast on performing activities of daily living and role responsibilities

▲ (Specify) Self-Care Deficit related to limitation of movement secondary to cast

* Risk for Ineffective Respiratory Function related to imposed immobility or restricted respiratory movement secondary to cast (body)

* Deficient Diversional Activity related to boredom and inability to perform usual recreational activities

▲ Risk for Ineffective Therapeutic Regimen Management related to insufficient knowledge of cast care, signs and symptoms of complications, use of assistive devices, and hazards

Cesium Implant

Postprocedure Period

Collaborative Problems

▲ PC: Bleeding
▲ PC: Infection
△ PC: Pulmonary complications
  PC: Vaginal stenosis
▲ PC: Radiation cystitis
▲ PC: Displacement of radioactive source
△ PC: Thrombophlebitis
▲ PC: Bowel dysfunction

Nursing Diagnoses

▲ Anxiety related to fear of radiation and its effects, uncertainty of outcome, feelings of isolation, and pain or discomfort

▲ Bathing/Hygiene, Toileting Self-Care Deficit related to activity restrictions and isolation

---

▲ This diagnosis was reported to be monitored for or managed frequently (75% to 100%).

△ This diagnosis was reported to be monitored for or managed often (50% to 74%).

* This diagnosis was not included in the validation study.

▲ Risk for Impaired Skin Integrity related to immobility
  secondary to prescribed activity restrictions
▲ Social Isolation related to restrictions necessitated by
  cesium implant safety precautions
△ Risk for Ineffective Therapeutic Regimen Management
  related to insufficient knowledge of home care, re-
  portable signs and symptoms, activity restrictions,
  and follow-up care

Chemotherapy
See also *Cancer (General)*.

Collaborative Problems
* PC: Necrosis/phlebitis at intravenous site
* PC: Thrombocytopenia
* PC: Anemia
* PC: Leukopenia
△ PC: Peripheral nerve toxicosis
▲ PC: Anaphylactic reaction
△ PC: Central nervous system toxicity
△ PC: Congestive heart failure
▲ PC: Electrolyte imbalance
▲ PC: Extravasation of vesicant drugs
△ PC: Hemorrhagic cystitis
▲ PC: Myelosuppression
▲ PC: Renal insufficiency

Nursing Diagnoses
* Risk for Deficient Fluid Volume related to gastrointestinal fluid losses secondary to vomiting
* Risk for Infection related to altered immune system secondary to effects of cytotoxic agents or disease process
* Risk for Interrupted Family Processes related to interruptions imposed by treatment and schedule on patterns of living

▲ This diagnosis was reported to be monitored for or managed
frequently (75% to 100%).

△ This diagnosis was reported to be monitored for or managed
often (50% to 74%).

* This diagnosis was not included in the validation study.

*   Risk for Ineffective Sexuality Patterns related to amenorrhea and sterility (temporary/permanent) secondary to effects of chemotherapy on testes/ovaries

*   Risk for Injury related to bleeding tendencies

▲ Anxiety related to prescribed chemotherapy, insufficient knowledge of chemotherapy, and self-care measures

▲ Fatigue related to effects of anemia, malnutrition, persistent vomiting, and sleep pattern disturbance

△ Risk for Constipation related to autonomic nerve dysfunction secondary to vinca alkaloid administration and inactivity

▲ Diarrhea related to intestinal cell damage, inflammation, and increased intestinal motility

▲ Acute Pain related to gastrointestinal cell damage, stimulation of vomiting center, fear, and anxiety

▲ Risk for Impaired Skin Integrity related to persistent diarrhea, malnutrition, prolonged sedation, and fatigue

▲ Imbalanced Nutrition: Less Than Body Requirements related to anorexia, taste changes, persistent nausea/vomiting, and increased metabolic rate

▲ Impaired Oral Mucous Membrane related to dryness and epithelial cell damage secondary to chemotherapy

△ Disturbed Self-Concept related to change in lifestyle, role, alopecia, and weight loss or gain

Corticosteroid Therapy

Collaborative Problems

△ PC: Peptic ulcer

*   PC: Pseudotumor cerebri

▲ PC: Steroid-induced diabetes

△ PC: Osteoporosis

△ PC: Hypertension

△ PC: Hypokalemia

▲ This diagnosis was reported to be monitored for or managed frequently (75% to 100%).

△ This diagnosis was reported to be monitored for or managed often (50% to 74%).

* This diagnosis was not included in the validation study.

Nursing Diagnoses

▲ Risk for Excess Fluid Volume related to sodium and water retention
▲ Risk for Infection related to immunosuppression
△ Risk for Imbalanced Nutrition: More Than Body Requirements related to increased appetite
△ Risk for Situational Low Self-Esteem related to appearance changes (e.g., abnormal fat distribution, increased production of androgens)
△ Risk for Ineffective Therapeutic Regimen Management related to insufficient knowledge of administration schedule, adverse reactions, signs and symptoms of complications, hazards of adrenal insufficiency, and potential causes of adrenal insufficiency

Electroconvulsive Therapy (ECT)

Postprocedure Period

Collaborative Problems

PC: Hypertension
PC: Dysrhythmias

Nursing Diagnoses

Risk for Injury related to uncontrolled tonic-clonic movements and disorientation, confusion post-treatment
Acute Pain related to headaches, muscle aches, nausea secondary to seizure activity and tissue trauma
Risk for Aspiration related to post-ECT somnolence
Anxiety related to memory losses and disorientation secondary to effects of ECT on cerebral function

---

▲ This diagnosis was reported to be monitored for or managed frequently (75% to 100%).

△ This diagnosis was reported to be monitored for or managed often (50% to 74%).

Electronic Fetal Monitoring (Internal)

See also *Intrapartum Period (General).*

Postinsertion

Collaborative Problems

PC: Fetal scalp laceration
PC: Perforated uterus

Nursing Diagnoses

Impaired Physical Mobility related to restrictions secondary to monitor cords

Enteral Nutrition

Collaborative Problems

▲ PC: Hypoglycemia/hyperglycemia
▲ PC: Hypervolemia
△ PC: Hypertonic dehydration
▲ PC: Electrolyte and trace mineral imbalances
△ PC: Mucosal erosion

Nursing Diagnoses

▲ Risk for Infection related to gastrostomy incision and enzymatic action of gastric juices on skin
▲ Acute Pain related to cramping, distention, nausea, vomiting related to type of formula, administration rate, temperature, or route
▲ Diarrhea related to adverse response to formula, rate, or temperature
▲ Risk for Aspiration related to position of tube and of individual
△ Risk for Ineffective Therapeutic Regimen Management related to insufficient knowledge of nutritional indications/requirements, home care, and signs and symptoms of complications

---

▲ This diagnosis was reported to be monitored for or managed frequently (75% to 100%).

△ This diagnosis was reported to be monitored for or managed often (50% to 74%).

External Arteriovenous Shunting

Collaborative Problems

▲ PC: Thrombosis
▲ PC: Bleeding

Nursing Diagnoses

▲ Risk for Ineffective Therapeutic Regimen Management related to insufficient knowledge of catheter care, precautions, emergency measures, prevention of infection, and activity limitations

Hemodialysis

See also *Chronic Renal Failure.*

Collaborative Problems

▲ PC: Fluid imbalances
▲ PC: Electrolyte imbalance (potassium, sodium)
▲ PC: Nausea/vomiting
△ PC: Transfusion reaction
* PC: Aneurysm
▲ PC: Hemorrhage
* PC: Disruption of vascular access
△ PC: Dialysate leakage
▲ PC: Clotting
* PC: Infection
* PC: Hepatitis B
* PC: Fever/chills
* PC: Hemolysis
△ PC: Seizures
▲ PC: Hypertension/hypotension
△ PC: Dialysis disequilibrium syndrome
▲ PC: Air embolism
▲ PC: Sepsis
△ PC: Hyperthermia

▲ This diagnosis was reported to be monitored for or managed frequently (75% to 100%).

△ This diagnosis was reported to be monitored for or managed often (50% to 74%).

* This diagnosis was not included in the validation study.

Nursing Diagnoses

* Risk for Injury to (vascular) access site related to vulnerability
* Risk for Infection related to direct access to bloodstream secondary to vascular access
△ Powerlessness related to need for treatments to live despite effects on lifestyle
△ Interrupted Family Processes related to the interruptions of role responsibilities caused by the treatment schedule
▲ Risk for Infection Transmission related to frequent contacts with blood and high risk for hepatitis B
* Risk for Ineffective Therapeutic Regimen Management related to insufficient knowledge of rationale of treatment, care of site, precautions, emergency treatments (disconnected, bleeding, clotting), pretreatment instructions, and daily assessments (bruit, blood pressure, weight)

Hemodynamic Monitoring
See also *Medical Conditions* for the specific medical diagnosis.

Collaborative Problems

* PC: Sepsis
▲ PC: Hemorrhage
* PC: Bleeding back
* PC: Vasospasm
* PC: Tissue ischemia/hypoxia
▲ PC: Thrombosis/thrombophlebitis
▲ PC: Pulmonary embolism, air embolism
△ PC: Arterial spasm

Nursing Diagnoses

▲ Risk for Infection related to invasive lines
△ Impaired Physical Mobility related to position restrictions secondary to hemodynamic monitoring

---

▲ This diagnosis was reported to be monitored for or managed frequently (75% to 100%).

△ This diagnosis was reported to be monitored for or managed often (50% to 74%).

* This diagnosis was not included in the validation study.

△ Anxiety related to impending procedure, loss of control, and unpredictable outcome

* Risk for Ineffective Therapeutic Regimen Management related to insufficient knowledge of purpose, procedure, and associated care

Hickman Catheter

Collaborative Problems

PC: Air embolism
PC: Bleeding
PC: Thrombosis

Nursing Diagnoses

Risk for Infection related to direct access to bloodstream
Risk for Impaired Home Maintenance related to lack of knowledge of catheter management

Long-Term Venous Catheter

Collaborative Problems

△ PC: Pneumothorax
▲ PC: Hemorrhage
△ PC: Embolism/thrombosis
▲ PC: Sepsis

Nursing Diagnoses

▲ Anxiety related to upcoming insertion of catheter and insufficient knowledge of procedure

▲ Risk for Infection related to catheter's direct access to bloodstream

△ Risk for Ineffective Therapeutic Regimen Management related to insufficient knowledge of home care, signs and symptoms of complications, and community resources

---

▲ This diagnosis was reported to be monitored for or managed frequently (75% to 100%).

△ This diagnosis was reported to be monitored for or managed often (50% to 74%).

* This diagnosis was not included in the validation study.

Intra-aortic Balloon Pumping

Intraprocedure/Postprocedure Period

Collaborative Problems

PC: Arterial insufficiency/thrombosis
PC: Sepsis/infection
PC: Peripheral neuropathy/claudication
PC: Thrombocytopenia
PC: Bleeding
PC: Emboli
PC: Gastrointestinal bleeding
PC: Disseminated intravascular coagulation
PC: Dysrhythmias

Nursing Diagnoses

Impaired Physical Mobility related to prescribed immobility and restricted movement of involved extremity
Risk for Infection related to direct access to bloodstream
Risk for Constipation related to immobility and restricted movement of involved limb
Fear related to treatments, environment, and risk of death
Interrupted Family Processes related to the critical nature of situation and uncertain prognosis

Mechanical Ventilation

See also *Tracheostomy.*

Collaborative Problems

* PC: Acidosis/alkalosis
* PC: Airway obstruction/atelectasis
* PC: Tracheal necrosis
* PC: Infection
△ PC: Gastrointestinal bleeding
* PC: Tension pneumothorax

△ This diagnosis was reported to be monitored for or managed often (50% to 74%).

* This diagnosis was not included in the validation study.

△ PC: Oxygen toxicity
▲ PC: Respiratory insufficiency
▲ PC: Atelectasis
△ PC: Decreased cardiac output

Nursing Diagnoses

▲ Impaired Verbal Communication related to effects of intubation on ability to speak
△ Disuse Syndrome
▲ Risk for Infection related to disruption of skin layer secondary to tracheostomy
* Interrupted Family Processes related to critical nature of situation and uncertain prognosis
△ Fear related to the nature of the situation, uncertain prognosis of ventilator dependence, or weaning
* Risk for Disturbed Sensory Perceptions related to excessive environmental stimuli and decreased input of meaningful stimuli secondary to treatment and critical care unit
▲ Risk for Ineffective Airway Clearance related to increased secretions secondary to tracheostomy, obstruction of inner cannula, or displacement of tracheostomy tube
△ Powerlessness related to dependency on respirator, inability to talk, and loss of mobility
△ Risk for Dysfunctional Ventilatory Weaning Response related to unsatisfactory weaning attempts, respiratory muscle fatigue secondary to mechanical ventilation, increased work of breathing, supine position, protein–calorie malnutrition, inactivity, and/or fatigue
* Risk for Disturbed Self-Concept related to mechanical ventilation, dependence on achieving developmental tasks, and lifestyle changes

▲ This diagnosis was reported to be monitored for or managed frequently (75% to 100%).

△ This diagnosis was reported to be monitored for or managed often (50% to 74%).

* This diagnosis was not included in the validation study.

Pacemaker Insertion

Postprocedure Period

Collaborative Problems

▲ PC: Cardiac
▲ PC: Pacemaker malfunction
△ PC: Rejection of unit
△ PC: Necrosis near pulse generator site
* PC: Site (hemorrhage)

Nursing Diagnoses

* Acute Pain related to insertion site and prescribed post-procedure immobilization
△ Disturbed Self-Concept related to perceived loss of health and dependence on pacemaker
△ Impaired Physical Mobility related to incisional site pain, activity restrictions, and fear of lead displacements
* Risk for Infection related to operative site
△ Risk for Ineffective Therapeutic Regimen Management related to insufficient knowledge of activity restrictions, precautions, signs and symptoms of complications, electromagnetic interference (microwave ovens, arc welding equipment, gasoline engines, electric motors, antitheft devices, power transmitters), pacemaker function (daily pulse taking, signs of impending battery failure), activity restrictions, and follow-up care

Peritoneal Dialysis

Collaborative Problems

* PC: Fluid imbalances
▲ PC: Electrolyte imbalances
△ PC: Hemorrhage

▲ This diagnosis was reported to be monitored for or managed frequently (75% to 100%).

△ This diagnosis was reported to be monitored for or managed often (50% to 74%).

* This diagnosis was not included in the validation study.

* PC: Negative nitrogen balance
△ PC: Bowel/bladder perforation
△ PC: Hyperglycemia
* PC: Peritonitis
▲ PC: Hypovolemia/hypervolemia
▲ PC: Uremia

Nursing Diagnoses

▲ Risk for Infection related to access to peritoneal cavity, catheter exit site, and use of high-dextrose concentration in dialysis solution
* Risk for Injury to catheter site related to vulnerability
△ Risk for Ineffective Breathing Pattern related to immobility, pressure, and pain
△ Acute Pain related to catheter insertion, instillation of dialysis solution, outflow, suction, and chemical irritation of peritoneum
△ Imbalanced Nutrition: Less Than Body Requirements related to anorexia
* Risk for Excessive Fluid Volume related to fluid retention secondary to catheter problems (kinks, blockages) or position
△ Risk for Interrupted Family Processes related to the effects of interruptions of the treatment schedule on role responsibilities
△ Powerlessness related to chronic illness and the need for continuous treatment
* Impaired Home Maintenance related to insufficient knowledge of treatment procedure
△ Risk for Ineffective Therapeutic Regimen Management related to insufficient knowledge of rationale for treatment, medications, home dialysis procedure, signs and symptoms of complications, community resources, and follow-up care

----

▲ This diagnosis was reported to be monitored for or managed frequently (75% to 100%).

△ This diagnosis was reported to be monitored for or managed often (50% to 74%).

* This diagnosis was not included in the validation study.

Radiation Therapy (External)

Postprocedure Period

Collaborative Problems

* PC: Increased intracranial pressure
▲ PC: Myelosuppression
△ PC: Fluid/electrolyte imbalances
△ PC: Inflammation

Nursing Diagnoses

▲ Anxiety related to prescribed radiation therapy and insufficient knowledge of treatments and self-care measures
△ Acute Pain related to stimulation of the vomiting center and damage to the gastrointestinal mucosal cells secondary to radiation
▲ Fatigue related to systemic effects of radiation therapy
  Acute Pain related to damage to sebaceous and sweat glands secondary to radiation
△ Risk for Impaired Oral Mucous Membrane related to dry mouth or inadequate oral hygiene
▲ Impaired Skin Integrity related to effects of radiation on epithelial and basal cells and effects of diarrhea on perineal area
▲ Imbalanced Nutrition: Less Than Body Requirements related to decreased oral intake, reduced salivation, mouth discomfort, dysphasia, nausea/vomiting, and increased metabolic rate
△ Disturbed Self-Concept related to alopecia, skin changes, weight loss, sterility, and changes in role, relationships, and lifestyle
△ Grieving related to changes in lifestyle, role, finances, functional capacity, body image, and health losses

---

▲ This diagnosis was reported to be monitored for or managed frequently (75% to 100%).

△ This diagnosis was reported to be monitored for or managed often (50% to 74%).

* This diagnosis was not included in the validation study.

△ Interrupted Family Processes related to imposed changes in family roles, relationships, and responsibilities

* Diarrhea related to increased peristalsis secondary to irradiation of abdomen/lower back

* Risk for Infection related to moist skin reaction

* Activity Intolerance related to fatigue secondary to treatments or transportation

* Risk for Ineffective Therapeutic Regimen Management related to insufficient knowledge of skin care and signs of complications

Total Parenteral Nutrition (Hyperalimentation Therapy)

Collaborative Problems

▲ PC: Sepsis

▲ PC: Hyperglycemia

△ PC: Air embolism

* PC: Osmotic diuresis

* PC: Perforation

△ PC: Pneumothorax, hydrothorax, hemothorax

Nursing Diagnoses

▲ Risk for Infection related to catheter's direct access to bloodstream

* Risk for Impaired Skin Integrity related to continuous skin surface irritation secondary to catheter and adhesive

* Risk for Impaired Oral Mucous Membrane related to inability to ingest food/fluid

△ Risk for Ineffective Therapeutic Regimen Management related to insufficient knowledge of home care, signs and symptoms of complications, catheter care, and follow-up care (laboratory studies)

▲ This diagnosis was reported to be monitored for or managed frequently (75% to 100%).

△ This diagnosis was reported to be monitored for or managed often (50% to 74%).

* This diagnosis was not included in the validation study.

Tracheostomy

Postoperative Period

Collaborative Problems

▲ PC: Hypoxemia
▲ PC: Hemorrhage
▲ PC: Tracheal edema

Nursing Diagnoses

▲ Risk for Ineffective Airway Clearance related to increased secretions secondary to tracheostomy, obstruction of inner cannula, or displacement of tracheostomy tube
▲ Risk for Infection related to excessive pooling of secretions and bypassing of upper respiratory defenses
▲ Impaired Verbal Communication related to inability to produce speech secondary to tracheostomy
* Risk for Ineffective Sexuality Patterns related to change in appearance, fear of rejection
▲ Risk for Ineffective Therapeutic Regimen Management related to insufficient knowledge of tracheostomy care, precautions, signs and symptoms of complications, emergency care, and follow-up care

Traction

See also *Fractures.*

Collaborative Problems

PC: Thrombophlebitis
PC: Renal calculi
PC: Urinary tract infection
PC: Neurovascular compromise

▲ This diagnosis was reported to be monitored for or managed frequently (75% to 100%).

* This diagnosis was not included in the validation study.

Nursing Diagnoses

Risk for Impaired Skin Integrity related to imposed immobility

Risk for Infection related to susceptibility to micro-organisms secondary to skeletal traction pins

Risk for Constipation related to decreased peristalsis secondary to immobility and analgesics

Risk for Ineffective Respiratory Function related to imposed immobility and pooling of respiratory secretions

Acute Pain Management Guideline Panel. (1992). *Acute pain management in infants, children, and adolescents: Operative and medical procedures.* Quick Reference Guide for Clinicians. AHCPR Pub No. 92-0020. Rockville, MD: Agency for Health Care Policy and Research, Public Health Service, U.S. Department of Health and Human Services.

Algase, D. L. (1999). Wandering: A dementia-compromised behavior. *Journal of Gerontological Nursing, 25*(9), 10–16.

American Academy of Pediatrics. (2000). Task force on infant sleep position and Sudden Infant Death Syndrome: Changing concepts of Sudden Infant Death Syndrome; Implications for infants sleeping environment and sleep position. *Pediatrics, 105*(3), 650–56.

American Psychiatric Association. (2000). *DSM IV-TR: Diagnostic and statistical manual of mental disorders* (4th ed., text revision). Washington, D.C.: Author.

American Psychiatric Association. (2000). *Diagnostic and statistical manual of mental disorders* (4th ed: text revision). Washington, DC: Author.

Anetzberger, G. J. (1987). *The etiology of elder abuse by adult offsprings.* Springfield, IL: Charles C. Thomas.

Bandura, A. (1982). Self-efficacy mechanism in human agency. *American Psychology, 37*(3), 122–147.

Barry, K. L. (1999). Brief Interventions and Brief Therapies for Substance Abuse. Center for Substance Abuse Treatment Protocol (TIP) Series 34. Rockville, MD: Dept. of Health & Human Services.

Bennett, C. (2003). Urgent Urological Management of the Paraplegic/Quadriplegic Patient. *Urologic Nursing, 23*(6), 436–7.

Blackburn, S. (1993). Assessment and management of neurologic dysfunction. In C. Kenner, A. Brueggemeyer, & L. Gunderson (Eds.), *Comprehensive neonatal nursing.* Philadelphia: W. B. Saunders.

Blackburn, S., & Vandenberg, K. (1993). Assessment and management of neonatal neurobehavioral development. In C. Kenner, A. Brueggemeyer, & L. Gunderson (Eds.), *Comprehensive neonatal nursing.* Philadelphia: W.B. Saunders.

Boyd, M. A. (2005). *Psychiatric nursing: Contemporary practice.* Philadelphia: Lippincott Williams & Wilkins.

Bozzette, M. (1993). Observations of pain behavior in the NICU: An exploratory study. *Journal of Perinatal and Neonatal Nursing, 7*(1), 76–87.

Brandt, P., Groth, G., Harman, E., Phillips, C., & Dunbar Jacob, J. (1997). Noncompliance. In M. Rantz & P. LeMone (Eds.), *Classification of nursing diagnosis.* Proceedings of the Twelfth Conference of North American Nursing Diagnosis Association. Glendale, CA: CINALI.

Breslin, E. (1992). Dyspnea-limited response in chronic obstructive pulmonary disease: Reduced unsupported arm activities. *Rehabilitation Nursing, 17*(1), 13–20.

Burkle, N. (1988). Inadvertent hypothermia. *Journal of Gerontologic Nursing, 14*(6), 26–29.

Burnside, I., & Haight, B. (1994). Reminiscence and life review: Therapeutic interventions for older people. *Nurse Practitioner, 19*(4), 55–60.

Carpenito, L. J. (2004). *Nursing diagnosis: Application to clinical practice* (10th ed.). Philadelphia: Lippincott Williams & Wilkins.

Carscadden, J. S. (1993). On the cutting edge: A guide for working with people with people who self injure (pp. 29–34). London, Ontario: London Psychiatric Hospital.

Carson, V. B. (1989). *Spiritual dimensions of nursing practice.* Philadelphia: W. B. Saunders.

CDC. (2004). www.cdc.gov/health/tobacco.htm.

Centers for Disease Control and Prevention: HIV/AIDS Surveillance. (2001) report US. HIV and AIDS case reported through December 2001, *13*(2). Atlanta, Georgia: Department of Health and Human Services.

Centers for Disease Control and Prevention: Youth Risk Behavior Surveillance. (2000). MMWR, *49*(ss-5): 1–94.

CDC. (2003). Male Batterers. www.cdc.gov/ncipc/factsheet/malebat.htm.

Cohen-Mansfield, J., & Werner, P. (1998). Determinants of the effectiveness of one to one social interactions for treating verbally disruptive behaviors. *Journal of Mental Health and Aging, 4*(3), 323–324.

Collins, S. K., & Kuck, K. (1991). Music therapy in the neonatal intensive care unit. *Neonatal Network, 9*(6), 23–26.

Comffort, M., Sockloff, A., Loverro, J., Kaltenbach, K. (2003). Multiple predictors of substance abuse, women's treatments and outcomes: A *Prospective Longitudinal study.* Addiction Behavior, *28*(2), 199–224

Cooley, M. E., Yeomans, A. C., & Cobb, S. C. (1986). Sexual and reproductive issues for women with Hodgkin's disease. II. Application of PLIS-SIT model. *Cancer Nursing, 9*, 248–255.

Cutcliffe, J.R. (2004). The Inspiration of Hope in Bereavement Counseling. *Issues in Mental Health Nursing, 25*(2). 165–190.

DeFabio, D. C. (2000). Fluid and nutrient maintenance before, during, and after exercise. *Journal of Sports Chiropractic and Rehabilitation, 14*(2), 21–24, 42–43.

Denison, B. (2004). Touch the Pain Away. *Holistic Nursing Practice, 18*(3), 142–151

Dennis, K. (2004). Weight Management in Women. *Nursing Clinics in North America, 39* (14), 231–41.

Durham, R. (1983). Long-stay psychiatric patients in hospital. In S. Spence, & G. Shephard (Eds.), *Development in social skills training.* New York: Academic Press.

Eakes, G. (1995). Chronic sorrow: The lived experience of parents of chronically mentally ill individuals. *Archives of Psychiatric Nursing, 9*(2), 77–84.

Eckert, R. M. (2001) Understanding anticipatory nausea. *Continuing Education, 28*(10) 1553–1560.

Edgerly, E. S., & Donovick, P. J. (1998). Neuropsychological correlates of wandering in persons with Alzheimer's disease. *American Journal of Alzheimer's Disease, 13*(6), 317–329.

Elsen, J., & Blegen, M. (1991). Social isolation. In M. Maas, K. Buckwalter, & N. Hardy (Eds.), *Nursing diagnoses and interventions for the elderly.* Redwood City, CA: Addison-Wesley Nursing.

Evans, L. K., Strumpf, N. E., & Williams, C. C. (1992). Limiting use of physical restraints: A prerequisite for independent functioning. In E. Calkins, A. Ford, & P. Katz (Eds.), *The practice of geriatrics* (2nd ed.). Philadelphia: W. B. Saunders.

Flandermyer, A. A. (1993). The drug exposed neonate. In C. Kenner, A. Brueggemeyer, & L. Gunderson (Eds.), *Comprehensive neonatal nursing.* Philadelphia: W. B. Saunders.

Yarbro, C. H., M. H. Frogge, M. Goodman, & S.L. Groenwald. *Cancer nursing: Principles and practice* (5th ed.). Boston: Jones and Bartlett.

Fleitas, J. (2000). Whe Jack fell down. . . . Jill came tumbling after. . . . Siblings in the web of illness and disability. MCN. Am J. Maternal. *Child Nursing, 25*(5) 267–73.

Fuhrman, M.P. (1999), Diarrhea and tube feeding. *Nutritional Clinical Practice, 14*(2), 83–84.

Larson, C.E. (2000). Evidence-based practice. Safety and efficary of oral rehydration therapy for treatment of diarrhea and gastroenteritis in pediatrics. *Pediatric Nursing, 26*(2), 177–179.

Gardner, D. L., & Campbell, B. (1991). Assessing postpartum fatigue. *Maternal Child Nursing Journal, 16*(5), 264–266.

Geisman, L. K. (1989). Advances in weaning from mechanical ventilation. *Critical Care Nursing Clinics of North America, 1*(4), 697–705.

Giger, J., & Davidhizar, R. (1999). *Transcultural nursing.* St. Louis: Mosby–Year Book.

Hall, G. R. (1991). Altered thought processes: Dementia. In M. Maas, K. Buckwalter, & M. Hardy (Eds.), *Nursing diagnoses and interventions for the elderly.* Menlo Park, CA: Addison-Wesley Nursing.

Hall, G. R., & Buckwalter, K. C. (1987). Progressively lowered stress threshold: A conceptual model for care of adults with Alzheimer's disease. *Archives of Psychiatric Nursing, 1*(6), 399–406.

Hall, G.R. (1994). Caring for people with Alzheimer's disease using the conceptual model of progressively lowered stress threshold in the clinical setting. *Nursing Clin-*

ics of North America, 29; 129–141.

Harrison, I., et al (1996). Effects of gentle human touch on preterm infants: Pilot study results. Neonatal Network, 15(2), 35–41.

Harkulich, J., & Brugler, C. (1988). Nursing Diagnosis—translocation syndrome: Expert validation study. Partial funding granted by the Peg Schiltz Fund, Delta Xi Chapter, Sigma Theta Tau International; Barnhouse, A. (1987). Development of the nursing diagnosis of translocation syndrome with critical care patients. Unpublished master's thesis. Kent, OH: Kent State University.

Hatton, C. L., & McBride, S. (1984). Suicide: Assessment and Intervention. Norwalk, CT: Appleton-Century-Crofts.

Herman-Staab, B. (1994). Screening, management and appropriate referral for pediatric behavior problems. Nurse Practitioner, 19(7), 40–49.

Hilliker, N. A. (1998). Sleep disorders. In M. A. Boyd & M. A. Nihart (Eds.), Psychiatric nursing: Contemporary practice. Philadelphia: Lippincott-Raven.

Hiltunen, E. (1987). Diagnostic content validity of the nursing diagnosis: Decisional conflict. In A. M. McLane (Ed.). Classification of nursing diagnoses: Proceedings of the seventh conference. St. Louis: C.V. Mosby.

Hinds, P. (1988). Adolescent hopefulness in illness and health. Advances in Nursing Science, 10(3), 79–88.

Hollander, D. (2000). Nix to Nonoxynol-9 to prevent HIV.

Family Planning Perspective, 32(6), 266.

Holmstrom, L., & Burgess, A. W. (1975). Development of diagnostic categories: Sexual traumas. American Journal of Nursing, 75, 1288–1291.

Hootman, J. (1993). Procedural manual of quality nursing intervention in school. Portland, OR: Multnomah Education Service District.

Jackson, D. B., & Saunders, R. B. (1993). Child health nursing. Philadelphia: J. B. Lippincott.

Janssen, J., & Giberson, D. (1988). Remotivation therapy. Journal of Gerontological Nursing, 14(6), 31–34.

Jenny, J. (1987). Knowledge deficit: Not a nursing diagnosis. Image: Journal of Nursing Scholarship, 19(4), 184–185.

Jenny, J., & Logan, J. (1991). Interventions for the nursing diagnosis Dysfunctional Ventilatory Weaning Response: A qualitative study. In R. M. Carroll-Johnson (Ed.), Classification of nursing diagnoses. Philadelphia: J. B. Lippincott.

Johnson, M., Maas, M., et al. (Eds.). (2000). Nursing Outcomes Classification (2nd ed.). St. Louis: Mosby.

Johnson-Crowley, N. (1993). Systematic assessment and home follow-up. In C. Kenner, A. Brueggemeyer, & L. Gunderson (Eds.), Comprehensive neonatal nursing. Philadelphia: W. B. Saunders.

Kavchak-Keyes, M.A. (2000). Autonomic hyperreflexia. Rehabilitation Nursing, 25(1), 31–35.

Kovalesky, A. (2004). Women with Substance Abuse Concerns. *Nursing Clinics of North America, 39*(1), 205–17.

Krieger, D. (1979). *The therapeutic touch: How to use your hands to help or to heal.* Englewood Cliffs, NJ: Prentice-Hall.

Ladd, L. A. (1999). Symptom management: Nausea in palliative care. *Journal of Hospice and Palliative Nursing, 1*(2): 67–70.

Landis, C. & Moc, K. (2004). Sleep and Menopause. *Nursing Clinics of North America, 39*(1), 97–115.

Levin, R. F., Krainovitch, B. C., Bahrenburg, E., & Mitchell, C. A. (1989). Diagnostic content validity of nursing diagnoses. *Image: Journal of Nursing Scholarship, 21*(1), 40–44.

Lindeman, M., Hokanson, J., & Batek, J. (1994). The alcoholic family. *Nursing Diagnosis, 5*(2), 65–73.

Little, D., Riddle, B., & Soule, C. (1994). The power in our hands: Integrating developmental care into neonatal transport. *Neonatal Network, 13*(7), 19–22.

Logan, J., & Jenny, J. (1991). Interventions for the nursing diagnosis dysfunctional ventilatory weaning response: A qualitative study. In R. M. Carroll-Johnson (Ed.), *Classification of nursing diagnoses: Proceedings of the ninth conference* (pp. 141–147). Philadelphia: J. B. Lippincott.

Lynch, C. S., & Phillips, M. W. (1989). Nursing diagnosis: Ineffective denial. In R. M. Carroll-Johnson (Ed.), *Classification of nursing diagnoses: Proceedings of the eighth conference.* Philadelphia: J. B. Lippincott.

Lyon, B.A. (2002). Cognitive Self-Care Skills: A Model for Managing Stressful Lifestyles. *Nursing Clinics of North America,* 37(2), 285–94.

Maas, M., & Specht, J. (1990). Bowel incontinence. In M. Maas, K. Buckwalter, & M. Hardy (Eds.), *Nursing diagnoses and interventions for the elderly.* Redwood City, CA: Addison-Wesley Nursing.

Macauley, M., Pettersen, L., Fader, M., Brooks, R., & Cottenden. (2004). A multicenter evaluation of absorbent products for children with incontinence and disabilities. *Journal of WOCN, 31*(4), 235–44.

Magnan, M. A. (1987). *Activity intolerance: Toward a nursing theory of activity.* Paper presented at the Fifth Annual Symposium of the Michigan Nursing Diagnosis Association, Detroit.

Maresca, T. (1986). Assessment and management of acute diarrheal illness in adults. *Nurse Practitioner, 11*(11), 15–16.

May, J. (1996). Fathers: The Forgotten Parent. *Pediatric Nursing, 22*(3), 243–71.

May, K. A., & Mahlmeister, L. R. (1998). *Maternal and neonatal nursing family-centered care* (2nd ed.). Philadelphia: Lippincott-Raven.

May, R. (1987). *The meaning of anxiety.* New York: W. W. Norton.

Maynard, C.K. (2004). Assess and Manage Somatization. *Holistic Nursing Practice,* 18(2), 54–60.

McClain, W., Sheilds, C., & Sixsmith, D. (1999). Autonomic dysreflexia presenting as a severe headache. *American Journal of Emergency Medicine*, 17(3). 238–240.

McCloskey, J., & Bulechek, G. (Eds.). (2000). *Nursing interventions classification (NIC): Iowa intervention project* (3rd ed.). St. Louis: Mosby.

McFarland, G., & Wasli, E. (2000). Manipulation in nursing diagnosis and process. In B. S. Johnson (Ed.), *Psychiatric-mental health nursing* (5th ed.) (p. 147). Philadelphia: J. B. Lippincott.

McLane, A., & McShane, R. (1986). Empirical validation of defining characteristics of constipation: A study of bowel elimination practices of healthy adults. In M. E. Hurley (Ed.), *Classification of nursing diagnoses: Proceedings of the sixth conference* (pp. 448–455). St. Louis: C. V. Mosby.

Meehan, T. G. (1991). Therapeutic touch. In G. Bulechek & J. McCloskey (Eds.), *Nursing interventions: Essential nursing treatments.* Philadelphia: W. B. Saunders.

Miller, C. (2004). *Nursing care of the older adult* (4th ed.). Philadelphia: Lippincott Williams & Wilkins.

Mina, C. (1985). A program for helping grieving parents. *Maternal-Child Nursing Journal, 10,* 118–121.

Moon, J. L., & Humenick, S. S. (1989). Breast engorgement: Contributing variables and variables amenable to nursing interventions. *Journal of Obstetric, Gynecologic, and Neonatal Nursing, 18*(4), 309–315.

Murray, J. S. (2000). A concept analysis of social support as experienced by siblings of children with cancer. *Journal of Pediatric Nursing, 15*(5), 313–322.

National Safety Council. (2000). Injury Facts. Ilaska: IL: National Safety Council.

Newman, D. K., Lynch, K., Smith, D. A., & Cell, P. (1991). Restoring urinary continence. *American Journal of Nursing, 91*(1), 28–36.

Norris, J., & Kunes-Connell, M. (1987). Self-esteem disturbance: A clinical validation study. In A. McLane (Ed.), *Classification of nursing diagnoses: Proceedings of the seventh NANDA national conference.* St. Louis: C. V. Mosby.

North American Nursing Diagnosis Association. (2001). *NANDA guidelines: Taxonomy 1 revised.* St. Louis: Author.

North American Nursing Diagnosis Association. (1992). *NANDA nursing diagnosis: Definitions and classifications.* Philadelphia: Author.

Overfield, T. (1995). Biologic variations in health and illness: race, age, and sex differences (2nd ed.). New York: CRC Press.

Ortiz, J., McGilligan, K. & Kelly, P. Duration of breast milk expression among working mothers enrolled in an employer-sponsored lactation program. *Pediatric Nursing, 30*(2), 111–19.

Petter, M. & Whitchill, D. L. (1998). Management of female assault. *American Family Physician, 58*(4), 920–29

Puterbough, C. (1991). Hypothermia related to exposure and surgical interventions. *Today's OR Nurse, 13*(7), 32–33.

Pillitteri, A. (2003). *Maternal and child health nursing* (4th ed.). Philadelphia: Lippincott Williams & Wilkins.

Polomeno, V. (1999). Sex and babies: Couples' postnatal sexual concerns. *Journal of Perinatal Education, 8*(4), 9–18.

Quinn, C. (1994). The four A's of restraint reduction: Attention, assessment, anticipation, avoidance. *Orthopaedic Nursing, 13*(2), 11–19.

Rakel, B. A. (1992). Interventions related to teaching. In J. Bulechek & J. McCloskey (Eds.), Nursing intervention. *Nursing Clinics of North America, 27*(2), 397–423.

Rantz, M. (1991). Diversional activity deficit. In M. Maas, K. Buckwalter, & M. Hardy (Eds.), *Nursing diagnoses and interventions for the elderly*. Redwood City, CA: Addison-Wesley Nursing.

Rateau, M.R. (2000). Confusion and aggression in restrained elderly persons undergoing hip repair surgery. *Applied Nursing Research, 13*(1), 50–54.

Reeder, S., Martin, L., & Koniak-Griffin, D. (1997). *Maternity nursing* (18th ed.). Philadelphia: Lippincott-Raven.

Rhoten, D. (1982). Fatigue and the postsurgical patient. In C. Norris (Ed.), *Concept clarification in nursing*. Rockville, MD: Aspen Systems.

Rolland, J. S. (1994). *Families, illness & disability*. New York: Basic Books.

Sarna, L. & Bialous, S.A., (2004). Why Tobacco is a Women's Health Issue. Nursing *Clinics of North America, 39*(1), 165–80.

Shields, C. (1992). Family interaction and caregivers of Alzheimer's disease patients: Correlates of depression. *Family Process, 31*(3), 19–32.

Shrago, L., & Bocar, D. (1990). The infant's contribution to breastfeeding. *Journal of Obstetric, Gynecologic, and Neonatal Nursing, 19*(3), 209–211.

Smith, B. (1990). *Role of orientation therapy and reminiscence therapy, Alzheimer's disease* (pp. 180–187). St. Louis: C. V. Mosby.

Smith, L. S. (1987). Sexual assault: The nurse's role. *AD Nurse, 2*(2), 24–28.

Smith, S. (1990). The unique power of music therapy benefits Alzheimer's patients. *Activities, Adaptation and Aging, 14,* 49–63.

Stanley, M., & Beare, P. G. (2000). *Gerontological nursing*. Philadelphia: W. B. Saunders.

Stanley, M., & Beare, P. G. (2000). *Gerontological nursing*. Philadelphia: F. A. Davis.

Stone, R., Cafferata, G., & Sang, L. J. (1987). Caregivers of the frail elderly: A national profile. *Gerontologist, 27*(5), 616–626.

Taylor, E. J. (2000). Spiritual and ethical end-of-life concerns. In C. H. Yarbro, M. H. Frogge, M. Goodman & S. L. Groenwald. *Cancer Nursing: Principles and Practice* (5th ed.) Boston: Jones and Bartlett.

Taylor, S. E., Klein, L. C., Lewis, B Petal, (2000). Biobehavioral Responses to stress in females: Tend and befriend, not flight or flight, *Psychology Review, 107*(3), 411–29.

Teel, C. S. (1991). Chronic sorrow: Analysis of the concept. *Journal of Advanced Nursing, 16*(11), 311–319.

Thomas, K. A. (1989). How the NICU environment sounds to a preterm infant. *MCN: American Journal of Maternal Child Nursing, 14*(4), 249–251.

Thomas, S. P. (1998). Assessing and intervening with anger disorders. *Nursing Clinics of North America, 33*(1), 121–134.

Townsend, M. C. (1994). *Nursing diagnosis in psychiatric nursing* (3rd ed.). Philadelphia: F. A. Davis.

Tusaie, K. & Dyer, J. (2004). Resilience: A Historical Review of Construct. *Holistic Nursing Practice, 18*(1), 3–8.

Vandenberg, K. (1990). The management of oral nippling in the sick neonate, the disorganized feeder. *Neonatal Network, 9*(1), 9–16.

Vincent, K. G. (1985). The validation of a nursing diagnosis. *Nursing Clinics of North America, 20*(4), 631–639.

Voith, A. M., Frank, A. M., & Pigg, J. S. (1987). Validations of fatigue as a nursing diagnosis. In A. McLane (Ed.), *Classification of nursing diagnoses: Proceedings of the seventh national conference* (p. 280). St. Louis: C. V. Mosby.

Willis, D. & Porche, D. (2004). Male Battering of Intimate Partners: Theoretical Underpinnings, Interventions, Approaches and Interventions. *Nursing Clinics of North America, 39*(1), 271–282.

Wong, D. L. (1998). *Whaley & Wong's essentials of pediatric nursing* (4th ed.). St. Louis: C. V. Mosby.

Zerwich, J. (1992). Laying the groundwork for family self-help: Locating families, building trust and building strength. *Public Health Nursing, 9*(1), 15–21.

HEALTH-PROMOTION/
WELLNESS DIAGNOSES

NANDA International's Diagnostic Review Process in 2002–2003 resulted in twelve new nursing diagnoses. Three diagnoses—*Nausea, Risk for Sudden Infant Death Syndrome,* and *Readiness for Enhanced Family Coping*—are found in the main body of this text. Nine of the diagnoses are health-promotion/wellness diagnoses and are contained in this appendix.

There is still considerable debate regarding the clinical usefulness of this type of diagnosis. This author takes the position that some of these health states can be strengthened and are clinically useful, for example, *Readiness for Enhanced Parenting.* Others are questionable to be clinically useful, for example, *Readiness for Enhanced Fluid Balance, Readiness for Enhanced Urinary Elimination,* and other similar diagnoses. If a person has a pattern of equilibrium between fluid volume and the chemical composition of body fluids that is sufficient for meeting physical needs, how can this be strengthened? Is this not an assessment conclusion? Given the multiple needs of clients, is this a reasonable use of nursing resources? In contrast, *Readiness for Enhanced Parenting* describes family functioning that is sufficient to support the well-being of family members. This could be strengthened.

Clinically, data that represent strengths can be important for nurses to know. These strengths can assist the nurse in selecting interventions to reduce or prevent a problem in another health pattern. If nurses want to designate a strength, delete "Readiness for" and use "Enhanced (insert pattern)." If the client desires assistance in promoting a higher level of function, "Readiness for Enhanced (specify)" could be useful. Interested clinicians can utilize these health-promotion/wellness diagnoses and are invited to share their work with NANDA and this author.

Readiness for Enhanced Family Processes (2002, LOE 2.1)

DEFINITION
A pattern of family functioning that is sufficient to support the well-being of family members and can be strengthened

DEFINING CHARACTERISTICS
- Expresses willingness to enhance family dynamics
- Family functioning meets physical, social, and psychological needs of family members
- Activities support the safety and growth of family members
- Communication is adequate
- Relationships are generally positive; interdependent with community; family tasks are accomplished
- Family roles are flexible and appropriate for developmental stages
- Respect for family members is evident
- Family adapts to change
- Boundaries of family members are maintained
- Energy level of family supports activities of daily living
- Family resilience is evident
- Balance exists between autonomy and cohesiveness

References

Bryan, A. A. (2000). Enhancing parent-child interaction with a prenatal couple intervention. *The American Journal of Maternal/Child Nursing, 25*(3), 139–145.

Carruth, A. K., & Tate, U. S. (1997). Reciprocity, emotional well-being, and family functioning as determinants of family satisfaction in caregivers of elderly parents. *Nursing Research, 46*(2), 93–100.

Edelman, C. L., & Mandle, C. L. (2002). Health promotion of the family. In *Health promotion throughout the lifespan* (5th ed., pp. 169–198). St. Louis: Mosby.

Readiness for Enhanced Fluid Balance (2002, LOE 2.1)

DEFINITION
A pattern of equilibrium between fluid volume and chemical composition of body fluids that is sufficient for meeting physical needs and can be strengthened

DEFINING CHARACTERISTICS
- Expresses willingness to enhance fluid balance
- Stable weight
- Moist mucous membranes
- Food and fluid intake adequate for daily needs
- Straw-colored urine with specific gravity within normal limits
- Good tissue turgor
- No excessive thirst
- Urine output appropriate for intake
- No evidence of edema or dehydration

References

Dabinett, J. A., Reid, K., & James, N. (2001). Educational strategies used in increasing fluid intake and enhancing hydration status in field hockey players preparing for competition in a hot and humid environment: A case study. *International Journal of Sport Nutrition and Exercise Metabolism, 11*(3), 334–348.

Holben, D. H., Hassell, J. T., Williams, J. L., & Helle, B. (1999). Fluid intake compared with established standards and symptoms of dehydration among elderly residents of a long-term-care facility. *Journal of the American Dietetic Association, 99*(11), 1447–1450.

Kleiner, S. M. (1999). Water: An essential but overlooked nutrient. *Journal of the American Dietetic Association, 99*(2), 200–206.

Readiness for Enhanced Knowledge (Specify) (2002, LOE 2.1)

DEFINITION
The presence or acquisition of cognitive information related to a specific topic is sufficient for meeting health-related goals and can be strengthened

DEFINING CHARACTERISTICS
- Expresses an interest in learning
- Explains knowledge of the topic
- Behaviors congruent with expressed knowledge
- Describes previous experiences pertaining to the topic

References

Crosby, R. A., & Yarber, W. L. (2001). Perceived versus actual knowledge about correct condom use among U.S. adolescents: Results from a national study. *Journal of Adolescent Health, 28*(5), 415–420.

Meischke, H., Kuniyuki, A., Yasui, Y., Bowen, D. J., Anderson, R., & Urban, N. (2002). Information women receive about heart attacks and how it affects their knowledge, beliefs and intentions to act in a cardiac emergency. *Health Care for Women International, 23,* 149–162.

Taylor, K. L., Turner, R. O., Davis, J. L., Johnson, L., Schwartz, M. D., Kerner, J., & Leak, C. (2001). Improving knowledge of the prostate cancer screening dilemma among African American men: An academic-community partnership in Washington, DC. *Public Health Reports, 116*(6), 590–598.

Readiness for Enhanced Nutrition (2002, LOE 2.1)

DEFINITION
A pattern of nutrient intake that is sufficient for meeting metabolic needs and can be strengthened

DEFINING CHARACTERISTICS
- Expresses willingness to enhance nutrition
- Eats regularly
- Consumes adequate food and fluid
- Expresses knowledge of healthy food and fluid choices
- Follows an appropriate standard for intake (e.g., the food pyramid or America Diabetic Association guidelines)
- Safe preparation and storage for food and fluids
- Attitude toward eating and drinking is congruent with health goals

References

Long, V. A., Martin, T., & Janson-Sand, C. (2002). The great beginnings program: Impact of a nutrition curriculum on nutrition knowledge, diet quality, and birth outcomes in pregnant and parenting teens. *Journal of the American Dietetic Association, 102*(3 Suppl. 1), S86–89.

Murphy, P. W., Davis, T. C., Mayeaux, E. J., Sentell, T., Arnold, C., & Rebouche, C. (1996). Teaching nutrition education in adult learning centers: Linking literacy, health care, and the community. *Journal of Community Health Nursing, 13*(3), 149–158.

Satia, J. A., Kristal, A. R., Curry, S., & Trudeau, E. (2001). Motivations for healthful dietary change. *Public Health Nutrition, 4*(5), 953–959.

Readiness for Enhanced Parenting (2002, LOE 2.1)

DEFINITION

A pattern of providing an environment for children or other dependent person(s) that is sufficient to nurture growth and development and can be strengthened

DEFINING CHARACTERISTICS

- Expresses willingness to enhance parenting
- Children or other dependent person(s) express satisfaction with home environment
- Emotional and tacit support of children or dependent person(s) is evident; bonding or attachment evident
- Physical and emotional needs of children/dependent person(s) are met
- Realistic expectations of children/dependent person(s) exhibited

References

Bell, R. P., & McGrath, J. M. (1996). Implementing a research-based kangaroo care program in the NICU. *Nursing Clinics of North America, 31*(2), 387–403.

Gielen, A. C., McDonald, E. M., & Wilson, M. E. (2002). Effects of improved access to safety counseling, products, and home visits on parents' safety practices: Results of a randomized trial. *Archives of Pediatric Adolescent Medicine, 156*(1), 33–45.

Long, A., McCarney, S., & Smyth, G. (2001). The effectiveness of parenting programmes facilitated by health visitors. *Journal of Advanced Nursing, 34*(5), 611–620.

Readiness for Enhanced Self-Concept (2002, LOE 2.1)

DEFINITION

A pattern of perceptions or ideas about the self that is sufficient for well-being and can be strengthened

DEFINING CHARACTERISTICS

- Expresses willingness to enhance self-concept
- Expresses satisfaction with thoughts about self, sense of worthiness, role performance, body image, and personal identity
- Actions are congruent with expressed feelings and thoughts
- Expresses confidence in abilities
- Accepts strengths and limitations

References

Carnevale, F. A. (1999). Toward a cultural conception of the self. *Journal of Psychosocial Nursing Mental Health Service, 37*(8), 26–31.

Cole, D. A., Maxwell, S. E., Martin, J. M., Peeke, L. G., Seroczynski, A. D., Tran, J. M., Hoffman, K. B., Ruiz, M. D., Jacquez, F., & Maschman, T. (2001). The development of multiple domains of child and adolescent self-concept: A cohort sequential longitudinal design. *Child Development, 72*(6), 1723–1746.

Walter, R., Davis, K., & Glass, N. (1999). Discovery of self: exploring, interconnecting and integrating self (concept) and nursing. *Collegian, 6*(2), 12–15.

Readiness for Enhanced Sleep (2002, LOE 2.1)

DEFINITION

A pattern of natural, periodic suspension of consciousness that provides adequate rest, sustains a desired lifestyle, and can be strengthened

DEFINING CHARACTERISTICS

- Expresses willingness to enhance sleep
- Amount of sleep and REM sleep is congruent with developmental needs
- Expresses a feeling of being rested after sleep
- Follows sleep routines that promote sleep habits
- Occasional or infrequent use of medications to induce sleep

References

Floyd, J. A., Falahee, M. L., & Fhobir, R. H. (2000). Creation and analysis of a computerized database of interventions to facilitate adult sleep. *Nursing Research, 49*(4), 236–241.

Mead-Bennett, E. (1990). Sleep promotion: An important dimension of maternity nursing. *Journal of National Black Nurses Association, 4*(2), 9–17.

Stockert, P. A. (2001). Sleep, health promotion. In P. A. Potter & A. G. Perry (Eds.), *Fundamentals of nursing* (5th ed., pp. 1268–1273). St. Louis: Mosby.

Readiness for Enhanced Therapeutic Regimen Management (2002, LOE 2.1)

DEFINITION
A pattern of regulating and integrating into daily living a program(s) for treatment of illness and its sequelae that is sufficient for meeting health-related goals and can be strengthened

DEFINING CHARACTERISTICS
- Expresses desire to manage the treatment of illness and prevention of sequelae
- Choices of daily living are appropriate for meeting the goals of treatment or prevention
- Expresses little to no difficulty with regulation/integration of one or more prescribed regimens for treatment of illness or prevention of complications
- Describes reduction of risk factors for progression of illness and sequelae
- No unexpected acceleration of illness symptoms

References

Bakken, S., Holzemer, W. L., Brown, M., Powell-Cope, G. M., Turner, J. G., Inouye, J., Nokes, K. M., & Corless, I. B. (2000). Relationship between perception of engagement with health care provider and demographic characteristics, health status, and adherence to therapeutic regimen in persons with HIV/AIDS. *AIDS Patient Care and STDs, 14*(4), 189–197.

Dodge, J. A., Janz, N. K., & Clark, N. M. (1994). Self management of the health care regimen: A comparison of nurses' and cardiac patients' perceptions. *Patient Education and Counseling, 23*(2), 73–82.

Schumann, A., Nigg, C. R., Rossi, J. S., Jordan, P. J., Norman, G. J., Garber, C. E., Riebe, D., & Benisovich, S. V. (2002). Construct validity of the stages of change of exercise adoption for different intensities of physical activity in four samples of differing age groups. *American Journal of Health Promotion, 16*(5), 280–287.

Readiness for Enhanced Urinary Elimination (2002, LOE 2.1)

DEFINITION

A pattern of urinary functions that is sufficient for meeting eliminatory needs and can be strengthened

DEFINING CHARACTERISTICS

- Expresses willingness to enhance urinary elimination
- Urine is straw colored with no odor
- Specific gravity is within normal limits
- Amount of output is within normal limits for age and other factors
- Positions self for emptying of bladder
- Fluid intake is adequate for daily needs

References

Kilpatrick, J. A. (2001). Urinary elimination, health promotion. In P. A. Potter and A. G. Perry (Eds.), *Fundamentals of nursing* (5th ed., pp. 1408–1411). St. Louis: Mosby.

Palmer, M. H., Czarapata, B. J. R., Wells, T. J., & Newman, D. K. (1997). Urinary outcomes in older adults: Research and clinical perspective. *Urologic Nursing, 17*(1), 2–9.

Pfister, S. M. (1999). Bladder diaries and voiding patterns in older adults. *Journal of Gerontological Nursing, 25*(3), 36–41.

INDEX

Page numbers followed by *t* indicate tables. Nursing diagnoses are in **bold**.